Markers for Diagnosis and Monitoring of Human Cancer

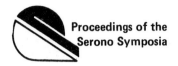 **Proceedings of the
Serono Symposia**

Recent Titles

*At the time of going to press these titles were in preparation.

Markers for Diagnosis and Monitoring of Human Cancer

Proceedings of the
Serono Symposia, Volume 46

Edited by

M.I. Colnaghi, G.L. Buraggi and M. Ghione

Istituto Nazionale per lo Studio e la Cura dei Tumori
Milan, Italy

*RC270
M37
1982*

1982

ACADEMIC PRESS

A Subsidiary of Harcourt Brace Jovanovich, Publishers

London New York
Paris San Diego San Francisco São Paulo
Sydney Tokyo Toronto

ACADEMIC PRESS INC. (LONDON) LTD.
24–28 OVAL ROAD
LONDON NW1

U.S. Edition published by
ACADEMIC PRESS INC.
111 FIFTH AVENUE
NEW YORK, NEW YORK 10003

British Library Cataloguing in Publication Data

Markers for diagnosis and monitoring of
  human cancer.–(Proceedings of the Serono
  symposia, ISSN 0308–5503; v. 46)
  1. Cancer–Diagnosis–Congresses
  I. Colnaghi, M. I. II. Buraggi, G. L.
  III. Ghione, M. IV. Series
  616.99′4 RC270

  ISBN 0–12–181520–X
  LCCCN 81 69582

Typeset in 10/11pt IBM (Typeface) by RDL., 26 Mulgrave Road, Sutton, Surrey.
Printed by T. J. Press (Padstow) Ltd., Padstow, Cornwall

CONTRIBUTORS

R. ACCINNI Istituto di Ricerche Cardiovascolari "G. Sisini", Università degli Studi di Milano, Via F. Storza, 35-20122 Milan, Italy

R. S. ACCOLLA Ludwig Institute for Cancer Research, 1066 Epalinges, Lausanne, Switzerland

A. ALBERTINI Istituto di Chimica della Facoltà Medica di Brescia, Brescia, Italy

K. D. BAGSHAWE Charing Cross Hospital Medical School, Fulham Palace Road, London W6 8RF, UK

M. A. BAILO Istituto di Ricerche Cardiovascolari "G. Sisini", Università degli Studi di Milano, Via F. Storza, 35-20122 Milan, Italy

A. BARGELLESI Ludwig Institute for Cancer Research, Epalinges, Switzerland

A. BARTORELLI Istituto di Immunologia Clinica, Università degli Studi di Milano, Via F. Storza, 35-20122 Milan, Italy

L. BASCHIERI Cattedra di Patologia Medica II°, Università di Pisa, Via Roma 67, 56100 Pisa, Italy

C. BIANCARDI Istituto di Ricerche Cardiovascolari "G. Sisini", Università degli Studi di Milano, Via F. Storza, 35-20122 Milan, Italy

E. BOMBARDIERI Department of Nuclear Medicine, Istituto Nazionale per lo Studio e la Cura dei Tumori, Via G. Venezian 1, 20133 Milan, Italy

G. BONORA I° Clinica Medica dell'Università di Bologna, Policlinico S. Orsola, Via Massarenti 9, Bologna, Italy

F. BUCHEGGER Institute of Biochemistry, University of Lausanne, 1066 Epalinges, Lausanne, Switzerland

P. BURTIN Institut de Recherches Scientifique sur le Cancer, Villejuif, France

B. BUSNARDO Istituto di Semeiotica Medica, University of Padua, Padua, Italy

N. A. CARPENTIER WHO Immunology Research and Training Centre, Hematological Division, Department of Medicine and Department of Surgery, University of Geneva, 1211 Geneva, Switzerland

S. CARREL Ludwig Institute for Cancer Research, 1066 Epalinges, Lausanne, Switzerland

V. CAVALCA Istituto di Ricerche Cardiovascolari "G. Sisini", Università degli Studi di Milano, Via F. Storza, 35-20122 Milan, Italy

M. CECCHETTIN Istituto di Chimica della Facoltà Medicà di Brescia, Brescia, Italy

P. CHOLLET WHO Immunology Research and Training Centre, Division of Oncohematology, Department of Medicine and Department of Surgery, University of Geneva, 1211 Geneva, Switzerland

J. COLLETTE Laboratory of Radioimmunology, University of Liège, Liège 1, Belgium

G. CORTE Institutes of Biochemistry and Microbiology, University of Genoa, Genoa, Italy

D. CUPPISSOL Laboratoire d'Immunopharmacologie des Tumeurs, INSERM U-236, ERA–CNRS No 844, Centre Paul Lamarque, B.P. 5054 34 033, Montpellier, Cédex, France

E. DINSDALE Ludwig Institute for Cancer Research, Royal Marsden Hospital, Sutton, Surrey SM2 5PX, UK

T. S. EDGINGTON Department of Molecular Immunology, Scripps Clinic and Research Foundation, 10666 North Pines Road, La Jolla, California 92037, USA

R. EGELI WHO Immunology Research and Training Centre, Hematological Division, Department of Medicine and Department of Surgery, University of Geneva, 1211 Geneva, Switzerland

C. FAVIER Laboratoire d'Immunopharmacologie des Tumeurs, INSERM U-236, ERA–CNRS No 844, Centre Paul Lamarque, B.P. 5054 34 033, Montpellier, Cédex, France

F. FAVIER Laboratoire d'Immunopharmacologie des Tumeurs, INSERUM U-236, ERA–CNRS No 844, Centre Paul Lamarque, B. P. 5054 34 033, Montpellier, Cédex, France

R. FERRARA Istituto di Ricerche Cardiovascolari "G. Sisini", Università degli Studi di Milano, Via F. Storza, 35-20122 Milan, Italy

G. L. FERRI I° Clinica Medica dell'Università di Bologna, Policlinico S. Orsola, Via Massarenti 9, Bologna, Italy

M. FORNI Clinique Médicale, Department of Medicine, University Hospital of Geneva, 1211 Geneva, Switzerland

P. FRANCHIMONT Laboratory of Radioimmunology, University of Liège, Liège 1, Belgium

F. GELDER Louisiana State University, Shreveport, Louisiana 71130, USA

C. GIANI Cattedra di Patologia Medica II°, Università di Pisa, Via Roma 67, 56100 Pisa, Italy

C. GIRARDET Institute of Biochemistry, University of Lausanne, 1066 Epalinges, Lausanne, Switzerland

M. E. GIRELLI Istituto di Semeiotica Medica, University of Padua, Padua, Italy

D. M. GOLDENBERG Division of Experimental Pathology, Department of Pathology, University of Kentucky Medical Center, Lexington, Kentucky, USA

R. B. HERBERMAN Laboratory of Immunodiagnosis, Building 10, Room 8B02, National Cancer Institute, National Institutes of Health, Bethesda, Maryland 20205, USA

J. C. HENDRICK Laboratory of Radioimmunology, University of Liège, Leige 1, Belgium

R. HUNTER Emory University, Atlanta, Georgia 30322, USA

G. LABO I° Clinica Medica dell'Università di Bologna, Policlinico S. Orsola, Via Massarenti 9, Bologna, Italy

P. H. LAMBERT WHO Immunology Research and Training Centre, Hematological Division, Department of Medicine and Department of Surgery, University of Geneva, 1211 Geneva, Switzerland

K. O. LLOYD Memorial Sloan-Kettering Cancer Center, 1275 York Avenue, New York, New York 10021, USA

J.-P. MACH Ludwig Institute for Cancer Research, 1066 Epalinges, Lausanne, Switzerland

S. MARIOTTI Cattedra di Patologia Medica II°, Università di Pisa, Via Roma 67, 56100 Pisa, Italy

P. MAURICE WHO Immunology Research and Training Centre, Division of Oncohematology, Department of Medicine and Department of Surgery, University of Geneva, 1211 Geneva, Switzerland

R. A. J. McILHINNEY Ludwig Institute for Cancer Research, Royal Marsden Hospital, Sutton, Surrey SM2 5PX, UK

K. R. McINTIRE Diagnosis Branch, Division of Cancer Biology and Diagnosis, Building 31, Room 3A10 National Cancer Institute, Bethesda, Maryland 20205, USA

W. B. MILLER Clinical Surgery, University Medical School, Edinburgh, UK

T. MING CHU Roswell Park Memorial Institute, Buffalo, New York 14263, USA

M. C. MINGARI Ludwig Institute for Cancer Research, 1066 Epalinges, Lausanne, Switzerland

P. MONAGHAN Ludwig Institute for Cancer Research, Royal Marsden Hospital, Sutton, Surrey SM2 5PX, UK

A. MORETTA Ludwig Institute for Cancer Research, 1066 Epalinges, Lausanne, Switzerland

L. MORRETTA Ludwig Institute for Cancer Research, 1066 Epalinges, Lausanne, Switzerland

V. MOSHAKIS Ludwig Institute for Cancer Research, Royal Marsden Hospital, Sutton, Surrey SM2 5PX, UK

A. R. MOOSSA University of Chicago, Illinois 60637, USA

R. M. NAKAMURA Department of Molecular Immunology, Scripps Clinic and Research Foundation, 10666 North Pines Road, La Jolla, California 92037, USA

A. M. NEVILLE Ludwig Institute for Cancer Research, Royal Marsden Hospital, Sutton, Surrey SM2 5PX, UK

Y. NIITSU Department of Internal Medicine, Sapporo Medical College, S-1, W16, Chuoku, Sapporo, 060 Japan

F. PACINI Cattedra di Patologia Medica II°, Università di Pisa, Via Roma 67, 56100 Pisa, Italy

S. PILOTTI Department of Pathology, Istituto Nazionale per lo Studio e la Cura dei Tumori, Via G. Venezian 1, 20133 Milan, Italy

A. PINCHERA Cattedra di Medicina Costituzionale e Endocrinologia, University of Padua, Padua, Italy

G. PIZZOCARO Section of Urological Oncology, Istituto Nazionale per lo Studio e la Cura dei Tumori, Via G. Venezian 1, 20133 Milan, Italy

J. E. PONTES Urologic Oncology, Roswell Park Memorial Institute, 666 Elm Street, Buffalo, New York 14263, USA

D. RAGHAVAN Ludwig Institute for Cancer Research, Royal Marsden Hospital, Sutton, Surrey SM2 5PX, UK

J. G. RATCLIFFE Department of Biochemistry, Royal Infirmary, Glasgow

G4 0SF, UK

J. RITSCHARD Division de Médecine Nucléaire, Department of Medicine, University Hospital of Geneva, 1211 Geneva, Switzerland

B. SERROU Laboratoire d'Immunopharmacologie des Tumeurs, INSERM U-236, ERA-CNRS No 844, Centre Paul Lamarque, B.P. 5054 34 033, Montpellier, Cédex, France

A. SULLIVAN Ludwig Institute for Cancer Research, Royal Marsden Hospital, Sutton, Surrey SM2 5PX, UK

D. M. P. THOMSON The Montreal General Hospital, 1650 Cedar Avenue, Montreal, Quebec, Canada H3G 1A4

I. URUSHIZAKI Department of Internal Medicine, Sapporo Medical College, S-1, W16, Chuoku, Sapporo, 060 Japan

U. VERONESI Istituto Nazionale per lo Studio e la Cura dei Tumori, Via G. Venezian 1, 20133 Milan, Italy

P. VEZZADINI I° Clinica Medica dell'Università di Bologna, Policlinico S. Orsola, Via Massarenti 9, Bologna, Italy

P. F. ZANGERLE Laboratory of Radioimmunology, University of Liège, Liège 1, Belgium

PREFACE

The scope of the Serono Symposium held in Milan, Italy, in April 1981, which originated this book, was to stress the interest in identifying reliable and reproducible test systems for early diagnosis and monitoring of tumours of clinical and epidemiological relevance in terms of incidence, severity and curability.

This book is intended to be not an all purpose review of the state of the art, but a selection of lectures and discussions specifically aimed at focalizing the marker problems in their function of early diagnostic and monitoring tools in tumours amenable to a therapeutic approach, i.e. breast, GI tract, lung, urogenital and blood tumours. Methods already described and relevant data are analysed in depth, as well as original approaches opening new lines of development in terms either of methodology or philosophy of research. In addition, basic technical and operational aspects of established or prospective test systems together with their practical implications are considered by renowned experts.

A relevant feature of the book is that a large part is devoted to discussion. Distinguished scientists, selected on the basis of their outstanding clinical or laboratory experience critically discuss the data presented by the lecturers with the aim of reaching a valid conclusion even from the point of view of clinical practice.

We would like to thank all the speakers of the Symposium who made it possible to realize successfully the programme as planned and who rapidly contributed to this book which, therefore, constitutes an up-to-date documentation in the field of tumour marker application.

We are also very grateful to the Serono Symposia for sponsoring this meeting and in particular to Dr S Rossetti and his staff.

April 1981   **M. I. COLNAGHI**
                                                               G. L. BURAGGI
                                                               M. GHIONE

CONTENTS

Contents

SURFACE MARKERS OF HUMAN LYMPHOCYTES:
PHENOTYPIC ANALYSIS OF FUNCTIONALLY DEFINED
T CELL SUBPOPULATIONS OR T CELL CLONES*

L. Moretta, G. Corte, A. Moretta, M. C. Mingari and A. Bargellesi

*Ludwig Institute for Cancer Research, Lausanne Branch, Epalinges,
Switzerland and Institutes of Biochemistry and Microbiology,
University of Genoa, Genoa, Italy*

Studies of cell surface markers and their ability to define subpopulations of lymphoid cells has been an area of most intensive investigation in human immunology.

This type of research has been further stimulated by the concept that lymphocyte surface markers may be directly involved in functional cell activities and/or interactions among cells. For example, surface immunoglobulin, the principal marker of mature B cells, is directly involved in the antigen induced B cell activation.

With respect to human T cell surface markers, they can be operationally divided into three different groups. (1) Those which define the whole T cell population, such as the receptor for sheep erythrocytes, heteroantisera rendered T specific after serial absorptions with different cell types, and, recently, monoclonal antibodies reported to bind to antigenic determinants uniquely expressed by T cells (Haynes *et al.*, 1980a; Moretta *et al.*, 1981d). (2) Those which are present only on a fraction of T cells, such as antigenic determinants recognized by the TH_1 or TH_2 heteroantisera (Evans *et al.*, 1977, 1978) or by monoclonal

* Partially supported by grants nos 99/78.02850.96 and 54/80.01525.96 awarded by CNR (PFCCN).

Serono Symposium No. 46, Markers for Diagnosis and Monitoring of Human Cancer, edited by M. I. Colnaghi, G. L. Buraggi and M. Ghione, 1982. Academic Press, London and New York.

antibodies, such as the OKT_4, OKT_5 (Reinherz and Schlossman, 1980), 3A1 (Haynes *et al.*, 1980a), 5/9 (Corte *et al.*, 1982), receptors for the FC fragment of different immunoglobulin isotypes (Moretta *et al.*, 1976, 1977), receptors for lectins (Hammaström *et al.*, 1973) and histamine (Saxon *et al.*, 1977). (3) A third group is represented by surface markers expressed only on activated T cells; among these are Ia antigens and a group of antigenic determinants recognized by monoclonal antibodies such as the 4F2 (Eisenbarth *et al.*, 1980) and the MLR 1–4 (Corte *et al.*, 1981).

Most of the presently familiar surface markers do not appear to be directly involved in T cell functions. An important exception is the surface FcR for IgG which is known to be involved in effector functions, such as the antibody dependent cellular cytotoxicity (ADCC) (Perlmann *et al.*, 1976; Perlmann and Cerottini, 1979) and in regulatory functions such as the inhibition of T or B cell proliferation in certain *in vitro* systems (Moretta *et al.*, 1977, 1979; Canonica *et al.*, 1980). FcR for all the different isotypes have been described, however FcR for IgG and IgM have been studied in greater detail. These receptors are virtually absent in thymocytes, whereas they are expressed on distinct sets of peripheral T cells. In addition, Fcγ R are detectable in a large fraction of activated T cells, especially after allogenic stimulation (Moretta *et al.*, 1981a,b).

Recent studies in several laboratories have focused on various activities displayed by isolated T cells bearing FcγR or FcμR (T_G and T_M cells, respectively). For example, in the *in vitro* B cell differentiation induced by pokeweed mitogen (PWM), a strictly T dependent phenomenon, it has been shown that T_G and T_M populations play an antithetical role, T_M cells being the helper cells and T_G the suppressor cells (Moretta *et al.*, 1977). Cells responsible for natural killer (NK) activity and ADCC are restricted to the T_G cell fraction (Pape *et al.*, 1979). T_G cells sharply inhibit the *in vitro* lymphoid colony formation (Canonica *et al.*, 1980). In addition, it has been shown that cells, with the T_G phenotype isolated from the bone marrow of patients with severe aplastic anaemia, suppress the *in vitro* myeloid colony formation in both autologous or allogeneic combinations (Bacigalupo *et al.*, 1980).

Taken together, the above functional analyses indicate that dissection of T cells according to their surface FcR may be useful for restricting some T cell activities to T_G or T_M populations. For example, it appears that naturally-occurring human suppressor cells frequently express surface FcγR (Moretta *et al.*, 1981d). However, identification of functional T cell subsets simply based on the use of FcR is not satisfactory. One of the main problems is the fact that only a small proportion of the cells in a given subset may be involved in the functional activity measured. Obviously, similar difficulties occur when T cell subpopulations are identified by other reagents such as monoclonal antibodies. Thus, the function of individual cells cannot be extrapolated simply by the presence of a given marker.

A more precise correlation between the surface phenotype and a given functional activity of the cell can be achieved by different experimental approaches, namely the combined use of different markers and the analysis of markers present on cloned T cells with defined functional properties.

COMBINED USE OF DIFFERENT MARKERS

The usefulness of this approach is demonstrated by two examples dealing with the phenotypical characterization of the T cells responsible for inducing B cell differentiation (helper T cells) and of the specific cytolytic cells (CTL), respectively.

Surface Phenotype of Helper T Cells

It has been reported that the T cells able to promote the PWM dependent B cell differentiation can be defined by their reactivity with a monoclonal antibody named OKT_4 (Reinherz and Schlossman, 1980). As mentioned above helper cells are also present in the T_M cell fraction. If all of the cells expressing these different phenotypes are indeed helper cells, this would imply that cells responsible for inducing B cell differentiation would represent a large fraction of peripheral T cells, since the antigens defined by OKT_4 and 3A1 monoclonal antibodies or the $Fc\mu R$ are all expressed in over 60% of E rosetting cells. However, recent experimental evidence has indicated that helper cells could be further restricted within a much smaller fraction of peripheral T cells, since all the helper cells appeared to be present, and highly enriched, in a T cell fraction reacting with 5/9 monoclonal antibody (Corte *et al.*, 1982; Moretta *et al.*, 1982). This antibody reacts with only 15-20% of peripheral T cells. In addition, not all of the $5/9^+$ cells express $Fc\mu R^+$ or $OKT4^+$. Therefore, human cells capable of inducing B cell differentiation can be defined more precisely by the simultaneous detection of different markers such as $Fc\mu R$, OKT_4, 3A1, 5/9. It should be noted that less than 10% of peripheral T cells simultaneously express all of these markers.

Surface Phenotype of Specific Cytolytic T Cells

As mentioned above, some surface markers are expressed on alloactivated T cells. Among these markers, Ia antigens and $Fc\gamma R$ are important in view of their direct involvement in certain immune reactions. $Fc\gamma R$ are expressed on 10-15% only of peripheral blood T cells (Moretta *et al.*, 1977), whereas Ia^+ cells represent 1-5% (Greaves *et al.*, 1979). Both of these markers, however, are expressed on high proportions of activated T cells (Moretta *et al.* 1981b; Winchester and Kunkel, 1980). In this context, 4F2 antibody (Eisenbarth *et al.* 1980) binds to activated but not to resting cells. $Fc\gamma R$, Ia and 4F2 antigens have been used for studying the surface phenotype of CTL generated in mixed lymphocyte culture (Moretta *et al.*, 1981b). Presence or absence of Ia antigens on alloactivated T cells did not select for specific CTL. In contrast, fractionation of alloactivated T cells in accordance to either surface $Fc\gamma R$ or 4F2 antigens showed that CTL were restricted to the $Fc\gamma R^-$ and to the $4F2^+$ cell populations, respectively. $Fc\gamma R^-$ and $4F2^+$ cell fractions are only partially overlapping as purified $4F2^+$ populations included up to 30% $Fc\gamma R^+$ cells, and $Fc\gamma R^-$ cells were up to 50% $4F2^-$. Further fractionation of

cells based on the combined use of the two markers showed that CTL activity
was restricted to the $4F2^+$, $Fc\gamma R^-$ subset. Such cell population usually accounts
for about 30% of alloactivated T cells (Moretta et al., 1981b).

ANALYSIS OF SURFACE MARKERS PRESENT IN CLONED T CELLS
WITH DEFINED FUNCTIONS

Another experimental approach leading to a precise correlation between cell
function and surface phenotype is based on the establishment of cloned T cells
with defined functions. T cell clones can be generated under limiting conditions in microculture systems in the presence of "filler" cells and T cell growth
factors (TCGF). TCGF, also referred to as "Interleukin 2", has been defined
as that material present in culture fluids obtained from lectin, or alloantigen,
stimulated lymphocyte cultures which is required for the continuous proliferation of cultured T cells (Smith, 1980).

By using these experimental devices, it is now feasible to analyse the phenotype of T cell clones previously selected for a given function. We have recently
used this approach for the phenotypical characterization of T cell clones with
different types of cytolytic activities (Moretta et al., 1981e). T cells stimulated
in secondary MLC were cloned under limiting conditions in microculture systems
using TCGF, derived from PHA stimulated human lymphocytes (Moretta et al.,
1981c), and irradiated allogenic cells as filler cells. T cell clones were selected for
their cytotoxic capacity against: (1) PHA activated target cells bearing the stimulating alloantigens (CTL activity) (2) L1210 mouse cells coated with rabbit
antibody (ADCC); (3) K562 human target cells (NK activity). Cells from micro-
cultures with lytic activity restricted to only one of the target cell types used were
expanded in macrowells, employing the culture conditions used for cloning and
analysed for different surface markers including rosette formation with sheep
erythrocytes (E rosettes), receptors for the Fc portion of IgG or IgM ($Fc\gamma R$ and
$Fc\mu R$), and a group of antigens recognized by monoclonal antibodies including
Ia, 4F2, OKT_8 and OKT_4 (Table I). All clones were E rosette positive with 73–
94% of the cells in individual clones forming rosettes. In 12 out of 14 cytolytic
clones, $Fc\gamma R$ were virtually absent, whereas 30–40% of the cells in two clones
with ADCC activity were $Fc\gamma R^+$. The percentage of $Fc\mu R^+$ cells in all cytolytic
clones was less than 10% but reached 26 and 50% respectively in two of the non-
cytolytic clones. Flow cytofluorometric analysis showed that all (cytolytic and
non-cytolytic) clones expressed relatively large amounts of Ia antigens. In addition,
virtually 100% of the cells in individual clones were Ia^+. Comparable results were
obtained when the clones were analysed for the expression of 4F2 antigen. In
contrast, only four of the cytolytic clones were $OKT8^+$. Among these clones,
three were cytolytic against K562 target cells, whereas only one had CTL activity.
Of the seven $OKT8^-$ CTL clones, three were $OKT4^+$. The latter antigen was also
expressed in two clones active in ADCC and two (out of four) non-cytolytic
clones. Flow cytofluorometric analysis of individual CTL clones indicated that
virtually 100% of the cells of a clone were positive or negative for OKT_4 or OKT_8
antigens.

Two clones selected for their high CTL activity were subcloned by limiting

Table I. Surface markers of human T cell clones with different cytolytic activities.

Clone number	Cytolytic activity	SRBC	FcγR	FcμR	Ia	4F2	OKT$_8$	OKT$_4$
1	NK (86)[a]	89[h]	1	0	+[c]	+[c]	+[c]	[c]
2	NK (46)	78	0	8	+	+	−	−
3	NK (75)	75	0	10	+	+	+	−
4	NK (80)	84	1	3	+	+	+	−
5	ADCC (35)	80	42	1	+	+	−	+
6	ADCC (41)	81	29	0	+	+	−	+
7	CTL (39)	93	2	1	+	+	−	+
8	CTL (82)	92	4	3	+	+	+	−
9	CTL (88)	94	0	1	+	ND	−	ND
10	CTL (51)	74	3	10	+	+	−	+
11	CTL (35)	83	0	4	+	+	−	−
12	CTL (27)	73	0	8	+	+	−	−
13	CTL (26)	75	0	8	+	+	−	−
14	CTL (60)	94	0	1	+	+	−	+
15	−	93	1	4	+	+	−	−
16	−	77	0	50	+	+	−	+
17	−	81	1	26	+	+	−	+
18	−	89	2	7	+	+	−	−

[a]Percentage of specific lysis at 30:1 lymphocyte/target ratio. [b]Percentage of rosette forming cells. [c]Presence or absence of surface antigens was analysed by fluorescence activated cell sorter.

dilution. All the subclones have been phenotypically and functionally identical to the parent cell clones suggesting a high degree of phenotypic stability, at least over the time period (2-3) weeks) needed for their isolation.

The fact that noticeable proportions, but not all, of the cells of the expanded clones formed E rosettes (or had detectable FcγR), is likely due to limitation of the techniques used. Alternatively, the possibility exists that cells at different stages of the cell cycle or with different metabolic activity vary in their expression of surface receptors. This possibility is supported by the finding that five individual subclones derived from the E rosette negative fraction of a putative clonal isolate were mostly E rosette positive.

It is of interest that FcγR were present in two clones active in ADCC but without lytic activity against K562 target cells. Conversely, the four clones reactive against K562 target cells were FcγR⁻ and devoid of K cell activity. Thus, although ADCC and NK activity are mediated by the same KcγR⁺ subset in peripheral blood lymphocytes, they can be dissociated in clones derived from alloreactive MLC populations.

Large amounts of Ia antigens were detected on the surface of all cloned cells analysed, including those with CTL activity. Studies at the population level gave conflicting results as to the expression of Ia antigens on human CTL. Reinherz *et al.*, (1980) reported that CTL activity was restricted to the Ia⁻ fraction of allo-

6 L. Moretta et al.

activated T cells. Earlier studies from our laboratory indicated that Ia^+ and Ia^- MLC cells exhibited similar levels of specific cytolytic activity. The procedure used in our studies for deriving expanded clones, including the use of TCGF, may favour the proliferation of Ia^+ cells. However, we can conclude that at least a fraction, if not all, of human CTL express Ia antigens. Previous studies on MLC T cell populations have shown that CTL activity was restricted to a $Fc\gamma R$ negative subpopulation expressing the 4F2 antigen (Moretta et al., 1981a). Although clonal analysis confirms that CTL are $4F2^+$, it is evident that this antigen cannot be used as a specific marker for CTL, as it is also expressed in non-cytolytic clones. These results are in agreement with our previous studies showing that CTL activity in MLC T cell populations is restricted to the $Fc\gamma R^-$ fraction of the $4F2^+$ populations.

Reinherz et al. (1980) have recently reported that CTL generated in MLC express the OKT_8^+, OKT_4^- phenotype. Such phenotype, however, was detectable in only one of eight CTL clones analysed. In addition, three of the OKT_8^- CTL clones expressed the OKT_4 antigen. These results clearly indicate that it is not possible to assign a given function to lymphocytes bearing either the OKT_4 or the OKT_8 antigen. Along this line, it is of note that three of four clones with NK activity were OKT_8^+, OKT_4^-, whereas the two clones active in ADCC expressed the opposite phenotype.

REFERENCES

Bacigalupo, A., Podestà, M., Mingari, M. C., Moretta, L., Van Lindt, M. T. and Marmont, A. (1980). *Journal of Immunology* 125, 1449.
Canonica, G. W., Pistoia, V., Ghio, R., Mingari, M. C. and Moretta, L. (1980). *Scandinavian Journal of Immunology* 12, 507.
Corte, G., Moretta, L., Damiani, G., Mingari, M. C. and Bargellesi, A. (1981). *European Journal of Immunology* 11, 162.
Corte, G., Mingari, M. C., Moretta, A., Damiani, G., Moretta, L. and Bargellesi, A. (1982). *Journal of Immunology*. (In press.)
Eisenbarth, G. S., Haynes, B. F., Schroer, J. A. and Fauci, A. S. (1980). *Journal of Immunology* 124, 1237.
Evans, R. L., Breard, J. M., Lazarus, H., Schlossman, S. F. and Chess, L. (1977). *Journal of Experimental Medicine* 145, 221.
Evans, R. L., Lazarus, H., Penta, A. C. and Schlossman, S. F. (1978). *Journal of Immunology* 120, 1423.
Greaves, M. F., Verbi, V., Festenstein, M., Papasteriadis, C., Garaquemada, D. and Hayward, A. (1979). *European Journal of Immunology* 9, 356.
Hammarström, S., Hellström, V., Perlmann, P. and Dillner, M. L. (1973). *Journal of Experimental Medicine* 138, 1270.
Haynes, B. F., Katz, P. and Fauci, A. S. (1980a). *Progress in Clinical Immunology* 4, 23.
Haynes, B. F., Mann, D. L., Hemler, M. E., Schroer, H. A., Shelhamer, H. H., Eisenbarth, G. S., Strominger, J. L., Thomas, C. A., Mostowski, H. S. and Fauci, A. S. (1980b). *Proceedings of the National Academy of Sciences of USA* 77, 2914.
Moller, G. (Ed.) (1979). *Immunological Review* 44.
Moretta, L., Ferrarini, M., Mingari, M. C., Moretta, A. and Webb, S. R. (1976). *Journal of Immunology* 117, 2171.

Moretta, L., Webb, S. R., Grossi, C. E., Lydyard, P. M. and Cooper, M. D. (1977). *Journal of Experimental Medicine* **146**, 184.

Moretta, L., Mingari, M. C. and Moretta, A. (1979). *Immunological Review* **45**, 163.

Moretta, A., Mingari, M. C., Colombatti, M. and Moretta, L. (1981a). *Scandinavian Journal of Immunology* **13**, 447.

Moretta, A., Mingari, M. C., Haynes, B. F., Sekaly, R. P., Moretta, L. and Fauci, A. S. (1981b). *Journal of Experimental Medicine* **153**, 213.

Moretta, A., Colombatti, M. and Chapuis, B. (1981c). *Clinical Immunology and Immunopathology* **44**, 262.

Moretta, L., Moretta, A., Canonica, G. W., Bacigalupo, A., Mingari, M. C. and Cerottini, J. C. (1981d). *Immunological Review* **56**, 141.

Moretta, L., Mingari, M. C., Sekaly, R. P., Moretta, A., Chapuis, B. and Cerottini, J. C. (1981e). *Journal of Experimental Medicine* **154**, 569.

Moretta, A., Corte, G., Mingari, M. C. and Moretta, L. (1982). *Journal of Immunology*. (In press.)

Pape, G. R., Moretta, L., Troye, M. and Perlmann, P. (1979). *Scandinavian Journal of Immunology* **9**, 291.

Perlmann, P. and Cerottini, J. C. (1979). *In* "The Antigens" (M. Sela, Ed.), p.173. Academic Press Inc., New York.

Perlmann, H., Perlmann, P., Pape, G. R. and Hallden, G. (1976). *Scandinavian Journal of Immunology* **5** (Suppl. 5), 57.

Reinherz, E. L. and Schlossman, S. F. (1980). *Cell* **19**, 821.

Reinherz, E. L., Hussey, R. E. and Schlossman, S. F. (1980). *Immunogenetics* **11**, 421.

Saxon, A., Morledge, V. D. and Bonavida, B. (1977). *Clinical and Experimental Immunology* **28**, 394.

Smith, K. A. (1980). *Immunological Review* **51**, 337.

Winchester, R. J. and Kunkel, H. G. (1980). *Advances in Immunology* **28**, 22.

CIRCULATING IMMUNE COMPLEXES AS MARKERS
FOR HUMAN NEOPLASIA

N. A. Carpentier, R. Egeli, P. Chollet, P. Maurice and P. H. Lambert

*WHO Immunology Research and Training Centre and Division of Oncology,
Department of Medicine, and Department of Surgery, University of Geneva,
Geneva, Switzerland*

INTRODUCTION

The formation of immune complexes is a normal part of the immune response
and occurs each time foreign antigenic molecules are available in extracellular
spaces when the corresponding antibodies appear. Since most of the immune
complexes appearing in circulating blood are cleared rapidly by the reticulo-
endothelial system, the formation of antigen-antibody complexes may be considered
as a physiological mechanism to clear antigens rapidly (Weigle, 1961). Immune
complexes can also participate in the regulation of the immune response
(Haakenstad and Mannik, 1977; Sedlacek, 1980).

Using sensitive methods for the detection of immune complexes (Lambert *et al.*,
1978), it has been found that, in some circumstances, immune complexes can
persist in large amounts in human biological fluids and produce pathological
manifestations when they localize in tissues (Zubler and Lambert, 1977). This is
particularly the case in immunological disorders and during some infectious
processes. In most of these diseases, the induction of inflammatory reactions is
usually considered as the major pathogenic consequence of the immune complex
formation.

More recently, circulating immune complexes (CIC) have been detected also in

Serono Symposium No. 46, Markers for Diagnosis and Monitoring of Human Cancer, edited
by M. I. Colnaghi, G. L. Buraggi and M. Ghione, 1982. Academic Press, London and New
York.

patients with various types of malignancy (Theofilopoulos and Dixon, 1979; Carpentier *et al.*, 1980a). In these patients, the biological consequences of the presence of CIC have yet to be defined. As suggested by data from clinical and experimental investigations, CIC might be involved in the pathophysiology of cancer. Several clinical studies have provided evidence for a temporal relationship of CIC with the activity of the malignancy and for their association with an unfavourable course of cancer (Amlot *et al.*, 1978; Brandeis *et al.*, 1978; Carpentier *et al.*, 1977, 1980b; Chollet *et al.*, 1980; Hoffken *et al.*, 1977; Hubbard *et al.*, 1981; Poulton *et al.*, 1978; Rossen *et al.*, 1977). Regardless of the nature of the complexed antigens, CIC could favour the progression of cancer by impairing the host's antitumour response, either at the afferent or efferent phase of the immune response. CIC may also represent the major part of humoral factors which inhibit cell mediated reactivity to tumour cells *in vitro*. Direct evidence for such a role of CIC in cancer patients has not yet been provided.

Over the past 5 years, we have investigated the presence of CIC in a large number of patients with leukaemia or malignant solid tumours, in particular breast and lung cancer (Carpentier *et al.*, 1977, 1979, 1980a,b; Heier *et al.*, 1977; Casali *et al.*, 1977; Chollet *et al.*, 1980). The method used for the detection of soluble IC was primarily the ^{125}I-C1q binding assay (Zubler *et al.*, 1976). In some cases, for comparison purposes, the Raji cell radioassay (Theofilopoulos *et al.*, 1976), and the conglutinin binding test (Casali *et al.*, 1977) were used. The identification of serum C1q binding material as immune complexes was demonstrated by physical and immunochemical analysis. On sucrose density gradient, this material sedimented as a 14–30 S molecular weight material which could be dissociated at acid pH with appearance of a 7 S peak containing IgG. The C1q binding ability of the material was abolished by removal of IgG by immunoabsorption or acid dissociation while it was not sensitive to DNase treatment.

The levels of CIC in the patients studied were examined in relation to clinical features, in particular the stage of cancer, the tumour size and the course of the disease in order to assess the clinical relevance of the detection of IC in cancer patients.

INVESTIGATION OF CIC IN LEUKAEMIA

A total of 492 patients with leukaemia were included in this study, 224 suffered from acute myeloid leukaemia (AML), 60 from acute lymphatic leukaemia (ALL), 64 from blastic crisis (BC) of chronic myeloid leukaemia (CML), 74 from CML and 70 from chronic lymphatic leukaemia (CLL). Whenever possible, serial serum samples were analysed and the level of IC was correlated to the stage and the course of the disease. In acute leukaemia (AML, ALL, BC) serum samples were taken from 187 patients at the time of diagnosis; the other samples corresponded to the period of complete remission or of relapse. Most of the patients were treated by chemotherapy according to the type and stage of leukaemia.

Incidence of CIC in Leukaemia

The C1q binding activity (C1q-BA) of 900 serum samples from the 492 patients studied was determined in parallel to that of sera from 375 healthy blood donors. The upper limit (mean + 3 SD) of the percentage of ^{125}I-C1q precipitated in the

Table I. Serum ^{125}I-C1q binding activity in 492 patients with leukaemia

Type of leukaemia (No. of sera)	C1q binding activity Mean ± 1 SD (%)	Patients with CIC[a]	
		No.	%
Acute myeloid (395)	8.3 ± 15.3	98/224	43.8
Acute lymphatic (100)	6.1 ± 16.1	17/60	28.3
Blastic crisis (110)	6.3 ± 10.0	26/64	40.6
Chronic myeloid (191)	2.1 ± 5.5	17/74	23.0
Chronic lymphatic (104)	7.5 ± 17.8	14/70	20.0

[a] Patients with serum C1q-BA > 3 SD above the mean normal value.

normal sera was 5.5%. Serum with a ^{125}I-C1q-BA exceeding this value was considered to contain IC. The incidence of CIC and the mean levels of serum C1q-BA in the patients grouped according to the type of leukaemia are shown in Table I. IC were found in 40.5% of patients with acute leukaemia and 21.5% of those with chronic leukaemia.

Serum samples from 48 leukaemic patients were tested simultaneously using the C1q binding test and the Raji cell radioimmunoassay. On a qualitative basis, the results obtained by the two methods were in agreement in 41 of the 48 cases (85.4%). In addition, sera from 24 patients with acute or chronic leukaemia were assayed simultaneously by the C1q binding test, the Raji cell radioimmunoassay and the conglutinin binding test. The results of the three tests, concordant in 59% of the cases, correlated significantly.

In most of the patients studied, the possible relationship of serum C1q-BA to the white blood cell count, haemoglobin and platelet levels, and erythrocyte sedimentation rate was investigated. No correlation was found. In patients with leukaemia in the acute stage, the presence of sepsis at the time of serum sampling did not correlate with the occurrence of CIC; IC were detected in 45% of the sera from patients with sepsis and in 40% of sera from patients with no evidence of such a complication. In 130 cases of acute leukaemia, the incidence and levels of CIC were analysed in terms of relationship to treatment. It was found that 58% of the sera from untreated patients were positive as compared to 34% of the sera from patients receiving chemotherapy. In the latter, the mean level of C1q-BA was significantly lower than that of untreated cases. In 30 patients who had received blood transfusions before serum sampling, the occurrence of complexes was investigated in relation to the presence of anti-HLA antibodies. Such antibodies were detected in ten cases, but no association was found with the presence of complexes (5/15 with CIC and 5/15 with C1q-BA within the normal range).

High Incidence of CIC During the Acute Stage of Leukaemia

In acute leukaemia (AML, ALL, BC), the incidence of CIC and serum C1q binding levels in patients tested during the blastic stage of the disease were compared with those observed in patients during complete remission. CIC were found more frequently in the 187 patients studied at diagnosis of leukaemia

Table II. High incidence of CIC during florid stage of acute leukaemia.

Stage of leukaemia	C1q binding activity	Patients with CIC[a]	
	Mean ± 1 SD (%)	No.	%
Diagnosis	15.1 ± 12.3	116/187	62.0
Complete remission	7.2 ± 11.2	34/112	30.4
Relapse	14.2 ± 12.2	42/64	65.6

[a] Patients with serum C1q-BA > 3 SD above the mean normal value.

and in the 64 patients at relapse than in the 112 patients in complete remission
(Table II). The mean values of serum C1q-BA were also significantly higher in
the patients during the acute phase than during complete remission. The pre-
valent association of CIC with the acute stage of leukaemia was also demonstrated by serial serum analysis. In several cases in which CIC were present
during the acute phase, CIC were no longer detectable after induction of complete
remission. Conversely, CIC were present at the time of relapse or of blastic transformation of CML respectively in patients who were negative during complete
remission of acute leukaemia, or during the chronic phase of CML.

Poor Response to Therapy in Patients with CIC

Low Incidence of Complete Remission

The incidence of complete remission was examined in relation to CIC in the
187 patients studied at diagnosis of AML, ALL or BC (Table III). The clinical
course in these patients correlated significantly with the presence or absence of
CIC at diagnosis. Complete remission was recorded in 75% of the 71 CIC-negative patients but in only 27% of the 116 CIC-positive patients ($P < 0.0005$).
Moreover, 61% of the patients with CIC at diagnosis who achieved remission
relapsed within 6 months. In contrast, relapse occurred during this period in
only four (8%) of the 53 CIC-negative patients who remitted.

Table III. Poor response to therapy in patients with CIC at diagnosis of acute
leukaemia.

Type of leukaemia	Patients with CIC[a]			Patients without CIC		
	No.	Complete remission		No.	Complete remission	
		> 6 mo.	< 6 mo.		> 6 mo.	< 6 mo.
Acute myeloid	88	10%	17%	53	70%	8%
Acute lymphatic	11	27%	27%	10	100%	—
Blastic crisis	17	—	6%	8	25%	—
TOTAL	116	10%	17%	71	69%	6%

[a] Patients with serum C1q-BA > 3 SD above the mean normal value.

Table IV. Combined prognostic value of age and CIC in patients with AML.

Patients	Incidence of complete remission					
	TOTAL		Patients with CIC		Patients without CIC	
	No.	%	No.	%	No.	%
More than 60-years-old	15/53	28	6/39	15	9/14	64
Less than 60-years-old	50/88	57	18/50	36	32/38	84
All patients	65/141	46	24/89	27	41/52	79

The poorer response rate to treatment of patients with CIC at diagnosis of leukaemia was unrelated to unfavourable prognostic features such as age, sex, haematological parameters or sepsis. For instance, analysis of response rate in AML patients separated into age groups showed that the incidence of complete remission decreased with increasing age, regardless of whether or not the patients had CIC (Table IV). Age and CIC appeared as two independent prognostic factors which could be combined to predict a high probability of achieving complete remission (84% complete remission in CIC-negative and age < 60 years) or a likelihood of failure (85% failures in CIC-positive and age > 60 years). However, the presence or absence of CIC at diagnosis appeared to be a more important prognostic factor than age.

In AML, the low incidence of complete remission in the patients with CIC at onset of disease was also unrelated to the cytological type of leukaemia. Analysis of the response rate in the patients grouped according to the cytological variety of AML, as defined by the French-American-British (FAB) classification, showed that the incidence of complete remission was much lower in all the groups of patients with immune complexes than in those without complexes regardless of the cytological type of the leukaemic cells (Table V).

Short Survival Time

The difference in response to chemotherapy in patients according to the presence or absence of CIC at diagnosis of acute leukaemia was reflected in the survival times. The median survival times within the 5-year period of study in the patients without CIC at onset of leukaemia were: 15.75 months in AML, 20 months in ALL, and 7 months in BC. The corresponding survival times in the patients with CIC at this time were much lower: 72, 140 and 100 days respectively in AML, ALL and BC.

CIC as Markers of Relapse During Complete Remission

Early Relapse in Patients with CIC at the Onset of Remission

Eighty patients were studied for the presence of CIC during their first complete remission. Of these 80, 45 were tested at least twice during the first 2 months of remission. CIC were found in 18 (40%) of these patients during this period. With one exception, all of the patients positive for CIC experienced a complete remission shorter than 6 months. On the contrary, in 27 patients without CIC at the onset of remission, only four (15%) relapsed within the first year of complete remission. The median duration of complete remission in the 18 patients with CIC during the first 2-month period of remission was 4 months, while it was 15.5 months in the 27 patients without such complexes.

Appearance of CIC During Maintained Remission May Predict Relapse

The significance of the appearance of CIC after several months of complete remission was examined in a population of 57 patients with an AML maintained in remission for more than 7 months. During the period of study, 35 (61%) of these patients relapsed. Of these 35, 23 had been tested repeatedly for the presence of CIC during the 6 months preceding relapse. CIC were detected in 18 (78%) of these patients 6 months to 3 weeks prior to overt haematologic relapse. CIC were not present more than 6 months prior to relapse in the patients studied.

INVESTIGATION OF CIC IN BREAST CANCER

The sera of 136 women with carcinoma of the breast were analysed by the C1q-binding assay for the presence of IC, 84 of these patients had localized tumours and 52 metastatic cancer at the time of the first sampling. The patients were studied sequentially for CIC during a follow-up period of 4 years. Most of the patients with regional disease were tested at the time of diagnosis and after initial treatment which consisted of tumour excision plus loco-regional radio-therapy in the case of lymph node involvement. These patients also received adjuvant chemotherapy during the 12 months following the local treatment. Patients with metastatic disease were treated with chemotherapy, even when complete remission was obtained, during 3 years. Clinical examinations including hepatic and bone scans were repeated at least every 6 months.

Incidence of CIC in Breast Cancer

The mean C1q-BA $\pm$ 1 SD of the 107 normal sera tested in this study was $0 \pm 2\%$. A serum C1q-BA exceeding 6% (3 SD of normal values) was found in 26.5% of the patients at the first sampling.

Table V. Combined prognostic value of cytological type and CIC in patients with AML.

Cytological subtype	Incidence of complete remission					
	TOTAL		Patients with CIC		Patients without CIC	
	No.	%	No.	%	No.	%
AML$_1$ (undifferentiated)	26/45	58	9/24	37	17/21	81
AML$_2$ (myeloblastic)	15/35	43	8/26	31	7/9	78
AML$_3$ (promyelocytic)	5/8	63	1/4	25	4/4	100
AML$_4$ (myelomonocytic)	6/12	50	3/9	33	3/3	100
AML$_5$ (monoblastic)	11/33	33	3/23	13	8/10	80
AML$_6$ (erythroleukaemia)	1/3	33	0/2	–	1/1	–

Table VI. High incidence of CIC in widespread breast carcinoma

Stage of cancer	C1q binding activity	Patients with CIC[a]	
	Mean ± 1 SD (%)	No.	%
Localized	2.9 ± 3.6	14/84	17
T1 or T2, N + or −	2.6 ± 3.1	7/49	14
T3 or T4,N + or −	2.4 ± 2.8	3/26	12
Bilateral	4.3 ± 5.9	4/9	44
Metastatic	5.8 ± 6.1	22/52	42
Evolutive	9.3 ± 7.2	14/23	61
Non-evolutive[b]	3.1 ± 4.0	8/29	28

[a] Patients with serum C1q-BA > 3 SD above the mean normal value. [b] Patients in complete or partial remission, i.e. with 100% or > 50% tumour regression.

In these patients, there was no evidence of sepsis or other infectious complication. No correlation was found between the level of CIC and the erythrocyte sedimentation rate in individual cases.

High Incidence of CIC in Widespread Breast Tumours

A comparative analysis of the serum C1q-BA and the clinical stage of cancer at the time of the first sampling indicated that CIC were much more frequently present in patients with disseminated than localized tumours ($P < 0.001$; Table VI). In addition, in the metastatic cancer group the incidence and levels of CIC were significantly higher in patients with evolutive disease than in those considered to be in complete (100% tumour regression) or partial (> 50% tumour regression) remission ($P < 0.025$). In the patients with localized disease, the level of CIC at diagnosis did not correlate with the size of the tumour. However, CIC were more frequent in patients with bilateral than unilateral tumours ($P < 0.05$).

Table VII. Poor prognosis in patients with CIC at diagnosis of localized breast cancer

	Incidence of long-term complete remission[a]			
	Patients with CIC[b]		Patients without CIC	
	No.	%	No.	%
T1, T2, N + or −	4/7	57	36/42	86
T3, T4, bilateral, N + or −	2/7	29	20/28	71
TOTAL	6/14	43	56/70	80

[a] Complete remission maintained 3 years or more. [b] Patients with serum C1q-BA > 3 SD above the mean normal value.

Table VIII. Incidence of CIC in bronchial cancer : relation to tumour burden

Stage of cancer	Patients with CIC			
	Raji cell assay		C1q binding assay	
	No.	%	No.	%
Low tumour burden:	2/14	14	6/24	25
I	2/11	18	2/4	50
II	0/3	0	4/20	20
High tumour burden:	9/19	47	13/29	45
III	7/14	50	9/18	50
Unresectable	2/5	40	4/11	36
TOTAL	11/33	33	19/53	36

Poor Prognosis of Breast Cancer in Patients with CIC

The prognostic value of the presence of CIC in patients with breast cancer was examined with regard to the course of the disease and patient's survival.

The incidence of long-term (3 or more years) complete remission was assessed in the patients with localized tumours at diagnosis. Among these patients, a persisting complete remission was recorded in 80% of the women without CIC at diagnosis but in only 43% of the patients with CIC during this period. The other patients had tumours which recurred and progressed early after the initial treatment. Analysis of the response in the patients grouped according to both the CIC levels and the extent of tumour at diagnosis revealed a poorer incidence of long-term complete remission in patients positive for CIC regardless of the initial tumour extent (Table VII). The tumour burden at diagnosis and the level of CIC appeared as two independent prognostic features. The survival times in the patients with localized breast cancer were also determined in relation to their initial levels of CIC. The median survival time was more than 5.5 years in the patients without CIC, and 3.33 years in those with CIC; all the patients positive for CIC at diagnosis died within 4 years.

In the patients with metastatic cancer, the course of the disease differed also in relation to the patient's level of CIC at the time of the first serum sampling. Cancer progression occurred in 91% of patients with CIC at this time as compared with 43% of those without such complexes.

CIC as Markers of Breast Cancer Progression

Serial serum analysis showed that in most of the patients whose cancer progressed during the period of observation, CIC appeared or their levels increased during the 6 month period preceding the clinical evidence of tumour progression (Fig. 1).

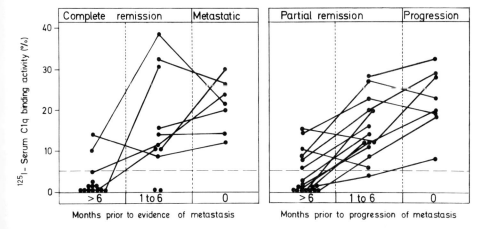

Fig. 1. IC and breast cancer progression. Serum C1q binding activity at various times before relapse among patients with breast cancer studied during remission and whose cancer progressed. Left: patients with localized breast tumours, right: patients with metastatic breast cancer.

INVESTIGATION OF CIC IN BRONCHIAL CANCER

Two series of patients with bronchial carcinoma were studied pre- and post-operatively for the presence of CIC. The first study was done at the Memorial Sloan Kettering Cancer Center in New York, USA, and included 33 patients*. Serum samples from these patients were analysed by the Raji cell radioimmuno-assay. The second study was done at the University Cantonal Hospital in Geneva, Switzerland. It included 53 patients whose sera were tested for IC using the ^{125}I-C1q binding assay. All of the patients were untreated at the time of the first sampling. Sixty-three had been treated by curative surgery at the time of the second sampling. The clinical staging of cancer at diagnosis was established in all cases according to the criteria of the American Joint Committee for Cancer Staging and End Results Reporting. All the metastatic cancer patients (stage III) included in this study had only loco-regional metastasis.

Incidence of CIC in Bronchial Cancer

Among the 33 patients tested by the Raji cell method, 11 (33%) had a pre-operative pathological level of CIC (> 16 g AHG equivalent/ml). A serum C1q-BA exceeding the upper normal limit (6%) was observed at diagnosis in 19 (36%) of the 53 patients studied by the C1q binding test.

Since acute or chronic infections of the lung are particularly frequent complica-tions of bronchial carcinoma, the levels of CIC at diagnosis in 35 documented cases

---

* In collaboration with Noorbibi K. DAY, Memorial Sloan-Kettering Cancer Center, 1275 York Avenue, New York, New York 10021.

were examined in relation to infection. The presence of a pulmonary infectious process at the time of the first sampling did not correlate with the presence of CIC, seven (54%) of 13 non-infected patients as compared to seven (32%) out of 22 infected patients had an increased serum C1q-BA.

High Incidence of CIC in Widespread Bronchial Cancer

The level of CIC in patients at diagnosis of bronchial cancer were examined in relation to the tumour stage (Table VIII). CIC were detected more frequently in patients with metastatic (stage III) or unresectable cancer than in those with localized disease (stage I and II), 46% of the 48 patients with high tumour-burden had CIC as compared to 21% of the 38 patients with low tumour burden.

In order to confirm the relationship between the level of CIC and the tumour load, individual pre-operative and post-operative levels of CIC were compared in patients which had curative surgery. All the eight patients positive for CIC with the Raji cell before surgery had a level of CIC within the normal range after tumour excision, of the 17 patients with increased serum C1q-BA before curative surgery, 71% had serum C1q-BA that decreased or returned within the normal values after tumour resection.

CIC and Histological Type of Bronchial Cancer

The incidence of CIC in patients with bronchial carcinoma was further examined in relation to the histological type of the tumour (Table IX). Most of the patients studied in the USA had adenocarcinoma, while the majority of European patients had epidermoid cancer. CIC were found at diagnosis in 29% of 28 patients with adenocarcinoma, 38% of 45 patients with epidermoid carcinoma and in four of nine patients with other histological types of bronchial cancer.

Poor Prognosis of Bronchial Cancer in Patients with CIC

The clinical course in individual patients was examined in relation to the detection of CIC at the time of diagnosis of cancer (Table X). The follow-up period for the patients studied by the Raji cell assay was 8–12 months and 3–15 months for those tested by the C1q binding assay. No evidence of disease during the period

Table IX. Incidence of CIC in bronchial cancer : relation to histological type

| Histological type | Patients with CIC | | | |
| | Raji cell assay | | C1q binding assay | |
	No.	%	No.	%
Adenocarcinoma	6/19	32	2/9	22
Epidermoid carcinoma	3/11	27	14/34	41
Oat cell carcinoma	1/1	–	0/2	–
Others	–	–	3/6	50

Table X. Poor prognosis in patients with CIC at diagnosis of bronchial cancer

Patients (no.)	Clinical course					
	Non-evolutive disease		Progressing disease		Death	
	No.	%	No.	%	No.	%
CIC-positive (26)	9	35	7	27	10	38
With Raji cell assay (11)	3	27	4	36	4	36
With C1q binding test (15)	6	40	3	20	6	40
CIC-negative (37)	27	73	4	11	6	16
With Raji cell assay (37)	14	70	3	15	3	15
With C1q binding test (17)	13	76	1	6	3	18

of observation was recorded after surgery in 73% of the 37 patients without CIC at diagnosis but in only 35% of the 26 patients with complexes at the time of diagnosis. Clinically progressing disease and death from cancer were observed in the other patients.

SUMMARY

The presence of circulating immune complexes in a large number of patients with leukaemia, breast or bronchial carcinoma was investigated, over a 5-year period, in relation to the activity, the extent and the clinical course of the malignancy. In acute leukaemia, circulating immune complexes were detected mostly in patients during the active stage of the disease. In patients with breast or bronchial cancer, the levels of circulating immune complexes correlated closely with the extent of the tumour. The presence of immune complexes at diagnosis proved to be an unfavourable prognostic factor in the three types of cancer studied. Most of the patients with circulating immune complexes at diagnosis failed to respond to initial therapy or experienced a short period of remission, and, consequently, had shorter survival times than patients without immune complexes. In patients with acute leukaemia, the presence of serum immune complexes at the beginning of complete remission was associated with early relapse. In these patients and in patients with breast cancer, an increase in the level of circulating immune complexes during maintained remission appeared as an indication of imminent recurrence or progression of cancer.

REFERENCES

Amlot, P. L., Pussell, B., Slaney, J. M. and Williams, B. D. (1978). *Clinical and Experimental Immunology* **31**, 166.
Brandeis, W. E., Helson, L., Wang, Y., Good, R. A. and Day, N. K. (1978). *Journal of Clinical Investigation* **62**, 1201.

Carpentier, N. A., Lange, G. T., Fière, D. M., Fournié, G. J., Lambert, P. H. and Miescher, P. A. (1977). *Journal of Clinical Investigation* **60**, 874.

Carpentier, N. A., Lambert, P. H. and Miescher P. A. (1979). *In* "Current Trends in Tumour Immunology" (S. Ferrone *et al.*, Eds), pp. 165–174. Garland Publishing, Inc., New York.

Carpentier, N. A., Louis, J. A., Lambert, P. H. and Cerottini, J. C. (1980a). *In* "Human Cancer Immunology" (B. Serrou *et al.*, Eds). North Holland Publication. (In press).

Carpentier, N. A., Fière, D. M., Schuh, D., Boye, J., Lambert, P. H. and Miescher, P. A. (1980b). *In* "New Trends in Human Immunology and Cancer Immunotherapy" (B. Serrou and C. Rosenfeld, Eds), pp. 465–477. Doin, Paris.

Casali, P., Bossus, A., Carpentier, N. A. and Lambert, P. H. (1977). *Clinical and Experimental Immunology* **29**, 342.

Chollet, P., Carpentier, N. A., Chassagne, J., Betail, G., Bidet, J. M., Lambert, P. H. and Plagne, R. (1980). *In* "New Trends in Human Immunology and Cancer Immunotherapy" (B. Serrou and C. Rosenfeld, Eds), pp. 496–503. Doin, Paris.

Haakenstad, A. O. and Mannik, M. (1977). *In* "Autoimmunity" (N. Talal, Ed.), p. 278. Academic Press, New York.

Heier, H. E., Carpentier, N. A., Lange, G., Lambert, P. H. and Godal, T. (1977). *International Journal of Cancer* **20**, 887.

Hoffken, K., Meredith, I. D., Robins, R. A., Baldwin, R. W., Davies, C. J. and Blamey, R. W. (1977). *British Medical Journal* **2**, 218.

Hubbard, R. A., Aggio, M. C., Lozzio, B. B. and Wust, C. J. (1981). *Clinical and Experimental Immunology* **43**, 46.

Lambert, P. H. *et al.* (1978). *Journal of Clinical and Laboratory Immunology* **1**, 1.

Poulton, T. A., Crowther, M. E., Hay, F. C. and Nineham, L. J. (1978). *Lancet* **2**, 72.

Rossen, R. D., Reisberg, M., Hersh, E. M. and Gutterman, J. V. (1977). *Journal of National Cancer Institute* **58**, 1205.

Sedlacek, H. H. (1980). *Klinische Wochenschrift* **58**, 543.

Theofilopoulos, A. N. and Dixon, F. J. (1979) *In* "Immunodiagnosis of Cancer" (R. Herberman, Ed.). Marcel Dekker, New York.

Theofilopoulos, A. N., Wilson, C. B. and Dixon, F. J. (1976). *Journal of Clinical Investigation* **57**, 169.

Weigle, W. O. (1961). *Advances in Immunology* **1**, 283.

Zubler, R. H., Lange, G., Lambert, P. H. and Miescher, P. A. (1976). *Journal of Immunology* **116**, 232.

Zubler, R. H. and Lambert, P. H. (1977). *In* "Recent Advances in Clinical Immunology" (R. A. Thompson, Ed.), Vol. I, 125. Churchill Livingston Press, New York.

CEA AND/OR CEA–LIKE GLYCOPROTEINS IN BREAST CANCER

A. Bartorelli[1] , C. Biancardi[2] , R. Ferrara[2] , M. A. Bailo[2] ,
V. Cavalca[2] and R. Accinni[2]

Istituto di Immunologia Clinica[1], Istituto di Ricerche Cardiovascolari
"G. Sisini"[2], Università degli Studi di Milano, Milan, Italy

Since first described by Gold 15 years ago, the carcinoembryonic antigen (CEA) has undergone several ups and downs. The interest of researchers and clinicians, initially very strong, weakened little by little, until it was subsequently broken down into different trends of biochemical and clinical research on particular problems.

All the researchers agree on the usefulness of monitoring the post-surgical follow-up period in patients with gastrointestinal tract cancer by this antigen. On the other hand, conflicting opinions have been reported concerning its use in the diagnosis of primary adenocarcinomas both of the gastrointestinal tract and other organs.

The use of this test for the screening and follow-up of breast cancers has raised many doubts, especially when considering the different results obtained by various laboratories — sometimes, even when employing the same assay techniques. Figure 1 reports a breakdown of some clinical investigations on breast carcinoma, performed with the different CEA techniques.

It is evident that the positivity percentages are rather similar for the metastases of breast adenocarcinoma, and above all for liver metastases. Contrary to this, a wide variability is shown by the positivity percentages of primary carcinomas and also, unfortunately, of the control cases.

Serono Symposium No. 46, Markers for Diagnosis and Monitoring of Human Cancer, edited by M. I. Colnaghi, G. L. Buraggi and M. Ghione, 1982. Academic Press, London and New York.

A. Bartorelli et al.

Several authors support the usefulness of CEA test for the follow-up of post-surgical patients (Reynoso *et al.*, 1972; Wang *et al.*, 1975; Laurence *et al.*, 1972). For example, Wang *et al.* (1975) suggest post-surgical measurements. According to his experiences, post-operatively raised CEA levels indicated faster recurrences.

Others (Franchimont *et al.*, 1977) recommended pre-surgical assays, since raised plasma CEA levels, at the onset of breast cancer, might be useful in the early recognition of non-clinically detectable metastases. On the other hand some authors (Wang *et al.*, 1975; Tormey *et al.*, 1977; Rimsten *et al.*, 1979) maintain that the pre-surgical assay does not show any relationship with the course of the disease. Laurence *et al.* (1972) go so far as to recommend the use of this test for the screening of primary breast cancers, while almost all the other researchers rule out this possibility.

All these results, though sometimes conflicting, fully justify different opinions. Now and then there is even complete disagreement on the usefulness of CEA test for breast pathology and, particularly, for the screening of primary carcinomas. Above all, the different positivity rates for primary breast carcinomas can be explained by different factors: among the variables of paramount importance are the cut-off level determined using non-neoplastic pathologies and the choice of the antigen or the antiserum.

The first established cut-off value was 2.5 ng/ml, employing the Roche CEA test; many case lists were based on this normal cut-off and, over a 7 year period, many conclusions were drawn by different authors on this assumption. It is very easily demonstrable that in the 2.6–5 ng/ml range (Table I) the Roche CEA test is unable to discriminate between neoplastic pathology and healthy donors (Bartorelli *et al.*, 1976; Bartorelli *et al.*, 1979). Even adopting 5 ng/ml as a normal cut-off value (Table II) the test is still affected by a high number of false positives (Bartorelli *et al.*, 1976; Bartorelli *et al.*, 1979).

When we consider that all the above authors (Fig. 1) agree in the assumption that primary breast carcinomas that are considered as positive, show values only slightly higher than the cut-off of their tests, we clearly realize which is the statistical and, above all, the diagnostic validity of these results.

Table I. Percentage of positives with Roche CEA test; samples are considered between the values 2.6 and 5 ng/ml.

Case no.	Type of disease	Cases between 2.6 and 5 ng/ml (%)
678	Colon, rectal and gastric carcinomas	24.4
696	Carcinomas of non-endodermic origin	26.0
1915	Other benign diseases	23.8
420	Emphysemas	36.7
120	Liver cirrhosis	44.2
194	Ulcerative colitis	17.8
320	Gastroduodenal ulcers	24.6
70	Polyps	14.4
92	Diverticulum	20.2
123	Pancreatitis, hepatitis, etc.	22.8

Table II. Comparison between our CEA test (six channels) and Roche CEA test.

Case no.	Type of disease	Six channels positive (%)	Roche 2.5 ng/ml (%)	Roche 5 ng/ml (%)
101	Gastrointestinal adeno-carcinomas	62.3	71.2	53.4
19	Malignant lung tumours	26.3	52.6	31.5
58	Other malignant tumours	24.1	41.3	20.6
15	Crohn's diseases	26.6	73.3	33.3
22	Gastroduodenal ulcers	0	45.4	18.1
45	Other benign gastrointestinal disorders	0	37.7	22.2
26	Various non-gastrointestinal disorders	4	38.4	26.9
20	Liver cirrhosis	10	65.0	50.0
40	Benign hepatic diseases	0	37.5	15.0
38	Healthy donors	0	23.6	5.2

In 1973 we developed a technique with a non-significant positivity for primary breast carcinomas (Bartorelli *et al.*, 1973; Mor *et al.*, 1977). This technique, confirming the abovementioned statements also has a very low number of false positives. It was clearly an improvement on the Roche test, with which it has been compared (Bartorelli *et al.*, 1976) (Table II). Thus, we expect that positivities higher than 10% in primary breast carcinomas may lead back to a more incorrect comparison with the different control pathologies, rather than to a real "specificity" of the CEA test for these tumours.

In addition to the variables due to the cut-off choice, or in any case, to those of methodological type, another major variation factor in the results could be the materials (antigen and/or antibody) employed for the assay.

Different CEA extracted from liver metastases of different donors, when labelled, react differently with different antisera. On the other hand, these antisera, when absorbed with normal human plasma, show further variability of response with the various labelled antigens (Vrba *et al.*, 1975) (Fig. 2). Different laboratories, which extract and label their own CEA, and raise their antisera, might get a different cut-off and probably different responses concerning the neoplastic and control pathology.

These observations not only explain the wide variability of the results of the case lists recorded by us (Fig. 1) but they also confirm that the CEA test, as it had been so far interpreted, is not useful in the screening of primary breast tumours— its usefulness for the follow-up of breast cancer is still a subject for discussion (Maxwell *et al.*, 1979).

All these findings, however, prompted some authors to study more thoroughly, and not only from a clinical point of view, the relationship between primary breast tumours and oncofoetal antigens (Pusztaszeri and Mach, 1973; Kuo *et al.*, 1973; Harvey *et al.*, 1976; Goldenberg *et al.*, 1976; Bartorelli and Accinni, 1977;

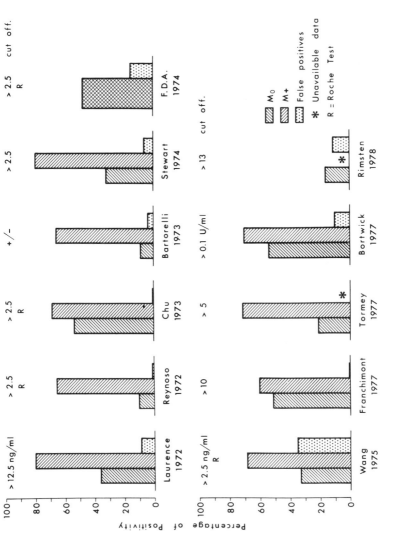

Fig. 1. CEA test in breast cancer: CEA positivity percentages obtained by the different researchers employing personal techniques or industrial kits (R). False positives were considered on non-neoplastic pathology used as control.

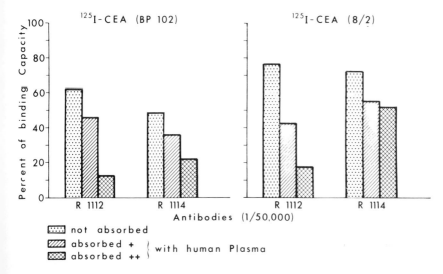

Fig. 2. ¹²⁵I-CEA from different source against different antibodies. CEA extracted in the same way from different liver metastases, after labelling, bind differently anti CEA antisera, raised with antigens obtained from different donors. These antisera, when absorbed with normal human plasma, differentiate even more.

Accinni *et al.*, 1977; Chism *et al.*, 1977; Wahren *et al.*, 1978; Shousha *et al.*, 1979; Bartorelli *et al.*, 1979; Cove *et al.*, 1979; Santen *et al.*, 1980).

These authors were faced with the following questions.

(1) Do primary breast carcinomas cells have CEA?

(2) If present, is it the CEA described by Gold, or a CEA-like glycoprotein with a more or less strong cross-reaction with CEA?

(3) Is it possible and useful to exploit this CEA or CEA-like glycoprotein for the diagnosis of primary breast carcinomas?

To the first question we may reply positively. In fact, several investigations prove it (Bartorelli *et al.*, 1977; Accinni *et al.*, 1977; Chism *et al.*, 1977; Wahren *et al.*, 1978; Shousha *et al.*, 1979; Bartorelli *et al.*, 1979; Cove *et al.*, 1979). These authors studied breast carcinoma cells by immunofluorescence (Wahren *et al.*, 1978), immunoperoxidase (Goldenberg *et al.*, 1976; Shousha *et al.*, 1979) or by extracting the antigen from primary carcinomas to test it by radioimmunotechniques (Bartorelli *et al.*, 1977; Accinni *et al.*, 1977; Chism *et al.*, 1977; Wahren *et al.*, 1978; Shousha *et al.*, 1979; Bartorelli *et al.*, 1979; Cove *et al.*, 1979). All these authors, except Goldenberg (1979), detected the presence of CEA or CEA-like substances in primary breast carcinomas, though in different percentages.

The ratio between the antigen which can be detected in these tumours and that which can be assayed in the plasma of the patients has varied considerably. In fact Wahren (1978) states that 22% of plasmas of the patients with primary breast cancers are positive to CEA test, while CEA can be detected by indirect immunofluorescence in 42% of primary carcinoma cells. Cove (1979) affirms that only 13% of plasmas of patients in stage I and II are positive, while it is possible to extract CEA from 68% of primary tumour cells. By the radioimmunological technique we developed (Bartorelli *et al.*, 1973) the number of false positives in the non-malignant control pathology, except cirrhoses, was very low (Table II). Therefore, by this technique, we obtained a very low percentage of positives in primary breast pathologies (Mor *et al.*, 1977).

On the other hand, in our experience, serial extracts of primary breast cancer tissue detect CEA or CEA-like antigens varying in quantity (or quality) from carcinoma to carcinoma (Fig. 3). The results are substantiated by immuno-fluorescence and immunoperoxidase investigations. Wahren (1978) pointed out that CEA-like containing cells were found at a frequency ranging from 5 to 80% of the tumour cell population, and that the presence of this antigen has no correlation with differentiation or cytological type of the cancer. Shousha (1979) obtained similar results, yet with an 80% positivity of the carcinomas tested. When we studied 46 primary breast carcinomas, employing the immunoperoxidase test, we found a 50% positivity. No immunological activity, except in one case of fibroadenoma, slightly positive to immunoperoxidase, was found in non-malignant tumour tissues.

Thus, the amounts of CEA or CEA-like substances seem to vary from tumour to tumour (Fig. 3) (Wahren *et al.*, 1978; Shousha *et al.*, 1979), and it is apparently impossible to correlate this variability with histological differences (Wahren *et al.*, 1978), in contrast to our knowledge on gastrointestinal CEA (Gold *et al.*, 1968).

Assuming that in primary breast carcinomas there exists a high molecular weight glycoprotein with immunological characteristics more or less similar to CEA, a second problem arises. Is this glycoprotein the CEA described by Gold, or an antigen similar to it?

From 1972 onwards, several research groups tried to extract glycoproteins, which they called CEA or CEA-like, from primary breast carcinomas or from their liver metastases. Kuo (1973) and Harvey (1976) did not find any detectable antigen in extracts of primary breast carcinomas. Both authors showed in the liver metastases of these tumours (with double diffusion and radioimmunoassay) some glycoproteins, which they assumed to be CEA-like. Pusztaszeri (1973) reported in one single case of primary breast carcinoma to have extracted a glyco-protein identical (with the double diffusion technique) to colon CEA. Santen (1980) demonstrated a "breast CEA", with physicochemical characteristics different from colon CEA. We feel, however, that this investigation has as its starting point a different assumption from all the others. In fact, this author exploits "a pool of primary and soft-tissues metastases of breast carcinomas" as starting material.

Some of these authors do not compare their pathological extracts with extracts of normal tissues. In addition, no one has ever tried to label the material, more or less purified, obtained from the extractions.

Chism (1977) reported the extraction of primary breast carcinomas which allowed him to label an antigen that, besides the classical "200,000 daltons colon CEA determinant(s)" also shows, to a remarkably greater extent, a "60,000 dalton determinant(s)". This antigen in the author's experience appears to be different from the colon CEA, in relation to many physicochemical parameters. The author identifies this antigen as a CEA-like substance.

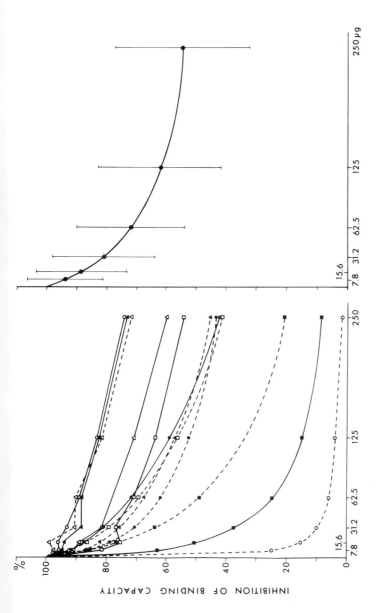

Fig. 3. Inhibition curves obtained with extracts of 12 primary breast cancers, against RIA ^{125}I CEA-anti CEA system (left). Mean and SD of inhibition curves obtained with extracts of 48 primary breast carcinomas (right).

In 1977 our group published a report on the extraction and the purification of CEA or CEA-like substances obtained from a pool of primary, non-preselected breast carcinomas (Bartorelli *et al.*, 1977; Accinni *et al.*, 1977). Likewise, autoptic normal breast glands from plastic surgery or non-malignant breast specimens were extracted and purified in the same way; subsequently, the corresponding antisera against all these extracts were raised. The cross-reaction between the antigen(s) extracted from primary breast carcinomas (BCA: breast cancer antigen(s)) and colon CEA was demonstrated (Bartorelli *et al.*, 1979). Normal and non-malignant tumour tissue does not seem to be endowed with CEA-like activity.

Further investigations, always on non-preselected pools of primary carcinomas, allowed us to label BCA and to point out further differences between BCA and CEA (Bartorelli *et al.*, 1979). Although it is extremely difficult and perhaps highly unlikely, with the techniques available nowadays, to state that two high molecular weight glycoproteins are equal or similar, the literature data and our

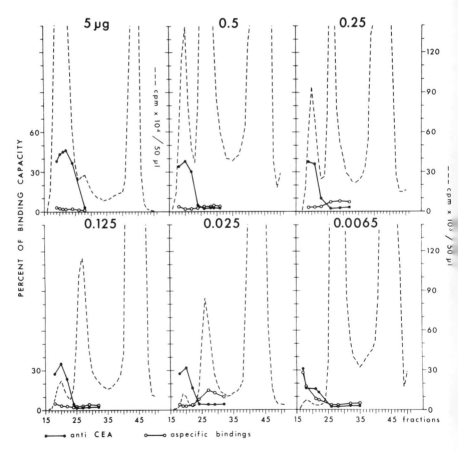

Fig. 4. CEA labelling at different concentrations. The real amounts of labelled antigen appear on the upper part of each graph. The third peak corresponds to the free iodine.

Table III. Extraction and purification of BCA.

	Total proteins (mg)	Specific activity (U/μg)	U tot. 10^3	% Yeld (U tot.)	Purification factor
Omogenization and 3 M KCl extraction	242	29	7018	100.00	1.00
Con A Sepharose chromatography (0.3 M α-methyl-glucoside)	23	140	3220	45.8	4.82
Bioabsorption chromatography	0.330	1400	462	6.58	48.2

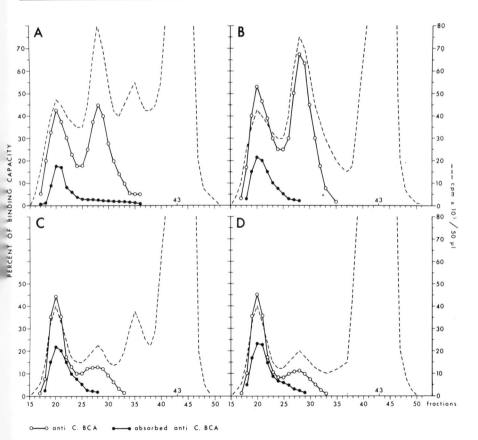

o——o anti C. BCA   ●——● absorbed anti C. BCA

Fig. 5. BCA labelling after Sephadex G-200 chromatography (A); after bioabsorption chromatography prepared with anti-human total serum γ-globulin (B); anti non-malignant breast tissue γ-globulin (C) and with both γ-globulins, contemporaneously employed (D). After bioabsorption chromatography, Sephadex G-200 chromatography was performed.

findings prompt us to conclude that the differences between these antigens, those extracted from colon adenocarcinoma liver metastases and those from primary breast tumour, are not only quantitative.

However, by extracting different pools of primary breast carcinomas, we did not obtain any reproducibility in the labelling with a loss, sometimes complete, of the immunological activity (unpublished data). In fact by labelling CEA, as a control at non-optimal concentrations (< 0.5 mg/ml), a remarkable loss of immunological activity is observed (Fig. 4).

Therefore, it is likely that the concentrations of CEA-like substances, which we obtained from the extracts of a non-preselected pool of breast carcinomas, were too low to be labelled. Consequently, we embarked upon studying each primary breast carcinoma adopting single extractions (Fig. 3). We did not detect any correlation between the immunological activity and the histological type (unpublished data); this is substantiated by the immunofluorescence and immunoperoxidase studies of other authors (Wahren et al., 1978; Shousha et al., 1979).

Following the indication of the radioimmunoassay and the immunoperoxidase tests, only the most immunologically active tumours were chosen. Table III records the extraction and purification of this pool with the specific activities considered as the ratio between the arbitrary unit (U) and the number of micrograms of protein required for a 50% inhibition in the RIA ^{125}I CEA- anti CEA system. The antigen(s) thus obtained can be labelled, though not, as yet, at optimal concentrations. The labelling is reproducible, both as specific and immunological activity. The labelling profile (Fig. 5) shows three peaks of labelled material, the first of molecular weight around 200,000 daltons and the second of about 60,000 daltons. These peaks are bound by the antiserum (anti-crude BCA) raised against a crude extract of a pool of non-preselected primary breast carcinomas (Fig. 5,A). When this antiserum is absorbed against normal human plasma and extracts of normal breast tissue, it recognizes only the material with the highest molecular weight (first peak) (Fig. 5,A).

When labelled material is studied by bioabsorption chromatography, prepared with anti-human total serum γ-globulin (Fig. 5,B), and anti non-malignant breast tissue γ-globulin (Fig. 5,C), the third and the second peak, respectively, drop considerably. A bioabsorption chromatography of both γ-globulins together causes a summation of these results (Fig. 5,D). This proves that, though BCA may be labelled and is reproducible, still it shows a marked contamination of serum and normal tissue components, which can be eliminated only by bioabsorption performed before labelling.

Unfortunately, as shown in Table III, which outlines the extraction of BCA, the bioabsorption chromatography, (prepared with anti-BCA γ-globulins) performed before labelling, even allowing a considerable increase of the specific activity, supplies very low yields. The amount of the antigen present in primary breast cancer tissue, very changeable due to the very morphology of the tumour and much lower than that obtainable from liver metastases, tends to decrease further.

The contamination of normal tissue components, so marked for BCA and absent at these purification levels for CEA, is well justified by the differences in the ratio healthy vs neoplastic tissue that we find when comparing a clump of colon adenocarcinoma liver metastases and breast primary adenocarcinoma.

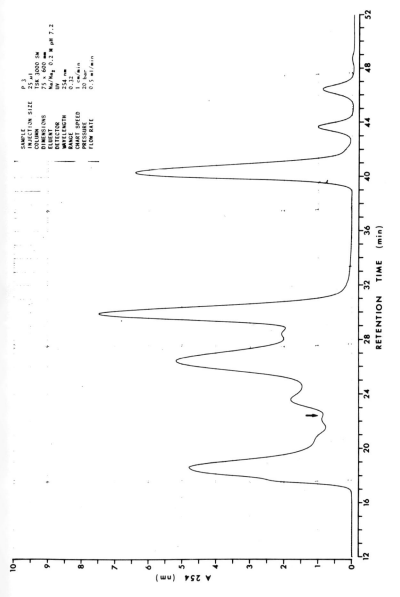

Fig. 6. High performance liquid chromatography (HPLC) performed on breast cancer patients plasma. The arrow shows the fraction of BCA activity detected by RIA.

The third question, concerning the usefulness of this glycoprotein for a possible early diagnosis of primary breast tumours, is the object of our present investigation: however, no definitive response has been obtained by us yet.

The data which we have shown clearly prove how, of primary breast tumour, only some show a satisfactory CEA-like activity. The question now arises whether the remainder of the tumours have less antigen or whether they possess antigens progressively shifting away from what we call BCA, by using CEA as a monitor. Should the quantitative hypothesis be the right one, the only possibility for a radioimmunological assay is, in our opinion, an extractive technique, which, by exploiting large amounts, succeeds in concentrating amounts of antigen sufficient for the assay.

This method, which we are now developing by also employing bioabsorption chromatography and HPLC (Fig. 6), will undoubtedly turn out to be expensive and difficult to manage. Should the qualitative hypothesis be the right one, the recently developed technique of monoclonal antibodies, recognizing single epitopes, represents a possible solution.

In any case, whatever this method will be, we feel it is highly unlikely that this test will allow a diagnosis of the site of the primary tumour. On the other hand, a very strong reason for continuing these investigations is that, undoubtedly, a high percentage of primary breast carcinomas are endowed with antigen(s)—though in variable and sometimes low concentrations but definitely higher than the norm.

All this prompts us to believe in the possibility of exploiting these antigens in screening a healthy population, though, at present, this kind of antigen, with the techniques available, has turned out to be useful only in monitoring tumour recurrences.

ACKNOWLEDGEMENTS

We wish to thank Dr G. Valcurone, Dr C. Zanchetti and Mr R. Sarri for the technical support in preparing the manuscript, Dr M. Sironi for the immunoperoxidase tests and Professor C. Mor, and Dr S. Orefice for clinical studies.

REFERENCES

Accinni, R., Bartorelli, A., Ferrara, R. and Biancardi, C. (1977). *Experientia* **33**, 88.

Bartorelli, A. and Accinni, R. (1977). *Experientia* **33**, 85.

Bartorelli, A. and Accinni, R. (1979). *In* "Current Trends in Tumour Immunology" (S. Ferrone, S. Gorini, R. B. Herberman and R. A. Reisfeld, Eds) pp. 233–252. Garland STPM Press, New York.

Bartorelli, A., Accinni, R., Golferini, A., Mistretta A. P., Tassi, G. C., De Barbieri, A., Mor, C., Leonetti, G., Orefice, S. and Rocco, F. (1973). *Bollettino dell'-Istituto Sieroterapico Milanese* **52**, 333.

Bartorelli, A., Accinni, R., Ferrara, R., Biancardi, C. and Dragoni, G. (1976). *La Ricerca in Clinica e in Laboratorio* **1**, 79.

Bartorelli, A., Biancardi, C., Ferrara, R. and Accinni, R. (1979). *In* "Compendium of Assays for Immunodiagnosis of Human Cancer" (R. B. Herberman, Ed.), Vol I, 17–25. Elsevier North Holland, New York.

Chism, S. E., Warner, N. L., Wells, J. V., Chrewther, P., Hunt, S., Marchalonis, J. J. and Fudenberg, H. H. (1977). *Cancer Research* 37, 3100.

Chu, T. M. and Nemoto, T. (1973). *Journal of National Cancer Institute* 51, 1119.

Cove, D. H., Woods, K. L., Smith, S. C. H., Burnett, D., Leonard, J., Grieve, R. J. and Howell, A. (1979). *British Journal of Cancer* 40, 710.

Franchimont, P., Zangerle, P. F., Hendrick, J. C., Reuter, A. and Colin, C. (1977). *Cancer* 39, 2806.

Gold, P., Gold, M. and Freedman, S. O. (1968). *Cancer Research* 28, 1331.

Goldenberg, D. M., Sharkey, R. M. and Primus, F. J. (1976). *Journal of National Cancer Institute* 57, 11.

Harvey, S. R., Girotra, R. N., Nemoto, T., Ciani, F. and Chu, T. M. (1976). *Cancer Research* 36, 3486.

Kuo, T., Rosai, J. and Tillack, T. W. (1973). *International Journal of Cancer* 12, 532.

Laurence, J. R., Stevens, U., Bettelheim, R., Darcy, D., Leese, C., Turberville, C., Alexander, P., Johns, E. W. and Neville, M. A. (1972). *British Medical Journal* 3, 605.

Maxwell Anderson, J., Stimson, W. H., Gettinby, G., Jhunjhunwala, S. K. and Burt, R. W. (1979). *European Journal of Cancer* 15, 709.

Mor, C., Orefice, S., Rocco, F., Ferrara, R., Biancardi, C., Accinni, R. and Bartorelli, A. (1977). *Neoplasma* 24, 345.

Pusztaszeri, G. and Mach, J. P. (1973). *Immunochemistry* 10, 197.

Reynoso, G., Chu, T. M., Holyoke, D., Cohen, E., Nemoto, T., Wang, J. J., Chuang, J. Guinan, P. and Murphy, G. P. (1972). *Journal of the American Medical Association* 220, 361.

Rimsten, A., Adami, H. O., Wahren, B. and Nordin, B. (1979). *British Journal of Cancer* 39, 109.

Santen, R. J., Collette, J. and Franchimont, P. (1980). *Cancer Research* 40, 1181.

Shousha, S., Lyssiotis, T., Godfrey, V. M. and Scheuer, P. J. (1979). *British Medical Journal* 1, 777.

Tormey, D. C., Waalkes, T. P., Snyder, J. J. and Simon, R. M. (1977). *Cancer* 39, 2397.

Vrba, R., Alpert, E. and Isselbacher, K. J. (1975). *Proceedings of National Academy of Sciences of USA* 72, 4602.

Wahren, B., Lidbrink, E., Wallgren, A., Eneroth, P. and Zajicek, J. (1978). *Cancer* 42, 1870.

Wang, D. Y., Bulbrook, R. D., Hayward, J. L., Hendrick, J. C. and Franchimont, P. (1975). *European Journal of Cancer* 11, 615.

MILK PROTEINS AND BREAST CANCER

P. F. Zangerle[1], J. Collette[1], J. C. Hendrick[1], W. B. Miller[2]
and P. Franchimont[1]

*Laboratory of Radioimmunology University of Liège, Liège, Belgium[1]
and Clinical Surgery, University Medical School, Edinburgh, UK[2]*

INTRODUCTION

The principal function of the breast is the synthesis of proteins, fats and carbohydrates, all components of milk. The proteins synthesized by the breast, during lactation, are the final products of highly differentiated glandular tissue. Therefore, they differ from the first tumour markers used such as CEA, AFP, HCG and its subunits, which are proteins secreted by young, most often embryonic or cancerous, cells. In contrast, milk proteins are synthesized by adult cells arrested at a complete stage of development. Mammary tissue from primates (Kleinberg and Todd, 1978) and humans (Bussolati *et al.*, 1975) has been shown to produce and contain lactalbumin and casein even in virgin, nulliparous and multiparous breasts. Thus, the breast cells are able to produce milk proteins at various times of life, other than during gestation and lactation.

Several examples exist of the use of tissue secretory products as an index of tumour activity (Laurence and Neville, 1977). The development of such systems for milk proteins produced by breast cancer, needs the maintenance of synthesis material in cancerous cells. Lactalbumin (Kleinberg, 1975; Kleinberg and Todd, 1978; Woods *et al.*, 1979), and casein (Bussolati *et al.*, 1975; Herbert *et al.*, 1978) have been observed in cancerous breast cells. Nevertheless, the frequency of lactalbumin production by cancer cells is lower than by normal cells and the

Serono Symposium No. 46, Markers for Diagnosis and Monitoring of Human Cancer, edited by M. I. Colnaghi, G. L. Buraggi and M. Ghione, 1982. Academic Press, London and New York.

induction of lactalbumin production by prolactin can be stimulated in normal but
not in malignant breast tissue (Wilson *et al.*, 1980). The milk proteins are produced
less by cancer cells. But these milk proteins could be an index, during the
woman's life, of breast activity and secretion. They are an index of, on the one
hand, a particularly favourable hormonal climate for the breast cells to synthesize
and secrete material in the mammary ducts, and, on the other hand, of their
mitotic activity. Petrakis *et al.* (1975) showed a correlation between breast
secretory activity and breast cancer risk. Furthermore, the breast secretion from
nipple aspirates could have mutagenic activity (Petrakis *et al.*, 1980).

Thus, the use of milk proteins in breast oncology may be of interest in two
potential areas: that in the cancer cells synthesize a protein which is biological
parameter of tumoral activity, or that this protein is an indication of a breast in
an hormonal condition of cancer transformation risk.

Two milk proteins are studied. Firstly, lactalbumin, with a molecular weight of
15,000 daltons (Brew *et al.*, 1970), has a biological role to provide a rapidly
responding control mechanism acting on the lactose synthetase in the milk
(Fitzgerald *et al.*, 1970). Lactalbumin is a major component of the milk (1-2 mg/
ml), and the final product of a highly differentiated adult tissue.

The second protein studied, the sweat α_2-globulin, was described by Jirka (1968).
This mucoprotein is present in a number of external secretions: saliva, tears,
cerumen, colostrum and milk. This product of the mammary and sweat glands
which have a similar embryological origin, has been purified from breast cyst
fluid of patients with breast cyst disease: GCDFP 15 (Haagensen *et al.*, 1979), and
GCDFP 70 (Zangerle *et al.*, 1981). It is a minor component of milk (1-2 μg/ml)
and a major one of breast cyst fluid and breast secretion (1-10 mg/ml); its biological role is still unknown.

We have refined and assessed a radioimmunoassay for lactalbumin and GCDFP
70. We used this assay to study these two milk proteins in serum from different
populations, in culture fluid from breast explants, in breast cyst fluid from breast
cystic disease patients, and in breast secretion from nipple aspirates.

MATERIAL AND METHODS

Radioimmunoassay

Lactalbumin Assay

Lactalbumin was purified, according to the method of Schultz and Ebner
(1977) from milk of lactating women collected between post-partum days
4 and 10. The protein obtained had a molecular weight of 15,000 daltons and
the enzymatic activity for lactose biosynthesis by transferring galactose, from
UDP-galactose, on glucose. This lactalbumin was used as a tracer after labelling with [125]I (Greenwood *et al.*, 1963) and as a reference preparation. Other
milk proteins, known tumour markers and egg lysozyme serum proteins from
children do not cross-react with human lactalbumin. The sensitivity of the assay
is 75 pg/ml and the interassay variation coefficient less than 4%. In the cases
where human immunoglobulins capable of binding the labelled lactalbumin were
present, we used the method of Woods *et al.* (1978) to neutralize them.

GCDFP 70

Gross cystic disease fluid protein was extracted from breast cyst fluid of women with breast cystic disease. In biological conditions the molecular weight is 70,000 daltons. This molecule was used as a tracer and as a reference preparation. Any other milk proteins, tumour markers such as CEA, HCG, β and α HCG or serum proteins from normal males do not cross-react in the immunological reaction. The sensitivity of the assay is 800 pg/ml, and the interassay variation coefficient is less than 5%.

Sera Studied

Normal Populations

Lactalbumin and GCDFP 70 were assayed in the serum of healthy subjects: 200 adult women, 200 adult men, 20 prepubertal boys and girls, five young women every 2 days during normal menstrual cycle, 55 gestating women and 19 lactating women during the 6 days post-partum.

Benign Disease Patients

Non-breast benign disease. There were 438 patients investigated with non-breast benign disease: 62 were bearing different digestive diseases (except viral hepatitis); 21, lung disease; 112, cardiovascular diseases; 23, infectious diseases; 36, endocrinological diseases; and 27, urogenital diseases.

Breast benign disease. There were 123 adult women investigated with breast benign disease: 74 were bearing non-cystic disease, such as fibroadenoma, and 49 had breast cystic disease.

Malignant Disease Patients

There were 105 patients investigated with breast cancer at different stages of evolution; 51 with lung cancer, 62 with digestive cancer, and 32 with different site cancers.

Breast Cyst Fluid

Forty-two breast cyst fluid samples were obtained by a needle aspiration of the cyst from women with breast cyst disease. Multiple cysts from the same patients were analysed in nine women.

Breast Secretion

Nipple aspirates (100–250 μl) gave breast secretion in 100 women without clinical evidence of breast disease.

Breast Culture

Tumours are cut into explants. Four weighed explants were placed on a lens paper, mounted on stainless steel grids in Petri dishes and cultured for 24 h at 37°C in 2 ml Waymouths 17β 725/1 medium, containing normal glutamine, 20 mM Hepes and insulin (10 μg/ml) with an atmosphere of 95% oxygen/5% CO_2. After culture, media are removed and deep frozen at -40°C until assayed for tumour markers. The explants are weighed, pulverized in liquid N_2, and extracted with a further 2 ml of culture medium. After centrifugation the resultant cytosol is removed and used for the estimation of milk proteins.

RESULTS

Sera from Normal Populations

Children

   GCDFP   None of the 20 male and 20 female children before puberty presented serum values of GCDFP higher than 5 ng/ml.

   Lactalbumin. Twelve of the 20 boys (60%) and eight (40%) of the girls did not have a detectable value of lactalbumin. No value exceeded 3 ng/ml.

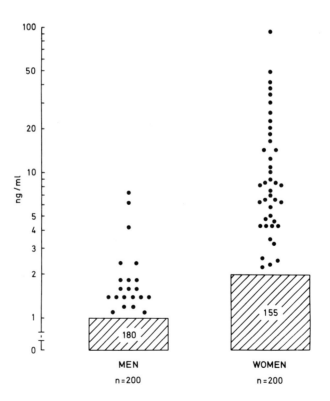

Fig. 1. Individual values of lactalbumin in healthy men and women.

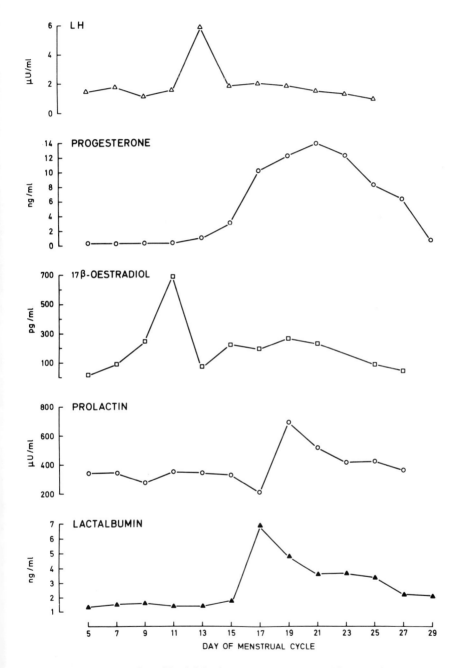

Fig. 2. Serum concentration of luteinizing hormone, progesterone, 17β-oestradiol, prolactin and lactalbumin throughout a menstrual cycle. Samples were withdrawn every 2 days from a 20-year-old fasting woman.

Healthy Adults

GCDFP.   Four of the 400 healthy males and females presented values of GCDFP higher than 5 ng/ml. There is no correlation between the detectable value and the sex repartition. No correlation has been found between blood groups.

Lactalbumin.   Lactalbumin was detected in the serum of 92/200 men (47.5%) with levels equal to or less than 4 ng/ml. Three of the 200 (1.5%) had levels higher than 4 ng/ml. No value exceeded 7.2 ng/ml (Fig. 1).

Out of 200 women, 124 (62%) had detectable values of lactalbumin with a wider range than in men (Fig. 1). Those women with values higher than 4 ng/ml represented 19.5% of the group. In this last group of women, the mean value of prolactin (694.32 μIU/ml ± 342) is higher than the mean value found in women without detectable values of lactalbumin (483 ± 268 μIU/ml). There was no statistical difference concerning the value of 17β-oestradiol, progesterone between the group of women with detectable lactalbumin values and the group without detectable lactalbumin values.

Menstrual cycle.   Of the five women studied throughout their menstrual cycle, three had detectable values of lactalbumin. Each presented a peak of LH between days 13 and 19 of the cycle (Fig. 2). In positive lactalbumin women, the lactalbumin values increased quickly at day 2 of the luteal phase, then decreased progressively. The mean value of lactalbumin was significantly higher during the luteal phase than during the follicular phase (Fig. 3).

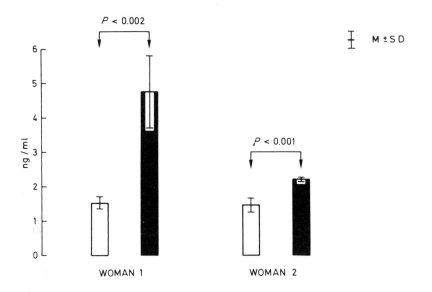

Fig. 3.   Mean lactalbumin levels, with standard deviation, during the follicular (open columns) and the luteal phase (closed columns) of two women normally cyclated.

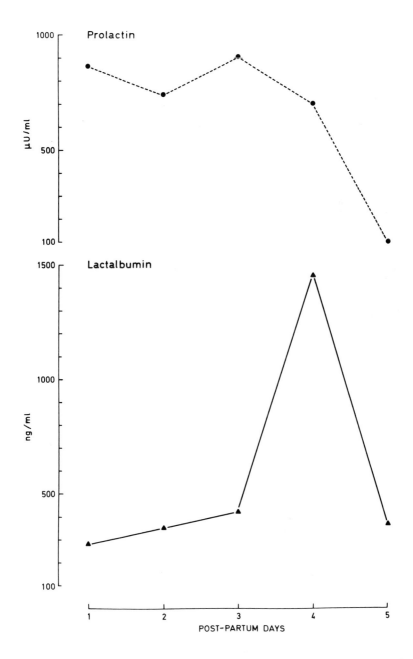

Fig. 4. Evolution of prolactin levels and lactalbumin levels in the post-partum period of a normal lactating woman.

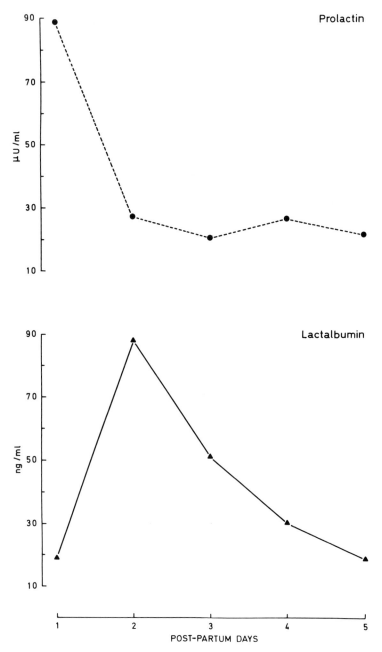

Fig. 5. Evolution of prolactin levels and lactalbumin levels in the post-partum period of a non-lactating woman with bromergocryptin (Sandoz).

Gestating women. No serum from gestating women had GCDFP values higher than 5 ng/ml. Lactalbumin was detected in all the sera of gestating women with a mean value of 120 ng/ml at the end of gestation.

Lactating women: normal lactation. In 17 women the prolactin and the lactalbumin levels were determined each morning, 15 min before the second suckling, during the first 6 days following delivery. Mean prolactin levels increased to reach their maximum on day 2 of the post-partum, then progressively decreased. The lactalbumin levels increasing during lactation, reached a maximum on day 4 after delivery and decreased thereafter (Fig. 4).

Non-lactating women. Two women who did not wish to breast feed, received bromergocryptine (Sandoz). Prolactin levels decreased to normal values after 3 days. Nevertheless, the lactalbumin levels remained low, although reaching a small peak on day 2 and then decreasing but with levels ten-times less than the levels found in lactating women (Fig. 5).

GCDFP was found only in one woman without fluctuation, according to the lactation time.

Patients with Benign Disease

Non-breast Benign Disease
In 315 patients with non-breast benign disease, the incidence of GCDFP higher than 5 ng/ml was 4/315 (1.2%) and the incidence of lactalbumin higher than 4 ng/ml was 5/315 (2.5%).

Benign Breast Disease
The incidence of pathological values of GCDFP ($>$ 5 ng/ml) was clearly different in patients with breast cyst disease (27/49, 55%) from the incidence found in patients with non-breast benign disease (1/74, 1.3%). The incidence of high lactalbumin levels in breast cyst disease patients (11/49, 22%) was also quite different from that in non-cystic breast disease (9/74, 12%) (Fig. 6).

Patients with Cancer
Non-breast cancer. The incidence of pathological values of GCDFP and lactalbumin in lung, digestive and different site cancer was 10/145 (6.9%) and 2/145 (1.4%), respectively.

Patients with breast cancer. Whatever the state of the disease, the incidence of lactalbumin values higher than 4 ng/ml was low—5%. In 105 women with breast cancer at different stages of the disease, the incidence of pathological values of GCDFP was 64/105 (61%).

Breast cyst fluid. The levels of GCDFP in cyst fluid were high ranging from 2 to 10 mg/ml. Multiple cysts were analysed in nine women and the concentration of GCDFP was in the same range in cysts of the same individual. The range of lactalbumin values was lower than in milk—from 0.1 to 150 μg/ml.

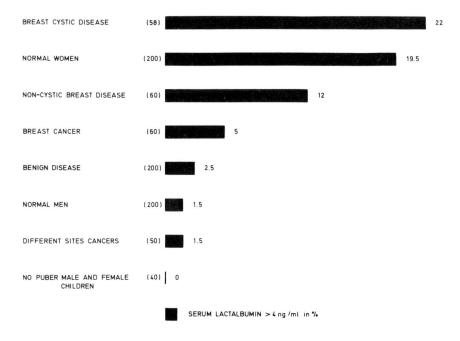

Fig. 6. Incidence of lactalbumin levels higher than 4 ng/ml (%) in the serum of healthy, with benign disease and with cancer populations.

Breast secretion. The breast secretions of nipple aspirates had the same range of GCDFP concentration as in breast cyst fluid. The values of lactalbumin were lower and never exceeded 125 ng/ml (Fig. 7).

Culture medium. Seventy-five out of 84 human breast cancer explants produced GCDFP in the culture fluid with an extremely wide range of levels, varying from 0.4 to 125 ng/ml. Of the remaining nine, five were equivocal and four had no evidence of GCDFP production (Fig. 8). Lactalbumin was present in eight only (9.5%). In cultures producing GCDFP the levels were always much lower in media on day 2 compared with those on day 1 and values in the explants after culture were also very low. The combined levels in the culture media exceeded those present in the explants before culture; this may be evidence of *de novo* synthesis during culture. The levels of GCDFP 70 in the culture fluid were not related to:

(1) the menopausal status of the patient,
(2) tumour oestrogen receptor (Fig. 9);
(3) whether the cancer tissue was derived from primary tumour or invaded node (Fig. 10); or
(4) from patients with early or late disease.

Three explants from normal breast tissue did not produce GCDFP or lactalbumin in the culture fluid.

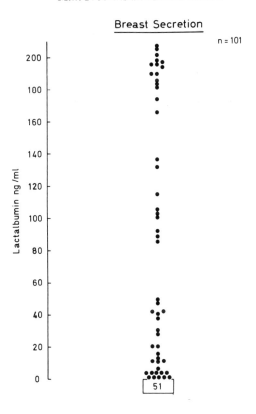

Fig. 7. Lactalbumin levels in breast secretion from nipple aspirates of 101 healthy women.

DISCUSSION

Lactalbumin

The purified molecule has the molecular weight and the biological enzymatic activity previously described (Schmidt and Ebner, 1971; Brew *et al.*, 1970; Fitzgerald *et al.*, 1970).

The levels found in the serum of normal population were similar to those assessed by Kleinberg (1975), Woods and Heath (1978) and Woods *et al.* (1978).

Lactalbumin can be considered as an index of the physiological activity of the breast.

(1) In lactating women, the serum lactalbumin level evolution is the same as the kappa casein evolution (Zangerle and Hendrick, 1976; Zangerle *et al.*, 1978; Franchimont *et al.*, 1979) with values comparable to those described by Martin *et al.* (1980). Like kappa casein, the lactalbumin does not follow exactly the evolution of prolactin.

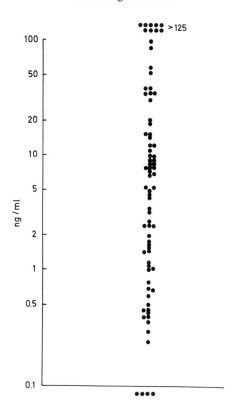

Fig. 8. GCDFP values in day 1 fluid of breast cancer explant cultures.

(2) During the menstrual cycle, when present (three out of five women), there is a cycle of lactalbumin with higher mean values during the luteal phase than those in the follicular phase, together with higher values of prolactin, 17β-oestradiol and progesterone.

(3) In a normal population, a sex difference, which does not exist among prepubertal girls and boys, appears between adult men and women (Fig. 1).

In women, the hormonal difference between the group with detectable lactalbumin and the group without detectable lactalbumin is only significant for prolactin.

Lactalbumin is not a marker of breast cancer since it is not found in breast cancer culture fluid and in breast cancer cell cytosols. The absence of lactalbumin in the culture could be attributed to the short time periods of culture and the complete absence of hormone in the fluid. Nevertheless, in the presence of cortisol (Ono and Oka, 1980), prolactin (Wilson *et al.*, 1980; Kleinberg and Todd, 1978) or oestrogen (Ip and Dao, 1978), cancerous cells do not product lactalbumin more than do normal cells.

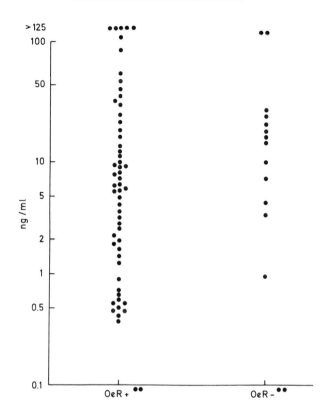

Fig. 9. GCDFP values repartition in day 1 fluid of breast cancer explant culture, following the presence (OeR⁺) or the absence (OeR⁻) of oestrogen receptor in the tumour.

In the serum of breast cancer patients, the incidence of lactalbumin values higher than 4 ng/ml is low—5%. The presence of lactalbumin in the serum could be related to the presence of high risk disease since 22% of patients with breast cyst disease have values higher than 4 ng/ml (Fig. 6). This cystic mastopathy has been associated with a tendency to hyperoestrogenism, frequently related to luteal insufficiency (Mahon *et al.*, 1973).

The presence of lactalbumin in normal breast secretion (→ 125 ng/ml) and in breast cyst fluid (→ 125 μg/ml) shows the persistence of secretory activity of the breast during normal and pathological conditions.

Following these results, lactalbumin could be considered as an index of mammary function, but not as a marker for breast cancer. As its production depends on multiple hormones, its presence in the serum indicates a prevalence of hormones such as prolactin, acting on the breast metabolism, synthesis, secretion and mitotic activity or a difference in the sensitivity of the tissue leading to the same activation. In this condition, the presence of high values of lactalbumin in the serum could be considered as an index of risk. This hypothesis is re-enforced

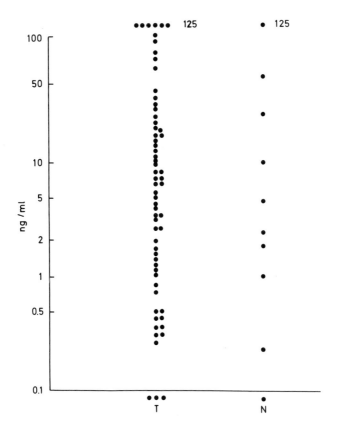

Fig. 10. GCDFP values repartition, in day 1 fluid of breast cancer explant culture from primary (T) or lymph node invaded (N).

by the studies of Patrakis (1973, 1980), which establish a relation between high secretion activity and breast cancer risk. Nevertheless, epidemiological studies are needed to confirm such an hypothesis.

GCDFP

GCDFP is quite different from lactalbumin: it has lower levels in milk and higher levels in breast secretion and in breast cyst fluid. GCDFP is not at all a marker of the function of the breast since it is absent in the serum of gestating or lactating women. Its level is not cyclated during the menstrual cycle.

GCDFP is produced essentially by cancer cells as shown by the 90% positive value in breast cancer culture medium and its presence in the cytosols of breast cancer cells. Normal mammary cells in culture do not seem to produce GCDFP.

In the blood, the presence of GCDFP can be correlated only with breast cyst disease (55%) and breast cancer (68%). It is not significantly found in any other benign disease or cancer from another origin. Therefore, GCDFP 70 can be considered as a marker of breast cancer. The reason why the mammary gland secretes this milk protein is still unknown.

It is interesting to note the association of pathological values for the two diseases: one benign with a high risk, the breast cystic disease, and the other, breast cancer.

The presence of blood values of GCDFP and lactalbumin in patients with GCDFP is an argument for the high metabolical activity of such a disease.

REFERENCES

Brew, K., Castellino, F. G., Vanaman, T. C. and Hill, R. L. (1970). *Journal of Biological Chemistry* **245**, 4570.

Bussolati, G., Pich, A. and Alfani, V. (1975). *Virchows Archiv. A Pathological Anatomy and Histology* **365**, 15.

Fitzgerald, D. K. Colvin, B., Mawal, R. and Ebner, K. E. (1970). *Analytical Biochemistry* **36**, 43.

Franchimont, P., Hendrick, J. C., Thirion, A. and Zangerle, P. F. (1979). *In* "Immunodiagnosis of Cancer" (R. Herberman and R. McIntire, Eds), pp. 499–512, Marcel Dekker Inc., New York, Basel.

Greenwood, F. C., Hunter, W. M. and Glover, G. (1963). *Biochemical Journal* **89**, 114.

Haagensen, D. E., Jr, Mazoujian, G., Holder, W., Jr, Kister, S. G. and Wells, S. A. Jr (1979). *Annals of Surgery* **3**, 279.

Herbert, D. C., Burke, R. E. and McGuire, W. L. (1978). *Cancer Research* **38**, 2221.

Ip, C. and Dao, T. I. (1978). *Cancer Research* **38**, 2077.

Jirka, M. (1968). *FEBS Letters* **1**, 77.

Kleinberg, D. L. (1975). *Science* **190**, 276.

Kleinberg, D. L. and Todd, G. (1978). *Cancer Research* **38**, 4318.

Laurence, D. G. R. and Neville, A. M. (1977). *In* "Immunology for Surgeons" (G. E. Castro, Ed.), pp. 135–173. MTP Press, Liverpool.

Martin, R. H., Glass, M. R., Chapman, C., Wilson, G. D. and Woods, K. L. (1980). *Clinical Endocrinology* **13**, 223.

Mahon, M., Cole, P. and Brown, J. (1973). *Journal National Cancer Institute* **50**, 21.

Ono, M. and Oka, T. (1980). *Science* **207**, 1367.

Petrakis, N. L., Mason, L. and Lee, R. E. (1975). *Journal National Cancer Institute* **54**, 829.

Petrakis, N. L., Maack, C. A., Lee, R. E. and Lion, M. (1980). *Cancer Research* **40**, 188.

Schmidt, D. V. and Ebner, K. E. (1971). *Biochemical Biophysical Acta* **243**, 273.

Schultz, G. S. and Ebner, K. E. (1977). *Cancer Research* **37**, 4489.

Wilson, G. D., Woods, K. L., Walker, R. A. and Howell, A. (1980). *Cancer Research* **40**, 486.

Woods, K. L. and Heath, D. A. (1978). *Clinical and Chemical Acta* **84**, 207.

Woods, K. L., Cove, D. H., Morrison, G. M. and Heath, D. A. (1979). *European Journal of Cancer* **15**, 47.

Zangerle, P. F. and Hendrick, J. C. (1976). *In* "Cancer Related Antigens" (P. Franchimont, Ed.), pp. 61–71. North-Holland, Amsterdam, New York.

Zangerle, P. F., Thirion, A., Hendrick, J. C. and Franchimont, P. (1978). *In* "Laboratory Testing for Cancer. Antibiotics and Chemotherapy" (S. Shönfeld, Ed.), Vol. 22, 141–148.

Zangerle, P. F., Collette, J., Hendrick, J. C. and Franchimont, P. (1981). *European Journal of Cancer*. (In press.)

TUMOR ASSOCIATED AND TUMOR SPECIFIC MARKERS
OF HUMAN MAMMARY CARCINOMA*

T. S. Edgington and R. M. Nakamura

Department of Molecular Immunology, Scripps Clinic and Research Foundation, La Jolla, California, USA

INTRODUCTION

There has been considerable interest in the identification of molecular and host response markers for neoplasms of the human breast. However, in spite of a substantial body of study, there is no generally accepted and well validated, highly effective, single marker for diagnosis, or monitoring or therapy on the basis of assay of serum or other body fluids. Clinical studies have explored onco-developmental antigens, differentiation products and, more recently, tumor associated markers. A few candidate tumor specific molecules have recently been described. These offer a possibility of elucidating the basic cell biology of mammary neoplasia, the specificity of the host response to this form of neoplasia, diagnosis and monitoring tumors, *in vivo* imaging with monoclonal hybridoma antibodies and perhaps, in the not so distant future, the treatment of neoplasia of the human breast. In this paper tumor associated markers of a variety of classes are considered, specifically omitting discussion of differentiation markers of the milk protein class which are addressed elsewhere in this volume. In addition, the study and application of estrogen receptors has received extensive attention with a large body of scientific study, such as to preclude brief discussion in this

* This is publication no. 2422 from the Immunology Departments and was supported by grants CA-28166 and CA-16600 from the National Cancer Institute.

Serono Symposium No. 46, Markers for Diagnosis and Monitoring of Human Cancer, edited by M. I. Colnaghi, G. L. Buraggi and M. Ghione, 1982. Academic Press, London and New York.

Table I. Candidate tumor specific markers.

References	Assays	Immune Response	Characteristics
Gentile and Flickinger (1972)	Hemagglutination	Serum antibody from breast carcinomas	(1) Antigens present in all (15) breast carcinomas (2) Antigens not present in normal tissues (3) Antibodies present only in breast carcinoma patients (4) Antigens < 80,000 daltons but not further characterised
Humphrey et al. (1974) Boehm et al. (1974)	Gel diffusion (ID) Immunoelectro-phoresis Complement fixation	Normal breast carci-noma serum antibody	(1) 0–0.9% antibody incidence in controls (ID) (2) 46% breast carcinoma sera antibody positive (3) 25% sera positive associated with fibroadeno-mas (4) 34% sera positive in fibrocystic disease (5) Antibody absent in advanced breast carcinoma (6) Not specific, react with other carcinomas (7) Probably at least two antigens, one may be breast carcinoma specific or associated
Hollinshead et al. (1974)	Delayed cutaneous hypersensitivity In vitro lymphocyte response	Host cellular response	(1) Tumor cell membranes intact and sonicated (2) A polyacrylamide gel electrophoresis fraction 2b elicited responses only in breast cancer patients
McCoy et al. (1974) Dean et al. (1975) Dean et al. (1977)		Host cellular response	(1) 3 M KCl extract to MCF-7 cells (2) Appeared specific for breast carcinoma patients (3) Antigens not present in normal or benign breast tissue
Acinni et al. (1977)			3 M KCl extract of tumors
Gorsky (1976)	Radioimmunoassay	Antibody isolated by affinity for immo-bilised malignant pleural effusion	Antigens present in pleural effusions produced by metastatic breast carcinoma Antibody or antigen capable of inhibition in 52% of breast carcinoma sera, 16% of sera from other malignancies and 5% of normal sera

Reference	Method	Source of antibody	Findings
Lopez and Thomson (1977)	Blocking tube leukocyte adherence test	Host cellular immune response	(1) Serum antigen(s) 80–150,000 daltons (2) Urine antigen(s) 40,000 daltons (3) Antigenically related to HLA
Nordquist et al. (1977)	Indirect immunofluorescence on viable tumor cells BOT-2	Serum antibody from breast carcinoma patients	Antibody induced capping and shedding of surface antigen from BOT-2 cells
Mesa-Tejada et al. (1978) Ohno et al (1979)	Immunoperoxidase on human breast carcinomas	Rabbit anti-MMTV Rabbit anti-MMTV gp52	Cross-reaction between a trypic peptide of MMTV gp52 and some breast carcinoma cells No characterisation of human tumor antigen molecule
Loisillier et al. (1978)	Indirect immunofluorescence	Heterologous antiserum to acid soluble extract of breast carcinoma	Antigen is organelle or membrane associated but is solubilised in acid buffer
Holton et al. (1978)	Indirect immunofluorescence	Sera antibody from breast carcinoma patients	Solubilised by 3 M KCl Approximately 20,000 daltons
Leung et al. (1978) Leung et al. (1979) Leung et al. (1981a) Leung and Edgington (1980a, 1980b, 1981b)	Immunodiffusion Electroimmunodiffusion Radioimmunoassay Immunohistochemical methods	Heterologous antiserum to isolated MTGP	20,000 daltons glycoprotein (MTGP) 37–58% carbohydrate pI, density and sedimentation velocity varies with tumor Breast carcinoma specific 53,000 daltons membrane MTGP
Schlom et al. (1980)	Immunoperoxidase on human breast carcinomas	Human hybridoma antibody	Antigens are uncharacterised

presentation. To facilitate orderly consideration of tumor cell markers they are taxonomically considered within classes: (1) candidate tumor specific markers; (2) oncodevelopmental markers, (3) differentiation markers, (4) other tumour associated markers, and (5) immune response markers.

CANDIDATE TUMOR SPECIFIC MARKERS

Within this class of markers are the still elusive tumor specific antigens, molecules that have long been recognised to exist from studies of syngeneic tumor transplantation in animals and a few studies in man. Since these have not yet been unequivocally identified in human breast carcinoma, or any other human or animal tumor, the following is a review of the search and the candidates (see Table I).

Gentile and Flickinger (1972) described a breast cancer antigen (BCA) in saline extracts of each of 15 carcinomas of the breast. This antigen, or indeed antigens, appeared to have a molecular weight of less than 30,000 daltons, from the published elution profiles by Sephadex G-200 chromatography. They were detected by an innovative approach of producing immune complexes by mixing the isolated serum immunoglobulin from breast carcinoma patients with saline extracts of their own tumours. The resultant immune complex fraction was isolated and heat dissociated to yield a putative specific antibody fraction by gel filtration. Positive reactions were obtained with sera from all of 15 breast carcinoma patients when analyzed by hemagglutination assay using extracts of autologous or homologous breast carcinomas, but not with extracts of control tissues. Antibodies appeared to be present only in breast carcinoma patients and were not observed in the serum of patients with other forms of neoplasia.

Humphrey *et al.* (1974) and Boehm *et al.* (1974) subsequently described antibody responses in breast cancer patients using agar gel double diffusion against a concentrated aqueous soluble extract of breast carcinomas. When analyzed by complement fixation, a higher frequency of positive reactions were observed for both controls and breast carcinoma sera. By immunodiffusion the sera of 0-0.9% of women without breast carcinoma gave positive reactions, 46% of breast cancer sera, 34% of sera from fibrocystic disease, and 25% of women with fibroadenomas had antibody to breast carcinoma antigen (BCA). This antibody appeared to be absent in most patients with advanced metastic carcinoma suggestive of *in vivo* absorption or suppression of synthesis. The specificity is, however, called into question by observations that the sera from these patients also reacted with extracts of ovarian carcinoma, a sarcoma, and a melanoma. Serum from patients with benign breast disease exhibited similar patterns of non-tumor specificity. Some resolution of the specificity has subsequently been suggested by Lee *et al.* (1978). Attempts at purification of BCA using gel chromatography, salt precipitation and hydrophobic chromatography suggested the presence of two different antigens. One was suggested to be specific for breast carcinoma tumor tissue, whereas the second appeared non-tissue specific. If verified it would appear that multiple antibody responses differing in specificity are clouding the interpretation of results; any attempt to use this as a marker system would first have to resolve this issue.

Utilising delayed cutaneous hypersensitivity (DCH) testing, Hollinshead *et al.* (1974), observed reactions of three of eight patients with autologous breast cancer cell membranes. Positive reactions were elicited in all eight with a solubilised fraction of sonicated cell membranes. It is notable that half of the patients who were tested with an equivalent solubilised fraction of non-cancerous breast tissue also gave positive skin tests. Reactivity may not be restricted to neither tumor nor autologous tissue since some patients also gave positive DCH responses with equivalent extracts of allogeneic benign breast. However, in view of the possibility of multiple immune responses these observations could reflect different specificities. When the solubilised breast cancer membranes were fractionated by polyacrylamide gel electrophoresis, one group of bands (2a) that were recovered and used in skin testing appeared to be associated with non-tissue specific reactivity; whereas, a second group of bands (2b) elicited positive DCH in most breast cancer patients. This fraction did not elicit DCH responses from control benign breast. Similarly, patients with other cancers or benign breast diseases did not respond to the region 2b fractions of solubilised breast cancer membranes.

A variety of studies have suggested the existence of a breast carcinoma specific or at least a tumor associated antigen capable of eliciting immune reactions *in vitro*. The studies of DCH described by Alford *et al.* (1973), are complemented by the report of Segall *et al.* (1972), describing a high frequency of positive leukocyte migration inhibition assay results with extracts of breast carcinomas. Studies by other groups (Cochran *et al.*, 1972, 1974; Wolberg and Goelzer, 1971; Andersen *et al.*, 1970; Black *et al.*, 1974a,b; McCoy *et al.*, 1974; Dean *et al.*, 1975, 1977). Although all of these studies suggested the presence of one or more tumor associated antigen, and even possibly tumor specific antigens, no discrete identification or characterisation of specific molecular entities has been forthcoming. In the studies of cellular immune responses *in vitro* by McCoy *et al.* (1974), and Dean *et al.* (1975, 1977), 3 M KCl extracts of breast carcinomas were used. A reasonably high degree of specificity for breast carcinoma patients was observed; and it appeared that normal or benign breast tissue did not possess the relevant antigens.

In a brief report, Accinni *et al.* (1977) suggested the presence in 3 M KCl extracts of breast carcinomas of not only a carcinoembryonic antigen (CEA)-like molecule but also the presence of an additional breast tumor associated antigen independent of CEA. This has not been further substantiated.

Gorsky *et al.* (1976) established a solid phase radioimmunoassay for the detection of breast cancer specific or associated antigen in serum and body fluids. The antibodies were purified from serum by binding to, and elution from, breast carcinoma pleural fluids immobilised as an immunoabsorbant in polyacrylamide gel. The purified antibodies, after radioiodination were analyzed for binding to the immobilised pleural fluid. Binding was inhibited by incubation of 52% of breast cancer sera and 16% of sera from patients with other malignancies with the antibody. About 5% sera of normal women also inhibited the antibody binding. The antigens with which these antibodies react remain to be characterised. At this point it is not known whether the antigens so detected are only present in breast carcinomas or possibly present in other types of neoplastic cells or normal cells.

Lopez and Thomson (1977), have used the blocking tube leukocyte adherence inhibition assay to detect and to monitor the isolation of an antigen present in

serum and in urine of individuals with carcinoma of the breast. In the serum it
appeared to have a molecular weight of 80,000–150,000 daltons and to have a
buoyant density similar to high density plasma lipoprotein (1.063–1.21 g/ml). In
the urine the tumor specific antigen appeared to have a molecular weight of c.
40,000 daltons, suggesting either cleavage of the larger serum antigen or an
entirely different antigen. The serum antigen appeared to possess antigeneic determinants related to HLA using xenoantisera; and HLA antigens also have been
independently demonstrated to associate with plasma high density lipoprotein.
These observations raised questions about the presence in these patients of a
modified HLA, or simply sensitisation to common framework epitopes of the
HLA molecule. Purification and structural analysis of these candidate tumor
specific antigens is clearly essential to resolve structural relationships to one
another and their biological significance.

Nordquist *et al*. (1977) described the presence of serum antibodies in breast
cancer patients. These antibodies were observed by indirect immunofluorescence
to react with viable cells in suspension, the line BOT-2 was derived from a human
breast carcinoma. Antibodies were not only demonstrated binding to the surface
of these BOT-2 cells, but could be demonstrated to "patch", cap and shed by following the fate of the fluorescein labeled second antibody in the reaction product
on the surface of the cells. It is an interesting possibility that this mechanism could
induce shedding of complexes of cell surface tumor associated antigen and autologous antibody, and as such represent the source of immune complexes in breast
cancer patients. The mechanism of induced transposition of breast tumor specific
antigens from the surface of the cell to the extracellular compartment has been
thought of as a property of the particular tumor specific or tumor associated
antigen. This may not be the case, as many plasmalemma molecules are not shed
to a significant degree. This mechanism, immune shedding, is intriguing. As yet,
characteristics of the antigens shed from BOT-2 have not been described.

A substantial advance in identifying a candidate tumor specific antigen in
human breast carcinomas has been provided by Spiegelman and colleagues (Mesa-
Tejada *et al.*, 1978; Ohno *et al.*, 1979). Based on previous observations of a slight
homology between the RNAs of human and murine mammary tumor particles
using assays of low stringency, they suspected the possibility of an immunochemical cross-reaction between proteins of the murine mammary tumor virus
particles and constituents of human mammary carcinomas. The possibility of this
was not entirely hypothetical since antibodies to constituents of murine mammary
tumor virus (MMTV) had been observed in the serum of a number of breast
cancer patients by Charney and Moore (1971) and others (Muller and Grossmann,
1972; Holder *et al.*, 1976; Bowen *et al.*, 1976). In addition, cellular immune
response assays as exemplified by leukocyte migration inhibition (Black *et al.*,
1976) describe responses to the gp52, the major surface glycoprotein, of MMTV
in breast cancer patients. The description of a possible cross-reaction between
MMTV and the human breast carcinoma derived cell line MCF-7 (Yang *et al.*,
1977) is similarly provocative. Using the IgG from a rabbit immunised with
MMTV which had been isolated from the milk of Paris RIII mice, immunohistochemical studies of human breast tumors were reported by Mesa-Tejada *et al*.
(1978). They observed reactions with various histological types of human breast
carcinomas in 39% of 131 cases. No reactions were observed with 119 benign

breast lesions, 18 normal breast tissues and only with one of 99 carcinomas from other tissue sites. It is notable that the reactions were not uniform in that only a minor portion of cells were positive by this assay. Whether this is a problem of sensitivity of the assay and the inability to detect a few molecules of antigen in the rest of the neoplastic cells is not clear. If this MMTV cross-reacting antigen is truly not expressed by most neoplastic cells of the mammary epithelium, then it may not play an essential role in the biology and immunobiology of the neoplastic cell. In addition, *in vivo* imaging with radiolabeled antibody and attempts at immunotherapy may be precluded from the outset.

The specificity of the MMTV cross-reaction was established by blocking of the reaction through prior absorption of the anti-MMTV antiserum with MMTV from three sources as well as gp52 from two differents strains isolated by two independent methods. A variety of tissues including human milk were not observed to block the reactions. The specificity of the reaction was further extended by demonstration that the gp52 polypeptide chain rather than the carbohydrate radicals was responsible for the specificity (Ohno *et al.*, 1979). Deglycosylated gp52 was equally effective in neutralising the anti-MMTV reaction with human cells, whereas the isolated polysaccharides were ineffectual. More recent studies have further defined a single tryptic peptide as possessing the cross-reacting antigeneic epitope. To date there is no characterisation of the molecule in human breast carcinoma cells that bears this cross-reacting epitope. With the available information and analytical approaches, it is reasonable to anticipate information regarding the biochemical characteristics of the human tumor specific molecule in the near future.

It should be noted in respect of the above observations that most antisera to MMTV, or to MMTV structural proteins such as gp52, have not reacted with human mammary carcinomas in other laboratories. If valid it may be an infrequent cross-reaction in heterologous antisera, thus only fortuitously encountered. Cardiff has confirmed the results of Mesa-Tejada *et al.* (1978) that the antisera used by Mesa-Tejada does cross-react with human mammary carcinoma cells by immunoperoxidase (pers. comm.). Another problem has been introduced recently by Dion *et al.* (1980). They have isolated a human milk protein that is structurally and antigeneically related to MMTV gp52 (referred to by this group as gp55). Immunoprecipitation analyses indicate the presence of an antigeneically cross-reacting protein of a molecular weight of about 58,000 daltons, 3000 daltons larger than the MMTV protein. In an extensive structural analysis they demonstrated that both had amino terminal serine. Further homology was demonstrated by tryptic peptide mapping. Although Mesa-Tejada *et al.* (1978) did not observe inhibition of their rabbit anti-MMTV or anti-MMTV gp52 by human milk assaying reactivity of their antisera by immunoperoxidase with human breast carcinomas, the studies of Dion *et al.* (1980) suggested the need for critical re-examination of this point. The possibility that the MMTV gp52 cross-reacting molecule observed in some human neoplastic mammary epithelial cells might represent a differentiation product present in only low concentration in human breast milk can not be safely dismissed without further study.

There are two brief descriptions of candidate tumor associated antigens of breast carcinomas. The first of these by Loisillier *et al.* (1978) evolved from the preparation of heterologous antiserum by immunisation with an acid buffer extract of the insoluble pellet of human mammary carcinomas. After extensive absorption, the antiserum gave a single precipitin line in gel diffusion with the immunising material, and the antiserum reacted only with human mammary carcinoma cells by immunofluorescence techniques. It appeared not to react with normal mammary gland epithelium nor with cells of benign mammary lesions. Although originally described as unreactive with other tumors, more recent observations suggest that it may react with some carcinomas of the colon (pers. comm.). At approximately the same time, Holton *et al.* (1978) using indirect immunofluorescence and serum from breast carcinoma patients observed reactions with a human mammary carcinoma cell line (SW527). Using 3 M KCl extracts, these workers have provided initial evidence for the isolation of a molecule of approximately 20,000 daltons that appears to neutralise homologous anti-tumor cell antibodies.

Leung *et al.* (1978) described a new trace glycoprotein in human breast carcinomas that has since appeared to be highly tumor specific. A variety of antibodies to normal tissues, blood group antigens, and known oncodevelopmental antigens such as CEA, were used to deplete the cytosol glycoprotein fractions of human breast carcinomas. What remained was fractionated by size. Following immunisation, a single rabbit produced antibodies to one fraction containing what is now designated mammary tumor glycoprotein (MTGP). Following absorption with a wide battery of tumors and non-neoplastic tissues, this single precipitin line was observed in agar gel diffusion against very high concentrations of glycoprotein from all of six breast carcinomas, but not other tumor or normal tissue that was analyzed. Using a quantitative electroimmunodiffusion assay, molecules were isolated from the cytosol fractions of human ductal carcinomas of the breast and were characterised by isoelectric point, sedimentation velocity, carbohydrate composition, buoyant density in cesium chloride, diffusion constant, estimated molecular weight and amino acid composition (Table II). Though bearing common antigenic determinants which were apparently identical by gel

Table II. Properties of cytosol and membrane forms of MTGP[a]

Characteristic	Cytosol MTGP	Membrane MTGP
Solubility	Water	Ionic detergent
$D_{20,w}^0$[b]	9.1×10^{-7} cm^2/s	5.6×10^{-7} cm^2/s
$S_{20,w}^0$	2.50	2.90
Density,[c] ρ	1.48 g/cm^3	1.32 g/cm^3
Molecular weight		
Svedberg equation	19,800	52,800
SDS polyacrylamide gel	41,000	64,000
Carbohydrate	58%	
Electrophoretic mobility	α_1	α_2
Isoelectric point	5.35	6.10

[a]Both forms derived from Type I tumors. [b]From molecular exclusion chromatography.
[c] From buoyant density in cesium chloride.

diffusion, the physical chemical properties and composition were very homogeneous for a single tumor but differed for different tumors. Although cytosol
MTGP was of approximately the same size (molecular weight: 19,000–19,800
daltons) significant differences were observed in sedimentation velocity, isoelectric
point of buoyant density as well as carbohydrate composition between
Type I tumors and Type II tumors. Further, the MTGP of Type II tumors lacked
tyrosine, whereas Type I tumors possess a single tyrosine residue with a reciprocal
difference in arginines. This antigen was demonstrated by immunohistochemical
techniques to be present in the cytoplasm of breast carcinoma cells in biopsies,
but could not be identified in benign breast cells. It was expressed both in the
cytoplasm of fixed breast carcinoma cells in culture as well as at the surface of
viable cells.

The frequency of association of this 19,000–20,000 daltons glycoprotein referred to as mammary tumor glycoprotein (MTGP 20), was assayed and found in
each of seven metastatic breast tumors in which 1g of tissue could be assayed.
MTGP 20 could not be demonstrated in 76 normal tissue samples or tumors
other than of breast origin, but was present in 79.5% of histologically confirmed
biopsies of ductal carcinomas of the breast or 76.2% of 101 breast carcinomas of
all types that were examined. The presence or concentration of MTGP 20 did not
significantly correlate with the presence or concentration of CEA or estrogen
receptor. It was also independent of a variety of histological features. It was
suggested that MTGP 20 represented an independent parameter simply reflecting
the neoplastic nature of the mammary epithelial cells.

Subsequently, Leung and Edgington (1980a), identified a second form of
MTGP in the plasmalemma of breast carcinoma cells. This highly insoluble form
of the molecule required SDS for solubilisation, being refractory to solubilization
by a variety of non-ionic detergents. This molecule segregated in parallel with
markers for plasmalemma and was recovered at high yield in the isolated plasma
membrane fraction. Subsequent studies (Leung *et al.* 1981a) have more carefully
delineated the physical chemical heterogeneity of both types of MTGP molecules
in different breast carcinoma cells. Using 15 cell lines of breast carcinoma origin,
MTGP molecules were identified in all by radioimmunoassay (Leung and
Edgington, 1980b). However, there was a marked variation in concentration,
some cells contained only membrane MTGP with no MTGP 20. Though, over
many years, each was highly homogeneous by physiochemical characteristics in
individual cell lines and their derivative clones, discrete and consistent differences
were observed in the MTGP molecules between different cell lines. This permitted
grouping breast carcinomas into four MTGP groups. These could be distinguished
by isoelectric point and buoyant density of both the cytosol MTGP 20 and
membrane form of the molecule. These studies further bear out the existence of
both common tumor specific antigenic determinants as well as structural variation that could accommodate hypothesised "variable" or individual tumor specific
structures and antigenic determinants.

Studies using highly sensitive radioimmunoassay confirm the absence of
MTGP from a variety of tissues, both neoplastic and benign. In many cases, the
level of confidence for the absence of MTGP in these tissues has been extended
to less than 100 pg for 5 mg of tissue or tumor glycoprotein or less than one
molecule of MTGP per tissue culture cell plasmalemma. Although variable in

concentration, the highest of cell lines (734-B, the parent culture from which MCF-7 was derived had approximately 10,000 molecules of MTGP per plasmalemma. Most tumor cells had considerably less. This membrane form of MTGP has recently been isolated to homogeneity (Leung *et al.*, 1981b). The membrane molecule from one tumor had a molecular weight of 52,000 daltons, estimated from sedimentation velocity, density and diffusion constant by Svedberg equation and approximately 30% carbohydrate as contrasted to 58% carbohydrate for the MTGP 20 in the cytosol (Table II). Preliminary studies suggest the existence of humoral antibody responses specific for the plasmalemma form of the molecule.

Schlom *et al.* (1980) have recently reported an entirely new approach to the identification of immunobiologically relevant tumor specific antigens of breast carcinomas. Cells from lymph nodes derived from mastectomies from 13 patients with breast carcinoma were fused with NS-1 murine myeloma cells to produce human-mouse hybrid cells that synthesise human monoclonal antibodies. Of the 52 hybridoma cultures synthesising human immunoglobulin, four were identified that react with tumor cells in sections of human breast carcinomas. Three of these did not react with normal mammary epithelium by the immunoperoxidase assay. They reacted with both primary and metastic cells, but gave different patterns of reactivity with breast carcinoma cells. One was able to discriminate between mammary carcinoma cells and benign cells from 55 of 59 tumors. With this approach, reasonably unlimited quantities of antibodies may become available for isolation of the responsible antigen to which the tumor bearing host has made the immune response. A wide variety of studies of the host of immune response to breast carcinomas as well as characterisation of the candidate tumor specific antigen are clearly possible.

ONCODEVELOPMENTAL MARKERS

Under this category of tumor markers are considered those that are present in higher concentration in fetal and developing embryonic tissues and reflect primary gene expression of that state of differentiation. Classical examples of this group of markers are α-fetoprotein, and carcinoembryonic antigen (CEA). In considering breast carcinoma, CEA has been of some interest, whereas α-fetoprotein is absent. β Onco fetal antigen (BOFA), and the isoferritins are a more specialised example. These oncodevelopmental products are not intrinsically tumor specific, but are frequently present at much higher concentrations in tumor cells than in the normal, well differentiated cells. This can be thought of as a biochemical mirror of the long recognised cytological features of tumor cells which suggest "dedifferentiation" and recapitulation of more embryonic cytology.

β Onco Fetal Antigen (BOFA)

This antigen, described by Fritsche and Mach (1975), was identified with heteroantisera raised against semipurified fractions of colon carcinomas. The antigen was observed to have a β electrophoretic mobility and was referred to as β onco fetal antigen or BOFA. The antigen was isolated by aqueous extraction, io exchange, chromatography of the ultracentrifugal supernatant and molecular exclusion chromatography. This antisera reacted with an apparently identical molecule in extracts of carcinomas of the breast, colon, lung, liver, pancreas and also melanomas. It was also observed to react with extracts from a variety of tissues of 16-week gestation from the human fetus, indicating its oncodevelopmental characteristic. It was estimated to have a molecular weight of 70,000 90,000 daltons and was pronase sensitive suggesting that it is protein. Its buoyant density of 1.30–1.32 g/ml suggests a modest carbohydrate content. BOFA was also demonstrated in the plasma of normal adults as well as the plasma of fetuses and of cancer patients. Attempts to apply this to serum diagnosis of cancer was unsuccessful. The plasma concentrations of BOFA in cancer patients or in fetuses was not significantly higher than in normal individuals.

Ferritin and Isoferritins

Ferritin is an iron storage protein that is found in most mammalian tissues. In many tissues ferritin exists in multiple molecular forms referred to as isoferritins, differing in structure and metabolism. The differing isoferritin forms result from different proportions of acid and basic subunits. In addition to the normal spectrum of isoferritins, variant forms have been observed in human and animal tumor cells. These observations have stimulated studies of isoferritins in human tumors, and because of the association of certain more acidic forms of ferritins in both fetal tissue and tumors, they have been considered by some as oncodevelopmental isoforms (see Drysdale and Singer, 1974).

Marcus and Zinberg (1974) described an antiserum to breast tumors that reacted strongly with neoplastic mammary epithelial cells but not with the normal breast. The responsible antigen, at first thought to be a tumor specific antigen, was purified by affinity chromatography using the responsible antibody, followed by molecular exclusion chromatography and ion exchange chromatography. It was also detected in human fetal serum (Burtin *et al.*, 1960) and had been referred to later as α-2-H protein (Buffe *et al.*, 1972). This was identified as an isoferritin by immunochemical criteria and binding of iron. Marcus and Zinberg (1974) observed acidic isoforms not observed in normal liver and these were referred to as "carcino-fetal" ferritins. Similar acidic isoferritins were observed in placenta and HeLa cells at about the same time by Drysdale and Singer (1974).

Using a radioimmunoassay for serum ferritin levels, Marcus and Zinberg (1975) described increased ferritin levels in the sera of 41% of women with mammary carcinomas and 67% of women with locally recurring or metastatic mammary carcinoma. The increases were not specific and were also observed in certain forms of hepatic and gastrointestinal inflammatory disease. Jacobs *et al.* (1976) confirmed the increased incidence of elevated ferritin in 229 women with early breast carcinoma; however, the assays that were utilised did not distinguish between normal and the more acidic isoferritin associated with breast tumors. Assay of ferritin, while statistically increased, was not comparable to that in acute leukemias where levels were far higher, 25-fold or more (Parry *et al.*, 1975).

The various isoferritins appear to differ to some degree immunochemically and this influences the quantitation by immunological assays. As a result, accurate

quantitative measurement of ferritin in tissues or serum with a single radioimmuno
assay is not entirely valid as it is influenced by the relative proportion of acidic and
basic isoferritin subunits and their assembly into the ferritin complex. In an
attempt to resolve these problems, Drysdale *et al.* (1977) resolved ferritin into
H and HL subunits and suggested a third or L subunit which is derived from the
HL subunit; Jones *et al.* (1980) developed assays for both adult splenic ferritin
and for acidic isoferritin which was purified from HeLa cells. They explored
the usefulness of assays for acidic isoferritin in parallel with assay relatively specific
for splenic ferritins. The study encompassed sera from 1,000 patients including
normals and individuals with cancer and leukemia. Of 149 patients with benign
breast disease, 146 with early breast-carcinoma and 148 with advanced breast-
carcinoma, the median concentration of splenic ferritin was higher in individuals
with advanced breast cancer and about one-half of these also had detectable levels
of acidic isoferritin in the serum. The acidic isoferritin was not detected in the
majority of normal sera (less than 2 μg/ml) though levels as high as 53 μg/ml were
observed in sera from some patients with malignant tumors. The acid isoferritin:
splenic ferritin ratio was, however, consistently very low; and the results were not
encouraging with regard to use, as either a diagnostic or prognostic marker in
breast cancer.

Carcinoembryonic Antigen (CEA)

Carcinoembryonic antigen was first identified and isolated in the search for
tumor specific antigens. Gold and Freedman (1965) demonstrated this glycoprotein by immunisation with extracts of human colonic carcinomas. It has
subsequently received wide attention and has been observed at elevated concentrations in the serum of individuals with a wide variety of malignant tumors, in
addition to colon carcinomas (Chu and Nemoto, 1973; Concannon *et al.*, 1973;
Steward *et al.*, 1974; and others) CEA has become useful primarily in recognising
recurrence of tumors or the existence of metastases due to the absence of the
decline to baseline of CEA following removal of primary tumors. It has not been
established as an effective diagnostic or detection method. Chu and Nemoto (197.
studied 136 patients with breast carcinoma for 2 years and found elevations of
CEA in 68% of 83 patients with metastases. The frequency of elevated levels
varied according to the site of metastases. Marked elevations of CEA were only
observed in association with hepatic metastasis. In these early studies, it was not
thought that serial CEA determinations could adequately distinguish between
tumor regression or progression. Steward *et al.* (1974) suggested that the elevations of the CEA in primary mammary carcinoma are infrequent and at low level,
requiring the use of a threshold of 2.5 ng/ml. In this study, only 27% of 22 patier
had elevations. In contrast, 79% of patients with metastatic disease had elevated
CEA. However, 6% of patients with benign cystic disease had CEA elevations
greater than 2.5 ng/ml. In contrast to Chu and Nemoto (1973), Steward *et al.*
(1974) suggested a trend of serial CEA values that correlated with the response to
treatment.

The use of serum CEA levels in the monitoring and prognosis of mammary
carcinoma had continued to receive considerable attention. The concentration of
CEA in mammary carcinomas is usually fairly low as compared to equivalent

colonic tumor burdens and, as for all tumors, may be absent. Thus, CEA cannot provide an accurate estimate of tumor burden. In those tumors that produce significant concentrations of CEA, serial monitoring may provide estimates of relative change in tumor burden. Some studies have been encouraging in regard to the use of serial CEA determinations, including the recent study of Lamerz *et al.* (1979), who observed that of 1,462 patients without metastases following mastectomy, 91% had normal serum CEA levels. In contrast, of 633 patients with metastases, only 45.7% had normal serum CEA following mastectomy. Thus, 54% of patients with metastatic breast cancer had significant serum CEA elevations after mastectomy; and the increases were most significant with metastases to the skin, lung, bone, and liver or with multiple organ involvement. They also observed a correlation between decreasing levels of CEA and remission and between persistent or fluctuating levels with stationary disease. Rising serum CEA antidated the clinical response by some weeks to months. In addition, this group used CEA derived from breast cancers in an attempt to improve the specificity of detection of this form of neoplasia. This did not appear to influence the result.

DIFFERENTIATION MARKERS

Differentiation markers represent discrete molecular entities that are a normal property of the cell type from which the tumor is derived. These are not *per se* tumor specific markers, but can be of considerable utility in identifying the histogenetic origin of a tumor, in assessing potential degree of differentiation of the tumor, and if released into the body fluids, in contrast to the normal tissue, they have potential utility as diagnostic or monitoring modalities. It is within this conceptual approach that attention has been addressed to the use of casein, the milk protein, as a marker. Increases in serum levels could be derived from neoplastic mammary epithelial cells that as a consequence of their invasive properties are anatomically displaced so as to preclude secretion into the normal mammary gland lumen. Similarly, for the other differentiation products that relate to lactation. These include as well: (1) α-lactalbumin, which has received some clinical evaluation, and more recently, (2) the proteins of the milk fat globule, markers associated with the functional lactating breast cell. Other differentiation products can be considered, including estrogen and progesterone receptors.

Mammary Gland Cyst Fluid Protein

Haagensen *et al.* (1977) described a new marker protein, a differentiation product found in high concentration in the fluid from gross cystic disease of the human breast. In this disease, considered as separate from fibrocystic disease, aspiration of cyst fluid is frequently performed. This fluid has been analyzed in detail by Haagensen *et al.* (1979) with the identification of four major proteins, one of a molecular weight of 15,000 daltons appeared to be specific for cyst fluid and not present in plasma by simple immunological analyses. It was found in human milk, saliva, and by radioimmunoassay the concentrations of this glycoprotein designated GCDFP 15 was 7–81 ng/ml. Of normal control women, 85% had plasma levels both below 50 ng/ml (Haagensen *et al.*, 1977). In contrast, 42% of patients with gross cystic disease of the breast had levels of GCDFP 15 greater than 50 ng/ml plasma. Among breast carcinoma patients, the frequency of elevation differed with the stage of disease. Elevations above 50 ng/ml plasma varied from 24% in localised carcinoma to 41% with extensive axilliary lymph node involvement, and 54% in patients with clinically evident metastases. Elevations above 150 ng/ml were observed in 30% of patients with clear evidence of metastases; and this was most pronounced in osseous metastases.

Two studies have correlated both CEA and GCDFP 15 plasma markers (Haagensen *et al.*, 1978, 1980). Of 216 patients under treatment for metastatic breast carcinoma, 111 (51%) had abnormally elevated plasma levels of CEA and/or of GCDFP 15. Abnormal plasma levels of CEA were present in 73 patients, whereas abnormal GCDFP levels were present in 67. Twenty-nine of the patients had increased plasma levels of both markers, whereas 44 had increased CEA only, and 38 had increased GCDFP 15 only. These two markers thus appear to vary independently of each other in 74% of the patients utilising both assays. Abnormal plasma levels of one or both markers were present in 79% of patients with bone metastases, 53% of patients with visceral metastases, but only 26% with soft tissue metastases. It was suggested that this assay may have utility in monitoring responsiveness to therapy. An increased concentration of either was indicative of disease progression, and a decreasing plasma level was indicative of regression.

In one study (Haagensen *et al.*, 1980), the utility of the dual CEA/GCDFP 15 assays in evaluating progression and response to therapy of patients with metastases to bone was emphasised. Responses to therapy are most difficult to evaluate in this group. Serial determination of plasma CEA and GCDFP 15 suggested that more objective indication of disease progression and regression could be achieved than with X-ray and bone scans.

OTHER TUMOR ASSOCIATED MOLECULES

This relatively unrestricted group of markers encompasses those that are not clearly tumor specific antigens, differentiation markers of the specific cells, oncodevelopmental markers or those related to the immune response. Such diverse entities as ectopic hormone production, synthesis of β_2-microglobulin or increased urinary polyamines are representative. Other markers, such as tissue polypeptide antigen (TPA), appear to be markers of the proliferating cell and may simply reflect the more rapid turnover associated with the tumor. Four examples are considered as representative of this group, and they have received wider interest.

Thomsen-Freidenreich (T) Antigen

The T antigen, first recognised on the erythrocyte surface, is now known to be the structural precursor of the human erythrocyte blood group MN antigen

$$0 \xrightarrow{\alpha \, Gal \, NAc} Tn \xrightarrow{\beta \, Gal} T \xrightarrow[\text{acid}]{\text{sialic}} N \xrightarrow[\text{acid}]{\text{sialic}} M$$

Fig. 1. Blood group M antigen and precursors.

(Springer and Desai, 1975). The MN carbohydrate structure has been well established. As illustrated in Fig. 1, omission of the two ultimate sialic acid residues results in the T antigen. The MN structures occur not only on erythrocytes but also on cells of the apocrine glands such as the salivary gland, as well as the kidney and liver. However, of more interest to the current topic is their expression by neoplasms of the breast, colon and lung as well (Springer *et al.*, 1975, 1976). Enzymatic desialation of the MN structure has been observed in association with bacterial and viral infections and this results in expression of the T antigen on cells such as erythrocytes but perhaps other cells also.

Virtually all adult individuals have anti-T antibodies, and, thus, the antibody response is not tumor specific. However, in a study of 15 carcinomas of the breast Springer *et al.* (1975) observed T antigen expression by all 15 using human serum anti-T antibody as the analytic reagent. Howard and colleagues (Howard and Taylor, 1979; Howard and Batsakis, 1980) have confirmed the T antigen expression using immunoperoxidase staining of breast carcinomas with human anti-T antibody. They demonstrated that in a small number of benign and malignant breast lesions one could distinguish the malignant mammary epithelial cells by reference to the positive binding of anti-T antibodies (Howard and Taylor, 1979). Subsequently, Howard and Batsakis (1980) utilised a long known specificity of peanut agglutinin for the T antigen, used immunoperoxidase staining and demonstrated a differential cytologic distribution of binding of peanut agglutinin which differed between benign and neoplastic mammary epithelial cells. The difference between the two reactions and the observed binding of peanut agglutinin to benign cells probably represents the less specific binding of peanut agglutinin, i.e., binding to other β-D-galactose $(1 \to 3)$-N-acetyl-D-galactosamine containing structures. Similarly, Springer *et al.* (1980) demonstrated T antigen specificity in all metastatic breast carcinomas and certain other carcinomas that they examined. It was, however, absent from four melanomas and a few other tumors. In addition, they demonstrated delayed cutaneous hypersensitivity skin reactions to purified T antigen in breast carcinoma patients, as well as *in vitro* evidence of cellular immunity to T antigen (Table III). Over 85% of ductal breast carcinoma patients and 77% of all breast carcinoma patients gave positive skin tests as compared to about 5% of patients with benign breast disease when tested with purified T antigen. It was also observed that serum anti-T antibody titers were depressed in 21% of 189 individuals with breast carcinoma as compared to 5% of 270 patients with benign breast disease or 3.6% of 470 other controls (Springer *et al.*, 1976), suggesting *in vivo* absorption of antibody or induction of immune suppression of this response. This was confirmed by observing increases of anti-T titer following removal of localised carcinomas.

In the case of the T antigen, we have a well demonstrated molecular structure, and evidence of systematic expression by breast carcinoma cells; however, this

Table III.   Cellular immune responses to Thomsen-Freidenreich (T) antigen in breast carcinoma.

Diagnosis	Delayed cutaneous hypersensitivity			Leukocyte migration inhibition		
	No.	Pos.	%Pos.	No.	Pos.	%Pos.
Normal	33	0	0	25	1	4%
Benign breast disease	74	4	5%	84	11	13%
Breast carcinoma	78	60	77%	69	25	30%

Data from Springer et al. (1980).

is clearly not a tumor specific antigen since it can be expressed under a variety of other circumstances, including desialation by infectious agents. There is a natural immunity to it, immune tolerance clearly not being established, and it can be expressed on certain other forms of cancer besides mammary carcinomas. Nevertheless, potential exists for exploitation in diagnosis and possibly in monitoring of patients with appropriate analytic methods.

Chorionic Gonadotrophin

Human chorionic gonadotrophin (HCG) is a product of normal placental metabolism. Ectopic hormone production has been described by a variety of neoplasms; among these HCG has probably been the most widely observed and certainly the most widely studied. Development of specific radioimmuno-assays for HCG as well as subsequent analyses for the α and β chains of HCG have facilitated the detailed analysis of HCG production by tumors, including breast carcinomas. Braunstein et al. (1973) utilised a radioimmunoassay specific for HCG and capable of distinguishing HCG from human luteinising hormone. The sera of 828 patients with non-testicular tumors were analyzed. Among these, four of 33 patients with breast carcinoma had elevated HCG. HCG has since been reported as elevated in the serum of approximately one-half of the patients with metastatic breast carcinoma and about one-third of these patients pre-operatively (Tormey et al., 1975). They suggested that HCG became elevated prior to other clinical evidence of recurrence of breast carcinoma; and changes in the serum concentrations appeared to reflect therapeutic response or failure. Metastasis to the liver was highly associated with elevated HCG, 63% of patients positive as compared to metastasis at other sites. These and other data indicate that a relatively high proportion of breast carcinomas are capable of ectopic synthesis of HCG. The synthesis of this molecule may reflect aberrant gene expression. In favor of this are the observations of Weintraub et al. (1974) and Rosen and Weintraub (1974)—that ectopic HCG synthesis may, in some circumstances, be associated with an abnormal product. Only synthesis of the α subunit of HCG has been demonstrated, since the β subunit is specific for HCG and the α subunit is nearly identical among four hormones, analyses of HCG have increasingly adopted assay of the β subunit.

Calcitonin

The ectopic production of calcitonin has been observed by several types of tumors besides Type C cell tumors of the thyroid. Production by breast carcinomas has been described (Coombes *et al.*, 1974). Serum calcitonin, measured by immunoassay, was observed in 22 of 28 patients studied with metastatic breast carcinoma. In contrast, only one of 13 patients with clinically localised breast carcinoma had elevated serum calcitonin. Elevations of calcitonin have also been observed in association with oat cell carcinomas of the lung, carcinoid tumors and pheochromocytomas.

β_2-Microglobulin

β_2-Microglobulin has a molecular weight of 11,800 daltons and is a single polypeptide chain molecule which is structurally homologous to the constant domain of immunologloglobulin light chains and may represent an evolutionary precursor as proposed by Poulik and colleagues (Poulik and Bloom, 1973; Poulik and Reisfeld, 1975). It is a co-associated chain in cell bound histocompatibility antigens, HLA in man, and is normally found in low concentration in biological fluids.

Three studies have demonstrated and confirmed that β_2-microglobulin occurs in serum at elevated concentrations in patients with advanced tumors (Evrin and Wibell, 1973; Kindt and van Vaerenbergh, 1976; Poulik, 1979). In the study by Evrin and Wibell, 216 patients were assayed for serum β_2-microglobulin. Because the level of serum β_2-microglobulin is known to increase with impaired renal function, only individuals with serum creatinine in the lower half of the normal range were studied. A normal range in control patients was 4–12 μg/ml serum. Most individuals with concentrations above 3 μg/ml had malignancy, though there were patients with immunologically mediated diseases and other immunological disorders. From these studies it was thought that perhaps β_2-microglobulin might have a role as a marker to monitor tumor growth or response to therapy; though clearly it provided neither the sensitivity nor the specificity to aid initial diagnosis.

More recently, Papaioannou *et al.* (1979) assessed the utility of this marker in 135 patients with breast cancer. Using a solid phase radioimmunoassay, they observed that there was a significant elevation of β_2-microglobulin associated with advanced metastatic breast cancer. Utilising an upper normal limit of 2.4 μg/ml, breast cancer patients with Stage I disease had a 30% incidence of elevated β_2-microglobulin; and in stage IV breast cancer, β_2-microglobulin was elevated in 50% of the individuals. Diagnostic application required age related correction of normal control values since there is a gradual rise in serum β_2-microglobulin with age; however, the ratio of serum β_2-microglobulin to creatinine clearance as an index of age dependent renal function could be used effectively. Whereas Stage I breast cancer patients had a ratio of less or equal to 3.1, Stage IV breast cancer patients had ratios of 6.4 or greater. This contrasted with most controls who did not exceed the ratio of 2.4. They concluded that β_2-microglobulin/creatinine ratio of greater than 3.8 was highly indicative of metastatic breast carcinoma.

Tissue Polypeptide Antigen

Tissue polypeptide antigen or TPA was described and characterised by Bjorklund and Bjorklund (1957) and Bjorklund *et al.* (1973). TPA is a single polypeptide chain with a molecular weight of 20,000 containing predominantly aspartic acid, glumatic acid and leucine. It is a structural component of cell membranes, apparently localised primarily within the endoplasmic reticulum and has been assayed by passive hemagglutination by several investigators including not only Bjorklund *et al.* (1973) but also, more recently, Holyoke and Chu (1979). TPA is not specific for given tissues, nor perhaps for the neoplastic cell *per se*. It appears to reflect increased proliferative rates in cells. It has been reported at elevated concentrations in the serum in association with a variety of neoplasms including carcinoma of the breast. Nemoto *et al.* (1979) described the use of dual assays for serum TPA and plasma CEA in 108 patients with breast carcinoma, 26 individuals with benign breast disease, and 40 normal women. TPA was elevated above 0.09 μg/ml in ten of 18 patients with primary localised breast carcinoma, whereas plasma CEA levels were elevated in only five. Both were increased significantly in 67 patients with metastatic breast cancer, i.e. 70% by TPA and 67% by CEA.

Among control healthy women, TPA was increased in 12% and CEA in 8% (Nemoto *et al.*, 1979). However, 27% of women with benign breast disease had increased levels of serum TPA whereas no elevation of plasma CEA was observed. TPA was most frequently increased in individuals with visceral metastases, and only a limited correlation was observed between the clinical course of the tumor and levels of TPA.

Urinary Polyamines

The polyamines putrescine, spermidine and spermine are excreted in increased concentrations in association with rapid proliferation of cells. Spermidine and spermine appear to be requisites for maximal DNA synthesis and they appear to increase intracellularly in an orderly sequential fashion as cells progress from the G_0 state to the mitotic phase of the cell cycle. The presence of abnormally increased levels of these polyamines in a variety of tumor cells and also in the blood and urine of a variety of tumor bearing patients was first described by DeVita (1971) and by Russell (1971), though only more recently has this been re-examined in the urine of breast cancer patients (Tormey *et al.*, 1975; Waalkes *et al.*, 1975). These three polyamines appear to derive from decarboxylation of ornithine. An additional polyamine of interest is cadaverine. This is produced by an independent metabolic pathway from lysine.

Tormey *et al.* (1975, 1980) assayed the concentration of these polyamines in urine using an amino acid analyzer. He observed that one-half of the patients with metastatic carcinoma of the breast had elevations of one or more individual polyamines; moreover, 38.5% of pre-operative patients with breast cancer had elevated urinary polyamines. About one-third of individuals 5–24 weeks following mastectomy but with evidence of tumor in regional lymph nodes, also had such elevations. They suggest that from sequential sampling of patients with metastatic breast cancer that the levels of urinary polyamines correlate with the clinical progression of the disease. Urinary polyamines increased in individuals refractory to therapy. The disease free period during the post-operative period was also somewhat shorter for individuals who had elevated urinary polyamines. These studies suggest application primarily as a prognostic parameter or in assessing changes in tumor burden.

IMMUNE RESPONSE MARKERS

Two general types of immune responses may be of significance in examining the basic biology of the neoplastic cell, elucidating the interaction between the host and neoplasms of the mammary gland, and in a clinical application to provide potential markers for diagnosis, prognosis, and potentially immunotherapy. The first of these, and clearly the most elusive, is the immune response to tumor specific or tumor associated molecules that are immunogeneic to the host. The second, is immune responses to potentially tumor associated markers of oncogeneic agents that may be implicated in the biology of the neoplasm. Current information regarding the host immune response to tumor specific antigens is limited owing to the lack of established tumor specific antigens of breast cancer as well as other tumors. In the absence of well established molecular entities, the described immune phenomena should be interpreted with caution. A number of studies purport to demonstrate immune responses to autologous or homologous breast cancer. Considerable interest and a body of data are available in regard to immune responses to structural proteins of the murine mammary tumor virus. Current data regarding the presence and association of circulating immune complexes in breast carcinoma will not be renewed. This has been addressed by others and, though of importance, cannot currently be defined in an adequately definitive fashion to represent a marker for breast carcinoma.

Humoral Immune Responses to MMTV

A number of investigators have reported the presence of antibody to MMTV in the serum of humans, and in elevated titer or frequency in the sera of patients with breast carcinoma. Charney and Moore (1971) observed neutralisation of infectivity of MMTV by human sera. The specificity of the reaction was not further confirmed and the number of sera examined in this initial study were too low to permit interpretation. Muller and Grossmann (1972) observed reactions of some breast cancer sera with MMTV-rich murine mammary tumor tissue sections. Specificity was in part demonstrated through absorption; however, this does not firmly establish specificity since neutralisation may have occurred as a result from contaminants of the MMTV preparation or be due to relatively non-specific interactions with the carbohydrate of MMTV. In a subsequent report (Muller *et al.*, 1976) it was shown that antibodies previously detectable in women with fibrocystic disease or breast cancer were directed to intracytoplasmic type A particles of MMTV. Immunofluorescence demonstrated that the human anti-bodies were bound only by tumors producing such type A particle clusters visible by light microscopy. The reaction was blocked by rabbit antisera to type A intracytoplasmic particles and much less of antisera to type B particles. It is notable that this group has not observed a diagnostically useful correlation of this anti-MMTV with breast carcinoma. Antibodies are frequently associated with benign breast disease and in normal women.

In the search for antibodies to structural proteins of MMTV, Zangerle et al. (1977) were unable to demonstrate antibodies in 100 sera from volunteers or patients with benign breast disease or breast cancer. Witkin et al. (1979) addressed the problem that apparent neutralisation of MMTV by certain human sera might reflect antibody independent but complement mediated reactions. They provide evidence that the type B retrovirus MMTV is not so disrupted by normal human serum. They have provided evidence that specific antibody was required for lysis of the viral particle. They developed an assay based on measurement of reverse transcriptase released from the disrupted virions to search for antibodies to MMTV in human sera. Significantly greater virolytic activity was detected in the sera of patients with breast cancer than in the sera of patients with benign breast disease or colorectal cancer or in sera from healthy individuals. Based on this apparent affirmation of the presence of antibody to MMTV, these investigators subsequently developed an enzyme linked immunoassay (Witkin et al., 1980) that was capable of detecting antibodies both to internal viral protein (p28) as well as to viral envelope components (gp52, gp34). Statistically, higher frequency of IgG binding MMTV is detected in the sera of breast cancer patients, 26% of which were positive. Ten per cent of sera from benign breast disease and 8% of normal sera were also positive. Their reactions were blocked well with rabbit antisera to MMTV gp34 and less well with anti gp52.

Cellular Mediated Immune Responses to MMTV

A number of studies have introduced the possibility of cellular immune reactivity to MMTV or some viral product in humans with an increased incidence in breast cancer patients. In an initial study, Black et al. (1974b) observed positive leukocyte migration inhibition, an indicator of cellular immunity, in one-third of breast cancer patients using milk from RIII mice as a source of MMTV. MMTV-free murine milk did not induce comparable responses. It was of interest to note that a high percentage of individuals who responded in the same assay to breast cancer tissue also responded to the MMTV positive milk. In a subsequent report (Black et al., 1975), these investigators suggested that diminished LMI responses correlated with tumor progression. This group (Black et al., 1976), further substantiated specificity for the major viral envelope glycoprotein gp55. The correlation between putative cellular immune responses in vitro to autologous or homologous breast cancer tissue and the structural protein of MMTV were addressed in some detail by Zachrau et al. (1978). In this detailed study, they concluded that reactivity was primarily to the major glycoprotein gp55 (or gp52 in other laboratories) and that this correlated very well with reactivity to autologous or homologous breast tissue. These workers also observed a high correlation with reactivity to MCF-7 extracts. These studies represent a substantial body of evidence linking a putative cross-reactivity between constituents of neoplastic mammary epithelium and structural proteins of MMTV. The full biological implications remain to be established. Application to clinical monitoring has not been widely adapted, most likely because of the requirements for the assay methodology.

Other Immune Responses

A variety of other immune responses have been described and some of these have included pertinent clinical correlations. A number of these are included in the section addressing candidate tumor specific antigens. The difficulty in reproducing many of these observations unquestionably lies in the poorly, if nonexistent, definition of the responsible antigen. As specific defined antigens are forthcoming, formal analysis or antibody responses in breast cancer patients and the correlations with disease may prove more informative.

CONCLUSIONS

In the present review, a variety of markers that have exhibited biological or clinical correlation with breast cancer have been considered. These reflect a variety of different approaches to the study of the malignant breast cancer cell, diagnosis of carcinoma of the breast or prognosis. No single marker is in wide clinical use. Perhaps, as the apparent relationship between murine mammary tumor virus and human breast carcinoma associated antigens are clarified and true tumor specific antigens are identified, a new era of understanding of the neoplastic cell of the mammary gland will emerge, as well as a far greater potential to accurately diagnose and perhaps treat these neoplasms.

ACKNOWLEDGEMENTS

The dedicated assistance of Alycia Bittick in the preparation of this manuscript is readily acknowledged, as are helpful suggestions by Dr Robert Cardiff.

REFERENCES

Accinni, R., Bartorelli, A., Ferrara, R. and Biancardi, C. (1977). *Experientia* **33**, 88.

Alford, C., Hollinshead, A. C. and Herberman, R. B. (1973). *Annals of Surgery* **178**, 20.

Andersen, V., Bjerrum, O., Bendixen, G., Schiodt, T. and Dissing, I. (1970). *International Journal of Cancer* **5**, 357.

Bjorklund, B. and Bjorklund, V. (1957). *International Archives of Allergy Application Immunology* **10**, 153.

Bjorklund, B., Bjorklund, V., Wiklund, B., Lundstrom, R., Ekdahl, P. H., Hagbard, L., Kaijser, I., Eklund, G. and Luning, B. (1973). *In* "Bjorklund Immunological Techniques for Detection of Cancer", pp. 133–187. Bonniers, Stockholm.

Black, M. M., Leis, H. P., Shore, B. and Zachrau, R. E. (1974a). *Cancer* **33**, 952.
Black, M. M., Moore, D. H., Shore, B., Zachrau, R. E. and Leis, H. P. (1974b) *Cancer Research* **34**, 1054.
Black, M. M., Zachrau, R. G., Shore, B., Moore, D. H. and Leis, H. P. (1975). *Cancer* **35**, 121.
Black, M. M., Zachrau, R. E., Dion, A. S., Shore, B., Fine, D. L., Leis, H. P. and Williams, C. J. (1976). *Cancer Research* **36**, 4137.
Boehm, O. R., Boehm, B. J. and Humphrey, L. J. (1974). *Clinical Experimental Immunology* **16**, 31.
Bowen, J. M., Dmochowski, L., Miller, M. F., Priori, E. S., Seman, G., Dodson, M. L. and Maruyama, K. (1976). *Cancer Research* **36**, 759.
Braumstein, G. D., Vaitukaitis, J. L., Cazbone, P. P. and Ross, G. T. (1973). *Annals Internal Medicine* **78**, 39.
Buffe, D., Rimbaut, C., Fuccaro, C. and Burtin, P. (1972). *Annals Institute Pasteur* **123**, 29.
Burtin, P., von Kleist, S. and Buffe, D. I. (1960). *Bulletin Society Chimica Biology* **49**, 1389.
Charney, J. and Moore, D. H. (1971). *Nature* **229**, 627.
Chu, T. M. and Nemoto, T. (1973). *Journal of the National Cancer Institute* **51**, 1119.
Cochran, A. J., Spilg, W. G. S., Mackie, R. M. and Thomas, C. E. (1972). *British Medical Journal* **4**, 67.
Cochran, A. J., Grant, R. M., Spilg, W. G., Mackie, R. M., Ross, C. E., Hoyle, D. E. and Russell, J. M. (1974). *International Journal of Cancer* **14**, 19.
Concannon, J. P., Dalbow, M. H. and Frich, J. C. (1973). *Radiology* **108**, 191.
Coombes, R. C., Hillyard, C., Greenberg, P. B. and MacIntyre, I. (1974). *Lancet* **1**, 1080.
Dean, J. H., Silva, J. S., McCoy, J. L., Leonard, C. M., Middleton, H., Cannon, G. B. and Herberman, R. B. (1975). *Journal National Cancer Institute* **54**, 1295.
Dean, J. H., McCoy, J. L., Cannon, G. B., Leonard, C. M., Perlin, E., Kreutner, A., Oldham, R. K. and Herberman, R. B. (1977). *Journal of National Cancer Institute* **58**, 549.
DeVita, V. T. (1971). *Cancer Chemotherapy Report* **2**, 23.
Dion, A. S., Farwell, D. C., Pomenti, A. A. and Girardi, A. J. (1980). *Proceedings of the National Academy of Sciences of USA* **77**, 1301.
Drysdale, J. W. and Singer, R. M. (1974). *Cancer Research* **34**, 3352.
Drysdale, J. W., Adelman, T. G., Arosio, P., Casareale, D., Fitzpatrick, P., Hazard, J. T. and Yokota, M. (1977). *Seminars in Hematology* **14**, 71.
Evrin, P. E. and Wibell, L. (1973). *Clinical Chimica Acta* **43**, 183.
Fritsche, R. and Mach, J. P. (1975). *Nature* **258**, 734.
Gentile, J. M. and Flickinger, J. T. (1972). *Surgery, Gynecology and Obstetrics* **135**, 69.
Gold, P. and Freedman, S. O. (1965). *Journal Experimental Medicine* **121**, 439.
Gorsky, Y., Vanky, F. and Sulitzeanu, D. (1976). *Proceedings of the National Academy of Sciences of USA* **73**, 2101.
Haagensen, D. E., Mazoujian, G., Holder, W. D., Kister, S. J. and Wells, S. A. (1977). *Annals of Surgery* **185**, 279.
Haagensen, D. W., Kister, S. J., Panick, J. Giannola, J., Hansen, H. J. and Wells, S. A. (1978). *Cancer* **42**, 1646.
Haagensen, D. E., Mazoujian, G., Dilley, W. G., Pedersen, C. E., Kister, S. J. and Wells, S. A. (1979). *Journal of the National Cancer Institute* **62**, 239.
Haagensen, D. W., Barry, W. F., McCook, T. A., Giannola, J., Ammirata, S. and Wells, S. A. (1980). *Annals of Surgery* **191**, 599.

Holder, W. D., Jr, Peer, G. W., Bolognesi, D. P. and Wells, S. A. (1976). *Surgery Forum* **27**, 102.

Hollinshead, A. C., Jaffurs, W. T., Alpert, L. K., Harris, J. E. and Herberman, R. B. (1974). *Cancer Research* **34**, 2961.

Holton, O. D., Fett, J. W., Alderman, E. M. and Lovins, R. E. (1978). *Federation Proceedings* **37**, 1485.

Holyoke, E. D. and Chu, T. M. (1979). *In* "Immunodiagnosis of Cancer" (R. B. Herberman and E. R. McIntire, Eds), p. 513. Marcel Decker, New York.

Howard, D. R. and Batsakis, J. G. (1980). *Science* **210**, 201.

Howard, D. R. and Taylor, C. R. (1979). *Cancer* **43**, 2279.

Humphrey, L. J., Estes, N. C., Morse, P. A., Jewell, W. R., Boudet, R. A. and Hudson, M. J. K. (1974). *Cancer* **34**, 1516.

Jacobs, A., Jones, B., Ricketts, C., Bulbrook, R. D. and Wang, D. Y. (1976). *British Journal of Cancer* **34**, 286.

Jones, B. M., Worwood, M. and Jacobs, A. (1980). *Clinica Chimica Acta* **106**, 203.

Kindt, R. and van Vaerenbergh, P. M. (1976). *Acta Clinica Belgium* **31** (Suppl. 8), 33.

Lamerz, R., Leonhardt, A., Ehrhart, H. and Lieven, H. V. (1979). *Oncodevelopmental Biology and Medicine* **1**, 123.

Lee, C. K., Humphrey, L. and Rawitch, A. B. (1978). *Federation Proceedings,* **37**, 1485.

Leung, J. P. and Edgington, T. S. (1980a). *Cancer Research* **40**, 316.

Leung, J. P. and Edgington, T. S. (1980b). *Cancer Research* **40**, 662.

Leung, J. P., Plow, E. F., Nakamura, R. M. and Edgington, T. S. (1978). *Journal of Immunology* **121**, 1287.

Leung, J. P., Bordin, G. M., Nakamura, R. M., DeHeer, D. H. and Edgington, T. S. (1979). *Cancer Research* **39**, 2057.

Leung, J. P., Nelson-Rees, W., Moore, G. C., Cailleau, R. and Edgington, T. S. (1981a). *International Journal of Cancer* (Submitted for publication.)

Leung, J. P., Moore, G. E. and Edgington, T. S. (1981b). *Federation Proceedings* (In press).

Loisillier, F., Metivier, D. and Burtin, P. (1978). *Comptes Rendu Academie des Sciences (Paris)* **287**, 1169.

Lopez, M. J. and Thomson, D. M. P. (1977). *International Journal of Cancer* **20**, 834.

Marcus, D. M. and Zinberg, N. (1974). *Archives of Biochemistry and Biophysics* **162**, 493.

Marcus, D. M. and Zinberg, N. (1975). *Journal National Cancer Institute* **55**, 791.

McCoy, J. L., Jerome, L. F., Dean, J. H., Cannon, G. B., Alford, T. C., Doering, T. and Herberman, R. B. (1974). *Journal of National Cancer Institute* **53**, 11.

Mesa-Tejada, R., Keydar, I., Ramanarayanan, M., Ohno, T., Fenoglio, C. and Spiegelman, S. (1978). *Proceedings National Academy of Sciences of USA* **75**, 1529.

Muller, M. and Grossmann, H. (1972). *Nature* **237**, 116.

Muller, M., Zotter, S. and Kemmer, C. (1976) *Journal National Cancer Institute* **56**, 295.

Nemoto, T., Constantine, R. and Chu, T. M. (1979). *Journal of National Cancer Institute* **63**, 1347.

Nordquist, R. E., Anglin, J. H. and Lerner, M. P. (1977). *Science* **197**, 366.

Ohno, T., Mesa-Tejada, R., Keydar, I., Ramanarayanan, M., Bausch, J. and Spiegelman, S. (1979). *Proceedings National Academy of Sciences of USA* **76**, 2460.

Papaioannou, D., Geggie, P. and Klassen, J. (1979). *Clinical Chimica Acta* **99**, 37.

74   *T. S. Edgington and R. M. Nakamura*

Parry, D. H., Worwood, M. and Jacobs, A. (1975). *British Medical Journal* i, 245.
Poulik, M. D. (1979). *In* "Compendium of Assays for Immunodiagnosis of Human Cancer" (R. B. Herberman, Ed.), p. 107. Elsevier, North Holland.
Poulik, M. D. and Bloom, A. D. (1973). *Journal Immunology* **110**, 1430.
Poulik, M. D. and Reisfeld, R. A. (1975). *In* "Contemporary Topics in Molecular Immunology" (F. P. Inman and W. J. Mandry, Eds), Vol. 4, 157–204. Plenum Publishing, New York.
Rosen, S. W. and Weintraub, B. D. (1974). *New England Journal of Medicine* **290**, 1441.
Russell, D. H. (1971). *Nature* **233**, 144.
Schlom, J., Wunderlich, D. and Teramoto, Y. A. (1980). *Proceedings National Academy of Sciences of USA* **77**, 6841.
Segall, A., Weiler, O., Genin, J., Lacour, J. and Lacour, F. (1972). *International Journal of Cancer* **9**, 417.
Springer, G. F. and Desai, P. R. (1975). *Carbohydrate Research* **40**, 183.
Springer, G. F., Desai, P. R. and Banatwala, I. (1975). *Journal National Cancer Institute* **54**, 335.
Springer, G. F., Desai, P. R. and Scanlon, E. F. (1976). *Cancer* **37**, 169.
Springer, G. F., Murthy, M. S., Desai, R. and Scanlon, E. F. (1980). *Cancer* **45**, 2949.
Steward, A. M., Nixon, D., Zamcheck, N. and Aisenberg, A. (1974). *Cancer* **33**, 1246.
Tormey, D. C., Waalkes, T. P., Ahmann, D., Gehrke, C. W., Zumwalt, R. W., Synder, J. and Hansen, H. (1975). *Cancer* **35**, 1095.
Tormey, D. C., Waalkes, T. P., Kuo, K. C. and Gehrke, C. W. (1980). *Cancer* **46**, 741.
Waalkes, T. P., Gehrke, C. W. and Tormey, D. C. (1975). *Cancer Chemotherapy Report* **59**, 1103.
Weintraub, B. D., Krauth, G. and Rosen, S. W. (1974). *Clinical Research* **22**, 352.
Witkin, S. S., Egeli, R. A., Sarker, N. H., Good, R. A. and Day, N. K. (1979). *Proceedings of the National Academy of Sciences of USA* **76**, 2984.
Witkin, S. S., Sarkar, N. H., Good, R. A. and Day, N. R. (1980). *Journal of Immunological Methods* **32**, 85.
Wolberg, W. H. and Goelzer, M. L. (1971). *Nature* **229**, 632.
Yang, N. S., Soule, H. D. and McGrath, C. M. (1977). *Journal National Cancer Institute* **59**, 1357.
Zachrau, R. E., Black, M. M., Dion, A. S., Shore, B., Williams, C. J. and Leis, H. P. (1978). *Cancer Research* **38**, 3414.
Zangerle, P. F., Carlberg-Bacq, C. -M., Colin, C., Franchimont, P., Gosselin, L., Kozma, S. and Osterrieth, P. M. (1977). *Cancer Research* **37**, 4326.

TUMOUR MARKERS AND HUMAN BREAST CANCER:
A DISCUSSION

A. M. Neville

Ludwig Institute for Cancer Research (London Branch),
Royal Marsden Hospital, Sutton, UK.

The range of markers which have been described to date as being expressed and/or produced by human breast cancers has been well covered and discussed by Edgington (this volume, p. 51). In addition the areas in which markers, in general, could provide useful clinical information have been discussed and illustrated by Veronesi (this volume, p. 81). The purpose, therefore, of this present discussion is to attempt to analyse critically just how closely the presently available markers, which occur and can be detected in the body fluids, approximate to those desired clinical needs and goals. Aspects of endocrine receptors as tissue markers with therapeutic and prognostic importance for breast cancer are not mentioned in this review.

HORMONES

Unlike many other tumours, such as those of the lung, breast cancers are seldom, if ever, associated with the inappropriate ("ectopic") production of hormones such as adrenocorticotrophin (ACTH), antidiuretic hormone (ADH) and parathormone (PTH). Two hormones, however, have been linked, particularly with breast cancers, mainly human chorionic gonadotrophin (HCG) and calcitonin (CT). Moreover, claims have been made for their assay in plasma having a useful clinical role.

Serono Symposium No. 46, Markers for Diagnosis and Monitoring of Human Cancer, edited by M. I. Colnaghi, G. L. Buraggi and M. Ghione, 1982. Academic Press, London and New York.

The most recent studies of HCG levels in the plasma in breast cancer cast doubt on this conclusion. It has been found that almost all those showing "elevated HCG" values are post-menopausal subjects. More detailed analysis of the radioimmunoassay results has shown that such "raised HCG values" can be totally accounted for by raised HLH levels. Other personal attempts to demonstrate HCG at a cellular level in breast cancer tissues have also been unrewarding so that the previous work purporting to show the prognostic importance of placental hormone and protein expression by breast cancers (Horne *et al.*, 1976) must also be questioned.

Calcitonin was also thought to be a common breast cancer product. While the occasional lesion may express it (Coombes *et al.*, 1975), the evolution of better radioimmunoassays has failed to confirm a high frequency for its production. Hypercalcaemia is a common complication of breast cancer, especially when osseous metastases are present. Its mechanistic aetiologies, however, have yet to be fully clarified. Certainly, parathyroid hormone is not, while prostaglandin may be, involved. However, to date, assay of plasma and/or urinary prostaglandins and their metabolites has not yielded a clinically valid result with respect to their use as markers.

IMMUNE COMPLEXES

Circulating immune complexes have been postulated to be of value as markers to monitor breast cancer and also as prognostic factors (Carpentier, this volume, p. 9); however, our own studies effected jointly with Cerrotini at the Lausanne Branch of the Ludwig Institute failed to confirm such conclusions. Nonetheless, immune complexes could be important sources of antibodies which could be used to probe biological and pathological aspects of breast cancer. It is possible that some of these antibodies could be directed to tumour specific or organ specific antigens. Moreover, others may be autoantibodies to normal tissue components. Such antibodies may arise as a result of normal cell death with release of their intracellular components as a result of tumour cell invasion. Hence, more data are needed before their utility can be assessed.

ANTIGENS AND RELATED MOEITIES

While a wide number of antigens and related moeities have been described few have been adequately tested at a clinical level. The best plasma marker tested to date in patients remains the carcinoembryonic antigen (CEA). In discussions at this meeting, Malkin has claimed that rising plasma CEA values can be found 1–2 years ahead of the overto development of metastases. Our own experience, however, suggests that such lead times are uncommon and values of the order of 3–6 months are more commonly the situation in about one-half of the subjects who develop metastases (Coombes *et al.*, 1980). Moreover, the measurement of nonspecific enzymes such as γ-glutamyl transpeptidase and alkaline phosphatase in plasma, in addition to CEA, can provide additional useful clinical data and can give a meaningful lead time in a higher number of patients. It is worth emphasizing that a not inconsiderable number of patients can develop metastases or recurrences without any significant change in the plasma levels of these parameters. CEA may also be a prognostic factor. Elevated levels persisting or evolving in the immediate post-operative period (1–3 months) are associated with a poorer outcome. Such data, together with steroid receptor status, may therefore be useful in the stratification of patients for various clinical therapeutic trials.

Other antigens of breast origin such as the mammary tumour glycoprotein (MTGP) (Edgington, this volume, p. 58–60) or the organ specific neoantigens (Thompson, this volume, p. 155) and breast gross cyst disease fluid protein or antigens of diverse origin, such as tissue polypeptide antigen (TPA), are in the process of being assessed in comparison to and with CEA and other diagnostic methods. The results are awaited with interest.

MILK PROTEINS

It was hoped by several workers that the ectopic breast products, i.e. milk proteins such as casein and lactalbumin, might serve as markers for breast disease. This was a most realistic concept and one highly analogous to hormone production by the endocrine system. After all, hormones have proved to be useful indices of disease activity. However, the present results stemming in large measure from the Belgian group (Zangerle *et al.*, this volume, p. 35) indicate that they are not of clinical value at present. Their expression, however, may be important to our understanding aspects of tumour biology and differentiation.

CONCLUSIONS

Although many "antigenic" moeities are being sought and their levels measured in body fluids to ascertain their relationship to breast cancer presence and extent, none, with the exception of CEA, has yet been examined in sufficient detail to enable valid conclusions to be drawn. In the present state of the art, therefore, it would appear that CEA is the only one with current clinical utility. Its role, however, is limited.

FUTURE APPROACHES

The endocrine system has shown that it is possible to measure secreted hormones in plasma or urine which may be used as a guide to disease activity, and, in the case of endocrine tumours, to disease extent. It is, therefore, not unreasonable to attempt to continue a search for materials unique to the breast and which are secreted products. In these contexts the data presented by Edgington and Thompson are of interest. Another approach to detect such breast specific moeities could involve the use of anti-breast monoclonal antibodies (Editorial, *Lancet*, 1981). Studies by Colnaghi reported in the discussion to this meeting, together with those by others, (Schlom *et al.*, 1980) appear promising. Tissue culture of normal and neoplastic breast cells might be a further approach which would enable the subsequent isolation and identification of products with biological and clinical importance (Westley and Rochefart, 1980; Bartorelli, this volume, p. 21).

However, it would be erroneous to direct all investigations towards finding plasma and/or urinary markers of clinical value in the detection of primary or metastatic disease. It could indeed be argued that at present no tumour derived material which is measured only in plasma allows the detection of minimal residual or metastatic disease. An alternative is to employ antibodies to breast associated antigens or related materials to detect disease either through their administration *in vivo* after radiolabelling (see Goldenberg, this volume, p. 141) or at the cellular level in biopsy material through the use of immunocytochemistry (Sloane *et al.*, 1980). In this latter context, Dearnaley *et al.* (1981) have made some progress in the detection of osseous micrometastases in breast cancer subjects.

Table I. Clinical state of breast cancer patients and detection of bone marrow infiltration using either antiserum to EMA or conventional methods[a].

	Total	EMA		Conventional histology	
	nos	Positive	Suspicious	Positive	Suspicious
Primary, no metastases	20	1	1	0	0
Post-primary, no metastases	10	1	0	0	0
Bone metastases	24	9	3	6	2
Metastases (not bone)	20	4	2	2	1
TOTAL	74	15	6	8	3

[a]After Dearnaley *et al.* (1981).

Table II. Relationship of number of EMA positive cells count compared to the detection of marrow infiltration by conventional Giemsa or Luke's preparations[a].

		Conventional methods	
No. EMA+ cells/smear	No.	Giemsa No. positive	Luke's No. positive
>100	5	5	4/4
5–100	3	0[b]	0
1–5	7	0[b]	0
0	1	1	0
Suspicious (<5)	6	0[b]	1

[a]After Dearnaley *et al.* (1981). [b]Suspicious sample.

Marrow aspirates were obtained, cytological preparations were made and then any breast cancer cells present were specifically demonstrated by immunocyto-chemical means using antibodies to the epithelial membrane antigen (EMA) (Heyderman *et al.*, 1979). As may be seen in Tables I and II, this results in a significant increased detection rate for subjects with micrometastases. Indeed, this approach allows the demonstration even of single isolated malignant cells in these preparations.

This approach is not applicable to every tissue, but may have relevance for the earlier detection of metastases in the liver or the presence of malignant cells in the peritoreum, pleural cavity or CSF.

SUMMARY

The best approach to find a plasma or urinary constituent to serve as a useful marker for the detection of primary and metastatic breast cancer may be to search for a cytoplasmically derived substance(s) with breast, but not necessarily tumour specificity. Until this objective is attained, the detection of small amounts of micrometastatic disease *in vivo* by radioimmunodetection or *in vitro* using biopsy materials and immunocytochemical methods seems to be a valuable avenue to explore.

REFERENCES

Coombes, R. C., Easty, G. C., Detre, S. A., Hillyard, C. J., Stevens, U., Girgis, S. I., Galante, L. S., Heywood, L., MacIntyre, I. and Neville, A. M. (1975) *British Medical Journal* **4**, 197–199.

Coombes, R. C., Powles, T. J., Gazet, J. -C., Nash, A. G., Ford, H. T., McKinna, A. and Neville, A. M. (1980). *Lancet* **1**, 296–298.

Dearnaley, D. P., Sloane, J. P., Ormerod, M. G., Steele, K., Coombes, R. C., Clink, H. Mc. D., Powles, T. J., Ford, H. T., Gazet, J. -C. and Neville, A. M. (1981). *British Journal of Cancer.* (In press.)

Editorial (1981). *Lancet* **3**, 421–423.

Heyderman, E., Steele. K. and Ormerod, M. G. (1979). *Journal of Clinical Pathology* **32**, 35–39.

Horne, C. H. W., Reid, I. N. and Milne, G. D. (1976). *Lancet* **2**, 279.

Schlom, J., Wunderlich, D. and Teramoto, Y. A. (1980). *Proceedings of the National Academy of Sciences of USA* **77**, 6841–6845.

Sloane, J. P., Ormerod, M. G., Imrie, S. F. and Coombes, R. C. (1980). *British Journal of Cancer* **42**, 392–398.

Westley, B. and Rochefart, H. (1980). *Cell* **20**, 353–362.

THE CLINICAL APPROACH TO BREAST CANCER
MARKERS: A DISCUSSION

U. Veronesi

Istituto Nazionale Tumori, Via G. Venezian 1, Milano, Milan, Italy

How can the biological markers contribute to the overall control of breast cancer? In which area of the general strategy of approaching breast cancer control can they be useful? Which priorities should be recommended to the investigators? In other words, what can the clinicians expect from the future development of markers and which directions should be indicated to the experimental researchers?

It is worth remembering that the present strategy of the fight against breast cancer rests on four main objectives: (1) to reduce the incidence through appropriate preventive measures, (2) to increase earlier detection, (3) to increase the survival rates, and (4) to improve the quality of life.

Very little can be expected from markers in regard to prevention. However, as one of the preventive measures is the control of morphological precancerous lesions, one possible development appears to be the research on gross cystic disease fluid protein (GCDFP) and lactalbumin.

Very important could be the role of markers in breast cancer detection. Although an improvement in early diagnosis has been observed in the last decade, still, the reluctance by most women to accept breast self-examination, the technical and economical difficulties of periodic mammography, and the limited value of thermography and echography mean a delayed diagnosis of breast cancer in most instances. Unfortunately, no markers are, at present, available for a mass screening programme of breast cancer. This area of research should enjoy the first priority as the one from which we can expect a drastic reduction in

Serono Symposium No. 46, Markers for Diagnosis and Monitoring of Human Cancer, edited by M. I. Colnaghi, G. L. Buraggi and M. Ghione, 1982. Academic Press, London and New York.

breast cancer mortality rates. MTGP antigen and antigenic determinants cross-reacting with oncogenic viruses like MMTV may appear interesting and promising areas of development, but the carcinoembryonic antigen (CEA) and other markers should also be investigated.

With regard to improvement of treatment, one of the main problems in breast cancer management today is the identification of subgroups of patients who may bear minimal residual disease after radical treatment of primary breast cancer and would need aggressive adjuvant treatments to eradicate the occult foci of metastases. The candidate marker in this sense seems to be the CEA: elevated levels are found mainly in breast cancer patients with metastatic disease, particularly with liver and bone metastases. Even more suggestive seems to be the association of elevated post-operative CEA levels with poor prognosis. Other candidates are: the pregnancy associated α-2-glycoprotein which was found in elevated values in all patients developing recurrent disease after mastectomy, before clinical detection of metastases; calcitonin, whose presence in the sera has been found to be stage related with high incidence in patients with metastatic disease; TPA (tissue polypeptide antigen), for which it has been reported that patients with repeatedly negative tests survived significantly longer than those with positive tests; T antigen, a precursor of MN blood group substances, against which antibodies are produced, whose decrease may be of prognostic value. And finally we can quote urinary polyamines (the disease-free post-operative period is shorter for individuals with elevated levels) and immune complexes whose increase during the disease-free period seems to indicate imminent recurrence or metastases.

Another important aspect of breast cancer treatment is the monitoring of therapy. Variations in the level of a tumour marker after therapy could provide indications of response to the therapy. Generally, decreasing levels correlate with a positive response as in the case of CEA or HCG (human chorionic gonadotrophin) useful in monitoring response to chemotherapy in patients with metastatic disease.

In addition, the combined use of two markers has been found of some use. With CEA and GCDFP used together, an increased concentration of one or the other was indicative of disease progression.

Finally, the recently developed technique of somatic cell hybridization, which gives rise to monoclonal antibodies, offers a great opportunity to obtain monospecific reagent and circumvent the problems connected with the use of alloantisera or xenoantisera whose polyspecificity can be reduced by appropriate absorption to take away unwanted antibodies, but cannot be rigorously eliminated. At our institute a monoclonal antibody has been isolated with a specificity for a structure which characterizes mammary epithelial cells and which is still present on breast carcinoma cells.

In the overall picture for a better control of breast cancer, the first priority should be the isolation of markers for detection (Table I) followed by the identification of markers for prognosis (Table II) as second priority. The marker candidate for clinical use should have characteristics as close as possible to the five major requirements for the "ideal" marker, quoted in Table III. From the methodological point of view, it is important that the clinical evaluation of the usefulness of a given candidate marker should be first conducted in patients with metastatic disease. If valuable in this category, one should proceed to evaluate it in localized cancer and, if positive, in the general population. A correct sequence of clinical testing of markers is reported in Table IV.

Table I. First priority: markers for detection of occult breast cancer in healthy women.

Diagnosis of breast cancer is late in most cases. Earlier diagnosis has been shown to be able to reduce mortality; no satisfactory and economically acceptable tests are available for screening programmes.

Table II. Second priority: markers for prognosis.

The identification in treated patients of subgroups at high risk of recurrence would enable the clinician to concentrate efforts in these subgroups in terms of aggressive adjuvant systemic treatments.

Table III. Characteristics of the ideal marker.

(1) Sensitivity, to detect *all* patients with (occult) breast cancer

(2) Specificity, to detect *only* patients with breast cancer

(3) Direct correlation with the tumour burden

(4) Ability to detect disease below the level of current detection methods

(5) Technically and economically applicable in most hospital clinical laboratories

Table IV. Sequence of clinical testing for evaluation of potential markers in breast cancer.

(1) Detection capability in metastatic disease

(2) Detection capability in localized cancer

    (a) Pre-operative
    (b) Post-operative, N+
    (c) Post-operative, N−

(3) Detection capability in women at high risk of developing breast cancer

(4) Detection capability in general healthy population

HORMONE MARKERS IN LUNG CANCER

J. G. Ratcliffe

Department of Biochemistry, Royal Infirmary, Glasgow, UK

INTRODUCTION

Recent interest in the clinical potential of hormone markers in lung cancer has stemmed from the following developments: (1) successful application of hormone measurements to routine diagnosis and management of endocrine tumours (e.g. chorionic gonadotrophin (CG) in trophoblastic tumours, pituitary hormones in pituitary tumours); (2) recognition that ectopic hormone production by lung tumours, especially small cell cancer, occurs more frequently than previously thought; (3) recent improvements in the chemotherapy of small cell lung cancer; and (4) wider availability of immunoassays for peptide hormones, which are commonly produced by lung cancer (e.g. ACTH, calcitonin).

The present review will distinguish the application of hormone measurements in lung cancer in patients with and without clinically overt hormonal syndromes. While the former application is limited to a relatively small proportion of patients with lung cancer, the latter may have potential relevance to the management of the majority of such patients. Brief consideration will also be given to the structure of hormones produced by lung cancer and their control. The wider topic of ectopic hormone production in malignant disease has been reviewed recently by Ratcliffe (1981).

LUNG CANCER WITH HORMONAL SYNDROMES

Clinical syndromes attributed to tumour hormone production (ectopic hormones) occur in about 10% of unselected patients with lung cancer (Azzopardi

Serono Symposium No. 46, Markers for Diagnosis and Monitoring of Human Cancer, edited by M. I. Colnaghi, G. L. Buraggi and M. Ghione, 1982. Academic Press, London and New York.

et al., 1970). The most common syndromes include hypercalcaemia (in the absence of overt metastatic disease), syndrome of inappropriate antidiuretic hormone (SIADH) production, and ectopic ACTH syndrome. Less common syndromes include gynaecomastia due to CG, acromegaly due to growth hormone and/or growth hormone releasing factor, galactorrhoea due to prolactin, and watery diarrhoea due to vasoactive intestinal peptide. However, virtually all known polypeptides may be produced by lung carcinoma though some do not give rise to clinically recognizable syndromes (e.g. calcitonin, placental lactogen).

Among lung tumours, small (oat) cell and carcinoid tumours are especially remarkable for their endocrine activity, both containing dense core granules characteristic of peptide producing endocrine cells. It is considered likely that these tumours arise from bronchial cells with apud features (Kultschitsky-type) which may have an endocrine or chemoreceptor role in normal lung (Corrin, 1980). These tumours are virtually always the histological types responsible for ectopic ACTH, ecotopic ADH, acromegaly or carcinoid syndromes. When other types of lung tumour are associated with these syndromes, careful review of the histology often leads to a revision of the original diagnosis. Squamous, glandular and large cell undifferentiated carcinomas of lung show no structural features of endocrine secretory activity, though their production of parathyroid hormone (PTH) and placental hormone-like peptides is well recognized. They are believed to arise from non-apud pulmonary epithelial cells.

DIAGNOSIS

Hypercalcaemia

This occurs in about 15% of patients with epidermoid (squamous cell) lung cancer (Bender and Hansen, 1974), but is rarely associated with other histological types. The biochemical basis remains elusive though several possibilities are under investigation. Tumour production of PTH-like peptides by lung cancer is well documented but appears to be an unusual cause. More commonly, the syndrome may be due to as yet uncharacterized peptide(s), which mimic certain actions of PTH (e.g. stimulation of renal adenylate cyclase, glucose-6-phosphate dehydrogenase and enhanced phosphaturia) (Stewart *et al.*, 1980). Other properties of these putative peptides differ from PTH (e.g. increased calcium excretion, absent PTH immunoactivity). Substances produced locally in bone by tumour cells may also cause hypercalcaemia e.g. prostraglandins and osteoclast activating factor. At present, it is not clear what proportion of lung tumours associated with hypercalcaemia produce PTH-like peptides, renal cAMP stimulating factor, prostaglandins or osteoclast activating factor. Because of these uncertainties and a lack of reliable assays, the measurement of these potential markers has not, so far, been of much value in the diagnosis and management of hypercalcaemia.

Syndrome of Inappropriate ADH Secretion (SIADH)

SIADH occurs in about 8% of patients with small cell lung cancer but rarely, if ever, in other histological types. Circulating ADH levels are distinctly elevated (>10 ng/l) in most patients with SIADH associated with lung cancer and provide a useful confirmatory test (Padfield *et al.*, 1976). The inappropriate negative relationship between elevated ADH and subnormal plasma osmolality clearly separates patients with tumour associated SIADH from normals, and when SIADH is due to other causes (e.g. bronchopneumonia, TB) plasma ADH levels are usually lower and, in contrast to ectopic ADH secretion, decrease as serum sodium normalizes during therapy.

Ectopic ACTH/LPH Syndrome

Ectopic ACTH/LPH syndrome occurs in about 3% of patients with small cell lung cancer but rarely, if ever, with other histological types. Assays for ACTH, LPH and "MSH" (i.e. cross reacting with β, γ LPH and β MSH) are useful in confirming the diagnosis of suspected ectopic ACTH syndrome since hormone levels are usually higher than found in pituitary driven Cushing's syndrome. A plasma ACTH or "β MSH" level greater than 200 ng/l in a patient with Cushing's syndrome is very suggestive of ectopic production and should lead to an intensive search for an extrapituitary tumour especially in the lung (Ratcliffe *et al.*, 1972). It is important to recognize that about one-half of the patients with ACTH producing bronchial carcinoids or thymomas, present with Cushing's syndrome before the tumour is diagnosed, so that hormone assays may be particularly useful in this context (Mason *et al.*, 1972). A high ratio of circulating β LPH (or "MSH")/ACTH and β LPH/γ LPH in a patient with elevated ACTH and LPH levels indicates an extrapituitary source (Gilkes *et al.*, 1977).

Tumour Localization and Monitoring

Rarely, selective venous sampling with hormone measurements may help in tumour localization. Serial hormone assays are sometimes useful in monitoring response to therapy and in detecting tumour recurrence before clinical diagnosis. However, circulating hormone levels correlate poorly with the stage of disease and variably with the clinical course, owing to selective effects of therapy on hormone synthesis with cloning out of non-hormone secreting tumour cells.

Rarer Hormonal Syndromes

Hormone assays may occasionally be useful in diagnosis and management of rarer hormone syndromes associated with lung cancer e.g. CG in gynecomastia, growth hormone in acromegaly, prolactin in galactorrhoea, vasoactive intestinal peptide in watery diarrhoea.

LUNG CANCER WITHOUT HORMONE SYNDROMES

In the last decade it has become clear that hormone production by lung tumours is more common than suggested by the prevalence of clinically apparent syndromes (Fig. 1). This has raised the possibility that detection of hormones in blood or tissue by immunological methods may serve as markers in diagnosis, prognosis and management of the generality of lung cancer patients, particularly as ectopic hormone secreting tumours often produce hormone-like peptides with immunological but not biological activity.

J. G. Ratcliffe

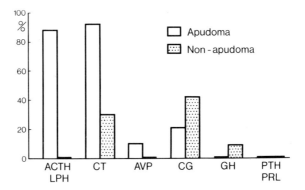

Fig. 1. Prevalence of significant levels of immunoactive hormones in lung cancer tissues. Apudoma includes small (oat) cell carcinoma and carcinoids: Non-apudoma includes epidermoid, adeno- and large cell undifferentiated carcinoma. Data taken from Ratcliffe and Podmore (unpublished) and from the literature. ACTH: adrenocorticotrophin; LPH: lipotrophin, AVP: arginine vasopressin, CG: chorionic gonadotrophin; GH: growth hormone; PTH: parathyroid hormone; PRL: prolactin. (Reproduced by courtesy of *Scottish Medical Journal*.)

Exploitation of this potential depends on the prevalence of hormone production and its relationship to tumour type, the relationship of circulating hormone levels to tumour mass, and the availability of assays for molecular forms of hormones which are relatively tumour specific. The clinical value of such assays is of course enhanced if effective therapy is available for tumours detected biochemically.

ACTH

Impaired suppression of corticosteroids is reported in about one-half of the patients with small cell lung cancer in the absence of the ectopic ACTH syndrome (Gilby *et al.*, 1975). Positive ACTH and LPH immunoactivity in tumour extracts and by immunoperoxidase staining is detected in the majority of small cell and carcinoid lung tumours at levels within the range found in proven cases of ectopic ACTH syndrome (>10 ng/g wet wt) (Bloomfield *et al.*, 1977). Tumour ACTH and LPH concentrations are well correlated, suggesting that both hormones are expressed together as in the normal pituitary. The ACTH content also correlates well with the presence of secretory granules in these lung tumours.

In contrast to small cell cancer, the production of ACTH by other types of lung cancer is less clearly established. Low tumour hormone levels may represent retained circulating hormone or non-specific effects in the assay. Occasionally, tumours which are classified as non-small cell cancer may contain carcinoid elements.

Estimates of the prevalence of elevating circulating ACTH levels in lung cancer vary widely. Elevated plasma ACTH levels were reported initially in the majority of patients with lung cancer of all histological types and in 20–30% of patients with non-malignant lung disease (Gewirtz and Yalow, 1974; Wolfsen and Odell, 1979). However, acute administration of dexamethasone suppresses ACTH levels by a similar proportion in patients with lung cancer, non-malignant lung disease and normal subjects, implying that the tumour is not the only source of elevated plasma ACTH (Torstensson *et al.*, 1980). We and others find elevated ACTH levels in a minority of lung cancer patients, mainly small cell cancer. Even in patients with small cell cancer, elevated levels occur in only 20-30%, and are poorly related to stage of disease (Hansen *et al.*, 1980a; Gropp *et al.*, 1980). The association of elevated levels only with small cell carcinoma appears to be more compatible with tumour hormone measurements discussed above and with pathological evidence, suggesting that ectopic ACTH production occurs in 19% of small cell tumours but not in other histological types (Singer *et al.*, 1978).

The explanation of these discrepancies is not yet clear but may be related to the selection of reference groups (patients with non-malignant lung disease vs healthy controls) and assay specificity, since the relative contribution of different molecular forms of ACTH to measured immunoactivity is poorly defined. In addition, sera from patients with small cell cancer may contain immune complexes comprising macromolecular IgG, complement and high molecular weight ACTH suggesting that HMW forms of ACTH released into the circulation are autoantigenic (Havemann *et al.*, 1979). The effect of such complexes on ACTH assays is not known.

Our data with an assay relatively specific for α^{1-39} ACTH suggest that, in general, there is no excessive secretion of regular ACTH in the absence of the ectopic ACTH syndrome (Ratcliffe and Podmore, 1980). This is compatible with the finding of normal plasma ACTH levels measured by radioreceptor assay in lung tumours. Using an assay for "total" ACTH immunoactivity (i.e. high molecular weight ACTH as well as α^{1-39} ACTH), elevated levels are found in 24% of patients with small cell lung cancer at the time of initial presentation (Ratcliffe and Stack, unpublished observations). The prevalence of elevated total ACTH levels is somewhat greater in patients with extensive than limited disease (32 and 12%, respectively), but the correlation with metastatic disease is too poor to be of much use in staging. The value of serial ACTH measurements for monitoring therapy is not yet clear. Gropp *et al.* (1980) found a good correlation between ACTH levels and the clinical course during therapy with increasing ACTH values before clinical evidence of tumour recurrence, but Hansen *et al.* (1980b) concluded that the relationship is too variable to allow treatment decisions to be based solely on changes in hormone concentrations. Plasma cortisol levels are, in general, higher in lung cancer patients than controls and are similar whether or not immunoactive ACTH levels are elevated. Highest cortisol values are found in patients with metastases and poor prognosis, but whether this is owing to tumour ACTH secretion or pituitary stimulation by non-specific stress mechanisms is not known.

ADH

Inappropriate ADH secretion occurs commonly in patients with small cell lung cancer but there is no definite proof that this is usually owing to tumour ADH secretion. In patients with small cell cancer, abnormal handling of a water load occurs in 40%, and urine ADH and plasma and urine osmolalities suggestive of inappropriate ADH secretion in 32% (Gilby *et al.*, 1975; Hansen *et al.*, 1980a).

The relationship between plasma ADH levels and urine: plasma osmolality after water loading is abnormal in most normonatraemic patients with small cell cancer. However, tumour ADH immunoactivity is detected only in small cell cancers associated with hyponatraemia, so that mechanisms other than ADH production by tumour may be the usual cause of raised ADH levels in normonatraemic lung cancer patients.

Thus, although subtle abnormalities in vasopressin control are commonly found in lung cancer, ADH assays are of marginal value in diagnosis or management. An alternative approach using assays for vasopressin and oxytocin associated neurophysin merits further investigation, since elevated plasma levels of one or other of these neurophysins is found in 62% of patients with small cell cancer but less than 15% with other histological types (North *et al.*, 1980).

Calcitonin (CT)

Although not associated with a clinical syndrome, calcitonin production occurs commonly in lung cancer. Positive tumour CT immunoactivity is reported in about 90% of small cell cancer and 43% of non-small cell tumours (Abe *et al.*, 1977). Estimates of the prevalence of elevated circulating calcitonin levels vary widely. Unequivocal hypercalcitoninaemia, sometimes into the range associated with medullary carcinoma of thyroid (MCT), is found in 25–72% of patients with small cell cancer (Silva *et al.*, 1979; Schwartz *et al.*, 1979). In an uncertain proportion of cases, elevated CT levels are due to thyroidal secretion possibly caused by tumour release of calcitonin secretagogues (e.g. prostaglandins). Calcitonin levels are increased after pentagastrin in over one-half of lung cancer patients though not to the same extent as in MCT (Samaan *et al.*, 1980).

Differences in assay specificity may account for some of the variations in prevalence noted above. Thus, the prevalence is higher using assays directed towards the C-terminal 22–32 peptide sequence (Roof *et al.*, 1979). Spuriously elevated circulating calcitonin levels may be common owing to non-specific artefacts in current assays (Roos *et al.*, 1980). CT immunoactivity in plasma from patients with non-small cell cancer differs from human CT in a variety of tests. The demonstration of high molecular weight CT which does not bind to CT receptors suggests that, as with ACTH, more specific assays for tumour CT-like material may have clinical value. In general, plasma CT levels are not closely related to tumour burden, though some authors report that serial levels are useful for monitoring therapy in lung cancer patients (Hansen *et al.*, 1980b). As with ACTH, present experience is too limited to allow definite recommendations for routine clinical practice.

CG

Positive levels of immunoactive CG and/or its subunits occur in up to one-third of sera and tumours from unselected patients with lung cancer (Vaitukaitis *et al.*, 1976). Tumour levels are higher in non-small cell cancers. However, serum levels are often only modestly elevated and there is no correlation between serum CG and testosterone levels with the stage of disease, suggesting a limited role for serum assays in the management of lung cancer (Gropp *et al.*, 1980).

Other Hormones

Elevated levels of somatostatin-like immunoactivity is found in 15% of small cell lung cancer (Roos *et al.*, 1981). Elevated levels of PRL, GH, PL occur too infrequently to be of much clinical value in lung cancer.

In summary, although production of ACTH, CT, CG and, possibly, ADH is common in lung cancer, circulating hormone levels by current assays are generally poorly related to tumour mass and the proportion of patients with clearly elevated (i.e. above those found in patients with non-malignant lung disease) is too low to be of much clinical value in early diagnosis and staging of lung cancer. ACTH and CT assays appear to have more promise in monitoring therapy. Further work is required using hormone assays of defined specificity especially for HMW, ACTH and CT.

STRUCTURE OF HORMONES PRODUCED BY LUNG CANCER

It has already been stressed that some of the differences in reports of the prevalence of hormone production by lung cancer are related to hormonal hetero-geneity. Present evidence suggests that, although the primary amino acid sequences of ectopic hormones closely resemble their normal counterparts, the relative abundance of the several molecular forms in tumour and blood differs from normal.

In general, ectopic hormones are more heterogeneous than eutopic hormones with a greater proportions of high molecular weight (HMW) forms, subunits and fragments in tumour tissue and blood. Precursor and fragment forms often predominate in hormone producing lung tumours. These observations can account for abnormal ratios of bio-to immunoactivities and C to N terminal immuno-activities in hormone producing lung tumours. They probably reflect changes in post-translational tumour hormone metabolism. Little is known, however, of the factors controlling the cascade of hormone metabolism in tumour tissue and blood.

Most information is available on ACTH and related peptides produced by extra-pituitary tumours. The following peptides have been partially characterized in tumours associated with ectopic ACTH production (Pullan *et al.*, 1980a).

(1) High molecular weight ACTH ("big" ACTH). This is the glycoprotein precursor of ACTH and LPH which is immunoactive but lacks significant steroidogenic activity. HMW ACTH is often the predominant form in lung tumours whereas it is a minor component in normal pituitary.

(2) α_h^{1-39} or α_h^{2-38} ACTH is uniformly present, though sometimes a minor component.

(3) small molecular weight fragments (e.g. α_h^{18-39} (CLIP) and N terminal fragments resembling α MSH) are often major components in tumours but are absent in normal pituitary tissue.

(4) LPH. Both $\beta(1-91)$ and $\gamma(1-58)$ LPH occur consistently, with γ LPH often predominating in contrast to the normal pituitary.

(5) LPH fragments ($\alpha(61-76)$ and $\beta(61-91)$ endorphins β and γ MSH-like peptides occur commonly, again in contrast to the normal pituitary.

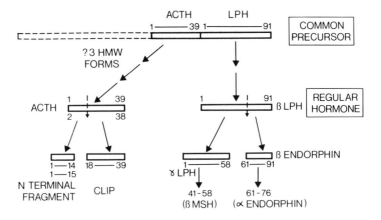

Fig. 2. Pattern of ACTH/LPH metabolism in tumours associated with ectopic ACTH syndrome, based on current evidence. (Reproduced by courtesy of *Scottish Medical Journal*.)

Met-enkephalin (61–65 LPH) also occurs frequently but appears to be synthesized separately from the ACTH/LPH family of peptides, suggesting that this gene is duplicated and capable of independent expression (Pullan *et al.*, 1980b). A summary of the mechanism of production of ACTH and LPH peptides by extra pituitary tumours is shown in Fig. 2.

The potential clinical use of assays for ACTH related peptides depends on identifying molecular species that are relatively tumour specific. Small cell lung tumours appear to secrete mainly HMW or fragment forms with immunological but little steroidogenic activity.

Similar evidence is accruing for the pattern of tumour hormone metabolism of other ectopic peptides such as calcitonin. An epidermoid lung cancer cell line secretes predominantly HMW forms (molecular weight: 40,000, and 10,000 daltons) in addition to monomeric calcitonin (molecular weight: 3,500), which is the major product of medullary carcinoma of thyroid (Ham *et al.*, 1980). Most of the plasma calcitonin immunoactivity from small cell and adenocarcinomas is also much larger than monomer, though a precursor relationship of HMW to monomeric calcitonin has yet to be established. Calcitonin-like peptides smaller than monomer have also been described in small cell lung cancer. Such molecular heterogeneity emphasizes the need to use assays of defined specificity and explains, in part, the variable results so far reported in lung cancer.

CONTROL OF TUMOUR HORMONE SECRETION

Ectopic hormone secretion is usually considered to be autonomous. It is now emerging that this is not always so. Thus, variations in plasma ACTH levels in ectopic ACTH syndrome may occur over weeks or months and responses to metyrapone and dexamethasone may occur acutely. Tumour corticotrophin releasing factor may play a role in these changes. Several other factors may also influence ACTH secretion. Thus, adenyl cyclase of ectopic ACTH producing tumours can be activated by TRH, GnRH, serotonin and prostaglandins as well as median eminence extracts (Hirata *et al.*, 1979). Inappropriate secretion of ectopic hormones may therefore be mediated by altered receptors on neoplastic cells. These observations suggest that tumour hormone secretion may be controlled by pharmacological means and anticipates the development of diagnostic dynamic tests of tumour hormone status. In this context, Samaan *et al.* (1980) report that circulating calcitonin levels increase after pentagastrin in patients with lung cancer, particularly small cell. This may have some clinical value in elucidating the cause of basal hypercalcitoninaemia since the CT response is greater in medullary carcinoma of thyroid than lung cancer.

CONCLUSION

Ideally, a tumour marker should have the following properties: (1) tumour specificity; (2) its level in blood or urine should reflect viable tumour mass and measurement should be sensitive enough to detect subclinical disease; (3) marker prevalence should be sufficiently high to make assay worthwhile; and (4) a simple and cheap assay should be available. None of the hormone markers meets all these requirements in lung cancer, not even in small cell cancer, so that their present clinical role remains unproven. Nevertheless, developments in chemotherapy, improved assay specificity and understanding of factors controlling hormone secretion may allow some exploitation of hormone markers such as ACTH and CT in monitoring small cell lung cancer. The detection of hormones in tumour tissue and blood may also be valuable in the functional classification of lung tumours with implications for the assessment of prognosis and selection of therapy.

ACKNOWLEDGEMENTS

I am grateful to the Scottish Hospitals Endowment Research Trust for financial support, To Drs B. H. R. Stack and J. Podmore for access to unpublished work, and to Miss Ann Gibson for secretarial help in preparing this manuscript.

REFERENCES

Abe, K., Adachi, I., Miyakawa, S., Tanaka, M., Yamaguchi, K., Tanaka, N., Kameya, T. and Shimosato Y. (1977). *Cancer Research* **37**, 4190.
Azzopardi, J. G., Freeman, D. and Poole, G. (1970). *British Medical Journal* **4**, 528.
Bender, R. A. and Hansen, H. (1974). *Annals of Internal Medicine* **80**, 205.
Bloomfield, G. A., Holdaway, I. M., Corrin, B., Ratcliffe, J. G., Rees, G. M., Ellison, M. L. and Rees, L. H. (1977). *Clinical Endocrinology* **6**, 95.
Corrin, B. (1980). *Investigation and Cell Pathology* **3**, 195.
Gewirtz, G. and Yalow, R. S. (1974). *Journal of Clinical Investigation* **53**, 1022.
Gilby, E. D., Rees, L. H. and Bondy, P. K. (1975). *Excerpta Medica Foundation International Congress Series* **375**, 132.

Gilkes, J. J. H., Rees, L. H. and Besser, G. M. (1977). *British Medical Journal* 1, 996.

Gropp, G., Havemann, K. and Scheuer, A. (1980). *Cancer* 46, 347.

Ham, J., Ellison, M. L. and Lumsden, J. (1980). *Biochemical Journal*. (In press.)

Hansen, M., Hansen, H. H., Hirsch, F. R., Arends, J., Christensen, J. D., Christensen J. M., Hummer, L. and Kuhl, C. (1980a). *Cancer* 45, 1432.

Hansen, M., Hammer, M. and Hummer, L. (1980b). *Cancer* 46, 2062.

Havemann, K., Gropp, C., Scheuer, A., Scherfe, T. and Gramse, M. (1979). *British Journal of Cancer* 39, 43.

Hirata, Y., Yoshimi, H., Matsukura, S. and Imura, H. (1979). *Journal of Clinical Endocrinology and Metabolism* 49, 317.

Mason, A. M. S., Ratcliffe, J. G., Buckle, R. M. and Mason, A. S. (1972). *Clinical Endocrinology* 1, 1.

North, W. G., Maurer, L. H., Valtin, H. and O'Donnell, J. G. (1980). *Journal of Clinical Endocrinology and Metabolism* 51, 892.

Padfield, P. L., Morton, J. J., Brown, J. J., Lever, A. F., Robertson, J. I. S., Wood, M. and Fox, R. (1976). *American Journal of Medicine* 61, 825.

Pullan, P. T., Clement-Jones, V., Corder, R., Lowry, P. J., Besser, G. M. and Rees, L. H. (1980a). *Clinical Endocrinology* 13, 437.

Pullan, P. T., Clement-Jones, V., Corder, R., Lowry, P. J., Rees, G. M., Rees, L. H., Besser, G. M., Macedo, M. M. and Galvao-Teles, A. (1980b). *British Medical Journal* 1, 758.

Ratcliffe, J. G. (1981). *In* "Recent Advances in Endocrinology and Metabolism" (J. L. H. O'Riordan, Ed.), No 2. Churchill Livingstone, Edinburgh. (In press.)

Ratcliffe, J. G. and Podmore, J. (1980). *In* "Cancer; Assessment and Monitoring" (T. Symington, A. E. Williams and J. G. McVie, Eds), pp. 324–343. Churchill Livingstone, Edinburgh.

Ratcliffe, J. G., Knight, R. A., Besser, G. M., Landon, J. and Stanfeld, A. G. (1972). *Clinical Endocrinology* 1, 27.

Roof, B. S., Weinsten, R., Vujic, I. and Burdash, N. M. (1979). *Biomedicine* 30, 82.

Roos, B. A., Lindall, A. W., Baylin, S. B., O'Neill, J. A., Frelinger, A. L., Birnbaum, R. S. and Lambert, P. W. (1980). *Journal of Clinical Endocrinology and Metabolism* 50, 659.

Roos, B. A., Lindall, A. W., Ells, J., Elde, R., Lambert, P. W. and Birnbaum, R. S. (1981). *Journal of Clinical Endocrinology and Metabolism* 52, 187.

Samaan, N. A., Castillo, S., Schultz, P. N., Khalil, K. G. and Johnston, D. A. (1980). *Journal of Clinical Endocrinology and Metabolism* 51, 237.

Schwartz, K. W., Wolfsen, A. R., Forster, B. and Odell, W. D. (1979). *Journal of Clinical Endocrinology and Metabolism* 49, 438.

Silva, O. L., Broder, L. E., Doppman, J. L., Snider, R. H., Moore, C. F., Cohen, M. H. and Becker, K. L. (1979). *Cancer* 44, 680.

Singer, W., Kovacs, K., Ryan, N. and Horvath, E. (1978). *Journal of Clinical Pathology* 31, 591.

Stewart, A. F., Horst, R., Deftos, L. J., Cadman, E. C., Lang, R. and Broadus, A. E. (1980). *New England Journal of Medicine* 303, 1377.

Torstensson, S., Thoren, M. and Hall, K. (1980). *Acta Medica Scandinavica* 207, 353.

Vaitukaitis, J. L., Ross, G. T., Braunstein, G. D. and Rayford, P. L. (1976). *Recent Progress in Hormone Research* 32, 289.

Wolfsen, A. R. and Odell, W. D. (1979). *American Journal of Medicine* 66, 765.

NON-HORMONE MARKERS OF HUMAN LUNG CANCER

K. R. McIntire

Diagnosis Branch, Division of Cancer Biology and Diagnosis, National Cancer Institute, Bethesda, Maryland, USA

INTRODUCTION

A number of investigative groups have described antigens associated with primary lung cancer in humans and most of them have attempted to establish sensitive quantitative assays that would allow for measurement of the antigen in blood or other body fluids. While several of these newly described antigens have shown some initial promise for eventual clinical utility, none as yet have more than very limited testing, usually only at the institution of origin. Therefore, these tumor associated antigens are not yet ready for consideration as lung cancer markers, but, in the near future, some will be evaluated sufficiently for a decision on their value in the clinical management of lung cancer. For the purpose of complete coverage, the lung cancer associated antigens will be briefly described in this chapter.

The most extensively studied marker for lung cancer is the carcinoembryonic antigen (CEA), originally described by Gold and Freedman. This will be discussed along with other oncofetal tumor markers. Great promise for developing useful markers for human lung cancer has been provided by a wide variety of circulating hormones. Lung cancer has long been known to be associated with the ectopic production of hormones more frequently than other forms of non-endocrine cancer. These hormones, which have correlated with changes

Serono Symposium No. 46, Markers for Diagnosis and Monitoring of Human Cancer, edited by M. I. Colnaghi, G. L. Buraggi and M. Ghione, 1982. Academic Press, London and New York.

in the disease status, have been of pituitary and placental as well as endocrine organ type. Recent recognition of functionally inactive precursor forms of many of these hormones has indicated that their occurrence in lung cancer is even more frequent than previously expected. The entire subject of hormones and lung cancer has been covered in the preceding chapter by Professor J. G. Ratcliffe.

There is a growing awareness that certain isoenzymes may be selectively synthesised by lung cancer cells or stimulated by their presence in the host and that they may serve as tumor markers. The isoenzymes found associated with lung cancer and abnormalities of certain serum proteins will also be covered since they can also be considered as potential markers. Other substances which may be affected by the presence of lung cancer will be briefly discussed; these include serum nucleosides and bases and carbohydrate containing complexes such as lipid associated sialic acid and protein bound carbohydrates.

It must be recognised that the lack of specificity for lung cancer of all the known tumor markers means that markers can only be used with caution to augment clinical judgements and decisions which are supported by other diagnostic procedures. It is also obvious that since all the known tumor markers lack ideal sensitivity, it will be necessary to identify the optimal marker(s) for each type of lung cancer and quite possibly, on an individual basis, for each patient with lung cancer. This might be accomplished by analyzing each patient's pretreatment serum with a panel or spectrum of assays to determine which marker(s) is abnormal and associated with the tumor. Frequent sampling of the patient's blood for quantitation of the selected markers will demonstrate the correlation with changes in tumor burden during the course of therapy. In patients who achieve clinical remission following therapy the previously selected markers can be used to monitor for the detection of recurrent tumor before the relapse becomes clinically apparent.

The extensive correlation of a number of markers with the clinical course of patients with lung cancer will provide a body of knowledge to choose markers more accurately for applications other than the monitoring of therapy. Examples of other applications are: (1) screening for and detection of lung cancer in asymptomatic individuals, primarily in populations that can be described as higher risk owing to factors such as age, family history, smoking, occupational exposure, etc.; (2) diagnosis of lung cancer in persons with symptoms or signs suggestive of lung cancer; (3) staging or estimation of the extent of tumor spread; (4) prognosis; (5) localisation of metastatic tumor by injection of radiolabeled antibody to tumor markers and allowing accumulation of radioactivity to be picked up by nuclear medicine scanning technology (Goldenberg *et al.*, 1978); and (6) classification of lung tumors by their biochemical and antigenic characteristics as well as by conventional morphology (Katoh *et al.*, 1979; DeLellis *et al.*, 1979).

In this chapter the definition of tumor marker will be broadly inclusive rather than restrictive and will cover any substance demonstrable in the blood or urine (as well as in the tumor) in abnormal amounts. This chapter will include those tumor associated antigens which are found circulating in body fluids and appear to offer some promise in helping to understand the dynamic biology of tumor growth and regression.

TUMOR ASSOCIATED ANTIGENS

The generation of antisera to immunogenic components in lung cancer extracts has been successfully achieved by many groups in the past decade. However, only a few of these endeavours have proceeded to the development of assays sufficiently sensitive to measure the putative antigen in the blood or other body fluids.

The group in Vancouver, British Columbia, used absorbed rabbit antiserum to purify a component which was found in many different lung cancer extracts but was virtually undetectable in normal tissues (Kelly and Levy, 1977). An enzyme linked immunoabsorbant assay capable of measuring antigenic activity in normal serum was developed and showed that sera from patients with primary lung cancer (squamous cell, adenocarcinoma and oat cell carcinoma) inhibited antibody binding in the test system while sera from patients with metastatic lung tumors of non-pulmonary origin had values in the normal range (Kelly and Levy, 1980).

The group in Bethesda, Maryland, also used absorbed rabbit antisera to identify, isolate and quantitate a cytoplasmic antigen which was present in extracts from 84 of 98 (86%) tumors of all histological types of primary lung cancer (Braatz *et al.*, 1978). Initial attempts to develop a double-antibody radioimmunoassay were frustrated by certain similarities between the tumor associated antigen and a normal protease inhibitor, α-1-antichymotrypsin (Gaffar *et al.*, 1980). Re-isolation of the antigen has facilitated the development of a radioimmunoassay which is not inhibited by α-1-antichymotrypsin. Preliminary data with this radioimmunoassay appear to distinguish over 50% of stage I and 80% of stage II lung cancers from a similar group of normal controls (Braatz *et al.*, 1981).

Several other laboratory groups have identified antigens associated with lung cancer which are not demonstrable or significantly less concentrated in normal tissues. These groups have not yet developed assays for determination of the antigens in serum, but any of them have potential for becoming lung cancer markers in the near future. Wolf (1978) has developed a preliminary radioimmunoassay for an antigen derived from pleural effusions but has been prevented from clinical evaluation of serum samples due to a non-specific inhibitor present in normal serum. Bell and Seetharam (1979) have described an endodermally derived antigen which is found in colorectal cancer as well as lung cancer of all types; they have also identified a neural crest derived antigen that appears specific for the oat cell type of lung cancer. Testing to date has been only with tissues and there has been no identification of either antigen in the circulation. Gennings *et al.* (1979) have discovered an antigen in extracts of all types of lung cancer so far examined as well as fetal lung; normal lung extracts have demonstrated no antigenic activity at concentrations eight times that of tumors. Attempts to develop a radioimmunoassay have been frustrated with various technical problems that have prevented measurements of the antigen in the circulation of patients with lung cancer and appropriate control conditions.

A group at the University of Marburg (Gropp *et al.*, 1979) have produced goat antisera to human lung cancer which, after absorption, still reacted with extracts of squamous, large cell and adenocarcinoma, but failed to react with

extracts of oat cell carcinoma, normal tissues or plasma proteins. An assay sufficiently sensitive for detection of circulating antigen has not been devised. Veltri
et al. (1980) have characterised a membrane antigen associated with 80% of
human lung cancers which is not present in normal or fetal tissues or in other
types of cancer. They have also not yet developed an assay for measuring circulating antigen. Ibrahim *et al.* (1980) have developed antiserum to human lung
cancer tissue which shares cross-reactivity with a number of epidermoid cancers,
but reacts only with serum from patients with lung cancer and not with the
serum of normal individuals or those patients with other types of cancer. Testing
of additional sera and developement of a quantitative assay will be necessary for
further evaluation of this and the other lung tumor associated antigens described
above.

ONCOFETAL PROTEINS

Carcinoembryonic Antigen (CEA)

The antigen described by Gold and Freedman, CEA, associated with adenocarcinoma of the large bowel (Gold and Freedman, 1965a,b) has also been
demonstrated in association with carcinomas of other organ sites, including
lung cancer (Thomson *et al.*, 1969; LoGerfo *et al.*, 1971; Reynoso *et al.*, 1972;
Vincent and Chu, 1973; Concannon *et al.*, 1974), of all histologic types (Plow
and Edgington, 1979). The frequency of elevated serum CEA appears to increase
with increasing extent of disease (Vincent *et al.*, 1975) and also appears greater
in association with adenocarcinoma and large cell undifferentiated than with
squamous cell and small cell types (Plow and Edgington, 1979). The correlation
of CEA elevation with the size of tumor cannot be used in an absolute sense
since there are many exceptions found in clinical experience (Vincent *et al.*, 1975).

Measurement of serum CEA as a screening technique for the early detection
of lung cancer is not worthwhile for the same reasons as for colorectal cancer:
a high proportion of patients with small or "early" cancers have normal CEA
(Vincent *et al.*, 1975). There is the further problem that about 10-20% of patients
with chronic obstructive pulmonary disease have a rise in serum CEA (LoGerfo
et al., 1971; Reynoso *et al.*, 1972), as do about 10% of chronic smokers (Hansen
et al., 1974; Cullen *et al.*, 1976; Alexander *et al.*, 1976) which appears to be
reversible with cessation of smoking.

Serum CEA may be useful in the evaluation of patients with lung cancer
since it is usually higher in those with metastic disease. Some studies have shown
that patients with serum CEA above a certain level have shorter survival after
resection of the tumor than those with CEA below that level (Concannon *et al.*,
1978; Dent and McCulloch, 1979). Since the CEA value in serum is the result
of not only the size of the tumor or number of cells, but also of the rates of
synthesis and degradation, it would seem unwise to rely entirely on the CEA
value as a prognostic indicator.

The clearest value of serum CEA in patients with lung cancer is for monitoring the effectiveness of therapy (Vincent and Chu, 1973; Vincent *et al.*, 1975;

Ford *et al.,* 1979) in those patients for whom CEA is an appropriate marker; initially to evaluate the completeness of surgical resection, later to anticipate the presence of recurrent tumor before it is clinically apparent and to determine the efficacy of adjuvant therapy. The studies of Vincent *et al.* (1979) have demonstrated that serial CEA determinations are not only helpful in judging the completeness of surgery but can also lead to repeated surgery where a postoperative progressive CEA elevation may be the only sign of recurrent cancer.

Recently, the serial study of patients with small cell carcinoma during therapy has shown a remarkable correlation between changes in serum CEA and response to therapy and a value greater than 10 ng/ml was frequently an indication of extrathoracic spread of the disease (Waalkes *et al.,* 1980; Goslin *et al.,* 1980).

α-Fetoprotein (AFP)

Despite the availability of sensitive radioimmunoassay methods capable of clearly measuring the normal serum AFP, there have been almost no reports of elevated values in association with primary lung cancer. In a series of 150 patients with lung cancer of all histologic types, ten had elevated serum AFP (Waldmann and McIntire, 1974) but only one had the degree of elevation which strongly suggested synthesis by the tumor (125,000 ng/ml). The nine other elevations of AFP were quite modest and could conceivably have been related to liver dysfunction. Other studies have indicated that an occasional patient with lung cancer may have elevated serum AFP (Corlin and Tompkins, 1972). At this time no studies have actually demonstrated synthesis of AFP by lung cancer cells.

It would appear that the oncofetal protein, AFP, may occasionally be a marker for lung cancer, but not with sufficient frequency to warrant routine serum AFP determinations on all patients with lung cancer.

Pancreatic Oncofetal Antigen (POA)

The POA, which was discovered by an antiserum developed against human fetal pancreas tissue (Banwo *et al.,* 1974), is now known to be elevated in the sera of many patients with pancreatic cancer and also in patients with other cancers, including lung cancer (Gelder *et al.,* 1979). Almost one-quarter of 53 patients with bronchogenic carcinoma had elevated serum POA and 15% were significant elevations, while only one of 12 patients with benign lung disease had an elevation of POA and this was not a significant elevation. The levels of POA found in lung cancer sera were comparable to those found in pancreatic cancer. Several patients were followed serially and POA was found to decrease following successful therapy and to increase as tumor mass grew (Gelder *et al.,* 1979).

POA has been proven antigenically distinct from CEA and AFP (Gelder *et al.,* 1979). Further work is now needed to determine the patterns of correlation with these two other oncofetal antigens. POA might prove helpful as a confirmation of CEA or as a marker to monitor tumor changes in patients who do not have elevated CEA.

SERUM PROTEINS

Immunoglobulins (Ig)

The synthesis and secretion of homogeneous immunoglobulins or their subunits is associated with most plasma cell neoplasma and by some tumors of the
B-lymphocyte such as lymphomas and chronic lymphocytic leukemia. Only
rarely has monoclonal immunoglobulin production been associated with a primary
lung cancer. Various reports have indicated a general change in serum immunoglobulins (Hughes, 1971; Zermoski et al., 1975; Nash, 1979; Plesnicar and Rudolf,
1979) or even a change for a specific class of immunoglobulins (Krant et al.,
1968; Mandel et al., 1973; LoGerfo and McLanahan, 1976), usually IgA.

In a study of patients suspected of having primary lung cancer where sera
were obtained before the confirmatory work-up, the mean serum IgA was significantly elevated over control values for all histological types of lung cancer, two-
thirds were more than 2 standard deviations above the normal mean value (Nash
et al., 1980). Interestingly, serum IgM was significantly decreased in these same
early lung cancer patients, indicating that this determination might also be useful
in aiding early detection. The pattern of simultaneously elevated IgA and depressed IgM could provide greater specificity than either protein by itself.

A study of 57 patients with non-metastatic epidermoid carcinoma of the
lung showed that all (100%) of those that lived longer than the mean survival
time had elevated serum IgA, and of those patients with elevated IgA over two-
thirds lived longer than the mean survival time (Plesnicar and Rudolf, 1979).
In the same study, 38 patients with small cell anaplastic carcinoma, 15 who
lived longer than the mean survival almost all had elevation of either serum
IgG or IgM, and the corrolary demonstration was, that the majority of patients
with either elevated IgG or IgM lived longer than the mean survival time (Plesnicar
and Rudolf, 1979). Serial studies would be helpful to show any correlation
between change in Ig levels and change in tumor size.

Ferritin

Ferritin, found in normal tissues and serum is iron containing protein that
has been found elevated in many tumor tissues and in the serum of patients
with various tumors (Marcus et al., 1979). There are over 15 different isomeric
forms of ferritin which are probably due to a number of changes in such things
as amino acid composition, subunit size, glycosylation, etc. (Marcus et al., 1979).
Organ specific isoferritin patterns have been recognized (Drysdale, 1970), and
a prevalence of acidic forms in fetal and tumor tissue was thought to be specific
for these conditions (Alpert et al., 1973) until it was recognised that several
normal adult tissues such as heart, kidney and placenta also had increased amounts
of acidic isoferritins (Drysdale and Singer, 1974).

Total serum ferritin, quantitated by various immunological assays has been
elevated in a high percentage of patients with lung cancer (Gropp et al., 1978;
Urushizaki et al., 1979; Ishitani et al., 1979; Maxim et al., 1980) and especially
in patients with stage I disease. There is also a preliminary report on the correlation of serum ferritin changes with change in lung tumor size during treatment
by either radiotherapy or chemotherapy (Urushizaki et al., 1979).

Despite certain antigenic differences between the acidic and basic forms of isoferritin, it has been difficult to develop specific immunoassays for each (Marcus *et al.,* 1979). With an assay reactive more for the acidic ferritins (Hazard *et al.,* 1977) it has been shown that the measurable serum ferritin level in patients with cancer is several times greater than when quantitated by an immunoassay for the basic ferritins (Hazard and Drysdale, 1977). This was specifically noted for lung cancer and indicates an area of necessary investigation to confirm the greater relative specificity of acidic isoferritins with lung cancer.

Ceruloplasmin

The quantitation of serum ceruloplasmin by immunoassay has indicated that 81% of 48 patients with lung cancer had elevated values (Linder, 1979b). While 55% of controls with benign lung disease also had elevated ceruloplasmin, the values were not as great as in the malignant disease patients. The level of ceruloplasmin was highly correlated with the stage of lung cancer and still was elevated in two-thirds of those patients with early or stage I disease (Linder, 1979b). Very preliminary data indicated that elevated serum ceruloplasmin levels reverted to normal when treatment was successful in providing remission.

In addition to quantitation as antigen, ceruloplasmin is also active as an oxidative enzyme involved in iron metabolism and serum can be quantitated specifically for the enzyme activity. The measurement of ceruloplasmin oxidase in human sera corroborates the findings of ceruloplasmin protein in that elevations are associated with lung cancer, greater in magnitude and incidence with increasing stage of disease (Linder, 1979a).

Since the synthesis of ceruloplasmin has not yet been demonstrated for tumor cells, it is most likely that the elevated serum levels reflect increased synthesis by the liver (Cohen *et al.,* 1979) as a response to tumor growth. However, the possibility that ceruloplasmin is responding simply as a non-specific acute phase reactant still needs to be ruled out by careful longitudinal studies covering a variety of stress situations in patients with lung cancer.

α-1-Antitrypsin (α1-AT)

The serum levels of α1-AT have been shown to be elevated in about two-thirds of the patients with primary lung cancer (Harris *et al.,* 1974; Micksche and Kokron, 1977) with the elevations evenly distributed among the various histological types of lung cancer (Nash *et al.,* 1980).

Due to the response of α1-AT as an acute phase reactant, it is crucial to develop data showing the degree to which α1-AT concentration correlates with change in tumor size and that it is independent of concurrent infection or other causes of increase in acute phase reactants.

β2-Microglobulin (β2-m)

The β2-m which is related to the immunoglobulin and histocompatibility locus A (HLA) molecules is elevated in the circulation of patients with impaired renal function and has also been shown to be elevated in many patients with neoplastic disease, including lung cancer (Kithier *et al.,* 1974).

In a study of β2-m levels in lung cancer, elevated values were found in 21% of 230 patients with confirmed lung cancer, but also elevated in 11% of 237 control patients with non-malignant pulmonary disease (Hallgren *et al.*, 1980). Elevations were found in both small cell and non-small cell carcinoma and appeared to increase with increase in tumor size. Unfortunately, there was no decrease in β2-m following surgical removal of the tumor (Hallgren *et al.*, 1980). Lung cancer patients with normal serum β2-m had a better prognosis than those with elevated levels.

Tissue Polypeptide Antigen (TPA)

The TPA, originally described by Bjorklund and colleagues (Bjorklund and Bjorklund, 1957; Bjorklund *et al.*, 1958), has been found in elevated amounts in sera from a majority of patients with cancer of various organ sites (including lung), but also in a high percentage of patients with benign disease, especially urinary tract infection (Holyoke and Chu, 1979).

Of 35 patients with lung cancer 80% had elevated serum TPA in a study by Manendez-Botet *et al.* (1978). Holyoke and Chu (1979) have noted that TPA and CEA were equally elevated in a study of 21 patients with bronchogenic carcinoma (57%) and that almost all elevations were coincidental. In patients with elevated TPA, the level fell after surgical resection of the tumor (Chu, pers. comm. 1980).

Further studies are needed to determine the accuracy of TPA in monitoring the effect of therapy and for the early detection of recurrent tumor. Studies should also be directed at the coincidence of CEA and TPA to see if this improves the reliability of both tests.

Circulating Immune Complexes (CIC)

The majority of studies of immune complexes in patients with cancer have dealt with the disadvantages and advantages of the complexes at the surface of malignant and normal cells and the filtration from the circulation by various organs (reviewed by Theofilopoulos and Dixon, 1979).

The detection and quantitation of CIC can be performed by several different methodologies which may give dissimilar results and which, at the present time, are not well understood. The methods and their interpretation are discussed by Theofilopoulos and Dixon (1979). It is accepted that the measurement of immune complexes is a non-specific assay and is, therefore, a non-specific cancer test since the antigen-antibody interaction can be the result of many different factors, some of which may be tumor related or even tumor specific. Identification of the component parts of the immune complexes requires further immunochemical determination. The diffferent assays for CIC may detect different components so that ideally a survey of lung cancer patients would utilise more than one assay.

Using the Raji cell assay, sera from 26% of 51 patients with lung cancer had elevated CIC, but this result was not significantly different from the 176 healthy controls (Theofilopoulos and Dixon, 1979). The C1q binding assay for CIC has been used in several studies and also showed elevations in lung cancer, but similar elevations in patients with benign lung disease (Rossen *et al.*, 1977; Baldwin *et al.*, 1979; Dent *et al.*, 1979). The C1q assay may have predictive value in that lung cancer patients with elevated CIC levels in the post-operative period have significantly shorter median survival (Dent, 1980).

Other Serum Proteins

Concentration of serum haptoglobulin, orosomucoid and C-reactive protein were measured by immunoassays in patients with lung cancer before and after radical resection of the primary tumor. The protein values correlated well with increasing tumor size; in those patients with higher than expected protein levels there was a significantly shorter survival time which was interpreted as an indication that these proteins might be indicators of undetected metastases (Bradwell *et al.*, 1979).

ENZYMES

Placental Alkaline Phosphatase

The Regan isoenzyme, a placental-type alkaline phosphatase, was originally detected in bronchogenic carcinoma (Fishman *et al.*, 1968), but has been demonstrated to be elevated in many different forms of cancer (Stolbach *et al.*, 1969). This isoenzyme is elevated in 6–14% of patients with lung cancer and the majority of these are minimal elevations. Placental alkaline phosphate might yet be useful in a battery of tests where it may corroborate other results despite the fact that by itself it has not yet proven to be of great value.

5′-Nucleotide Phosphodiesterase Isozyme-V (5′-NPD-V)

This enzyme appears to be more specific for liver metastases from any primary tumor site than it is for any certain organ cancer. Nevertheless, in sera of 36 lung cancer patients over 60% were positive for 5′-NPD-V while 14/40 (35%) of heavy smokers has positive sera (Tsou *et al.*, 1980). The positives in lung cancer sera were found in all histological types but were more frequent in patients with liver metastases (87%) than in patients without (38%).

This represents another assay where quantitative capability will allow easier comparison of serial samples. If there is no correlation with changes in the tumor, the enzyme may simply be an aid in confirming metastases to the liver.

Amylase

Case reports of elevated serum amylase in patients with lung cancer have appeared sporadically for almost three decades (Weiss *et al.*, 1951; McGeachin and Adams, 1957; Ende, 1961; Ammann *et al.*, 1973; Yokoyama *et al.*, 1977). The histological type most frequently associated with this condition is adenocarcinoma and there is evidence that the isoenzyme form is chemically different from that produced by the normal pancreas or salivary gland (Yokoyama *et al.*, 1977).

In a study of the frequency of elevated serum amylase and characterisation of the enzyme, it was found that the heat labile form of amylase occurred in all patients with primary lung cancer but not in those with benign lung disease or in healthy controls. The heat labile form accounted for 12–70% of the total serum amylase; 55% of the lung cancer patients had elevated levels of total amylase

(Sirsat *et al.*, 1979). There was a rapid fall in the heat labile amylase of three patients following surgical resection of their tumor.

Further studies are needed to define the correlation of the heat labile isozyme of amylase with the histology and stage of cancer. An immunoassay specific for this form would facilitate such studies.

Creatine Kinase BB

The isoenzyme CK–BB has been found elevated in the serum of various patients with adenocarcinoma of different organ sites (Hoag *et al.*, 1978) and this includes 40% of 32 patients with lung cancer while none of the 56 patients with non-malignant disease had elevated isoenzyme (Paris *et al.*, 1980). Serum CK–BB has also been elevated in patients with small cell carcinoma of the lung (Coolen, 1976).

With the development of a sensitive radioimmunoassay for CK–BB (Silverman *et al.*, 1979) it is now possible to determine the frequency in a larger series of patients with lung cancer and to test for a correlation with change in clinical status. The definite advantage of the immunoassay is that it no longer requires the isoenzyme to retain biological activity to enable identification and quantitation; even native, inactive forms (such as pro-enzyme, if they exist, might be measurable as a useful tumor marker (Silverman *et al.*, 1979).

Galactosyltransferase

Recently Podolsky *et al.* (1978) have described an electrophoretic variant of galactosyltransferase that appeared to be elevated in the sera of many patients with a variety of neoplasms which included 65% of 20 patients with broncho-genic carcinoma. This isoenzyme, called galactosyltransferase II, has also been shown to correlate with progression of malignant disease and is rarely found in benign disease control sera. Further work in other laboratories is needed to confirm these findings.

Sialytransferase

In a careful study of a large number of patients with cancer, serum elevations of sialyltransferase activity was found in the majority of patients with lung cancer (Henderson and Kessel, 1977). There was evidence that declining levels of sialyltransferase correlated with response to therapy and also that the elevations were more frequent in patients with liver metastases.

OTHER SUBSTANCES

Tennessee Antigen (TA)

This tumor associated antigen has been studied exclusively by a single group. While TA has some similarities to CEA it is antigenically distinctive from CEA and several other known tumor associated antigens, but has not been definitively compared with many others (Jordan *et al.*, 1979).

Positive TA assays have been reported in the sera of two-thirds of patients with lung cancer and one-third of patients with benign lung disease (Potter *et al.,* 1979). Improvement in the methods for quantitation of TA may be helpful in discriminating benign from malignant disease. Serial studies to demonstrate TA correlation with change in tumor size would be useful in deciding whether this glycoprotein will be of value in the management of therapy in patients with lung cancer.

Carbohydrate Markers

For almost 10 years there have been scattered reports of increased sialic acid in the serum of patients with various types of malignant disease, including lung cancer (Lipton *et al.,* 1979). Recently the measurement of serum sialic acid has been studied in a serial fashion during periods of therapy and remission and was shown to correlate with both disease progression and the onset of recurrent tumor (Chen *et al.,* 1979). The extraction and measurement of lipid associated sialic acid had indicated that a very high percentage of patients with lung cancer have values above the controls (Hirshaut, 1981, pers. comm.).

The careful measurement of serum fucose by gas–liquid chromatography has demonstrated a close correlation with the extent of disease (Gehrke *et al.,* 1979). Patients with lung cancer whose sera were obtained after successful treatment while they were in clinical remission were found to have fucose values in the normal range (13/16). When sera were obtained before therapy or after recurrent tumor had appeared, the majority of patients had elevated fucose.

Further studies are obviously essential to evaluate the clinical usefulness of serum carbohydrates in the management of lung cancer.

Nucleosides and Bases

The pioneering work of Borek, Gehrke and Waalkes in demonstrating abnormalities in urinary excretion of nucleosides and bases has indicated a very real potential for use as a guide to monitoring therapy. Analysis of sera from 16 patients with lung cancer by high performance liquid chromatography identified profiles that were significantly different from those of normal controls (Hartwick *et al.,* 1979). Further studies are necessary to identify all peaks and ascertain whether any of the abnormalities may be helpful for early diagnosis or if this technique will have its greatest utility in monitoring therapy.

REFERENCES

Alexander, J. C., Silverman, N. A. and Chretien, P. B. (1976). *Journal of American Medical Association* **235**, 1975.
Alpert, E., Coston, R. L. and Drysdale, J. W. (1973). *Nature* **242**, 194.
Ammann, R. W., Berk, J. E., Fridhandler, L., Ueda, M. and Wegmann, W. (1973). *Annals of Internal Medicine* **78**, 521.
Baldwin, R. W., Pimm, M. V., Illes, P. B. and Webb, R. J. (1979). *In* "Compendium of Assays for Immunodiagnosis of Cancer" (R. B. Herberman, Eds.), p. 325. Elsevier/North Holland, New York.
Banwo, O., Versey, J. and Hobbs, J. R. (1974). *Lancet* **1**, 643.

Bell, C. E., Jr and Seetharam, S. (1979). *Cancer* **44**, 13.

Bjorklund, B. and Bjorklund, V. (1957). *International Archives of Allergy and Applied Immunology* **10**, 153.

Bjorklund, B., Lundblad, G. and Bjorklund, V. (1958). *International Archives of Allergy and Applied Immunology* **12**, 241.

Braatz, J. A., McIntire, K. R., Princler, G. L., Kortright, K. H. and Herberman, R. B. (1978). *Journal of the National Cancer Institute* **61**, 1035.

Braatz, J. A., Scharge, T. R., Princler, G. L. and McIntire, K. R. (1981). (Submitted for publication.)

Bradwell, A. R., Burnett, D., Newman, C. E. and Ford, C. H. (1979). *Protides of the Biological Fluids Colloquium* **27**, 327.

Chen, Y. Q., Zhou, Y. Q. and Yu, S. Y. (1979). *Zhonghua Zhongliu Zazhi* **1**, 29.

Cohen, D. I., Illowsky, B. and Linder, M. C. (1979). *American Journal of Physiology* **236**, E309.

Concannon, J. P., Dalbow, M. H., Liebler, G. A., Blake, K. E., Weil, C. S. and Cooper, J. W. (1974). *Cancer* **34**, 184.

Concannon, J. P., Dalbow, M. H., Hodsson, S. E., Headlings, J. J., Markopoulos, E., Mitchell, J., Cushins, W. J. and Liebler, G. A. (1978). *Cancer* **42**, 1477.

Coolen, R. B. (1976). *Clinical Chemistry* **22**, 1174.

Corlin, R. F. and Tompkins, R. K. (1972). *Digestive Diseases* **17**, 553.

Cullen, K. J., Stevens, D. P., Frost, M. A. and Mackay, I. R. (1976). *Australian and New Zealand Journal of Medicine* **6**, 279.

DeLellis, R. A., Sternberger, L. A., Mann, R. B., Banks, P. M. and Nakane, P. K. (1979). *American Journal of Clinical Pathology* **71**, 483.

Dent, P. B. (1980). *Cancer* **45**, 130.

Dent, P. B. and McCulloch, P. B. (1979). *In* "Compendium of Assays for Immunodiagnosis of Human Cancer" (R. B. Herberman, Ed.) p. 273. Elsevier/North Holland, New York.

Dent, P. B., McCulloch, P. B., Louis, J. A. and Cerottini, J.-C. (1979). *In* "Compendium of Assays for Immunodiagnosis of Cancer" (R. B. Herberman, Ed.), p. 329. Elsevier/North Holland, New York.

Drysdale, J. W. (1970). *Biochimica et Biophysica Acta* **207**, 256.

Drysdale, J. W. and Singer, R. M. (1974). *Cancer Research* **34**, 3352.

Ende, N. (1961). *Cancer* **14**, 1109.

Fishman, W. H., Inglis, N. R., Stolbach, L. L. and Krant, M. J. (1968). *Cancer Research* **28**, 150.

Ford, C. H., Newman, C. E., and Anderson, I. G. (1979). *In* "Carcino-Embryonic Proteins" (F. -G. Lehmann, Ed.), Vol. 2, 169. Elsevier/North Holland, Amsterdam.

Gaffar, S. A., Princler, G. L., McIntire, K. R. and Braatz, J. A. (1980). *Journal of Biological Chemistry* **255**, 8334.

Gehrke, C. W., Waalkes, T. P., Borek, E., Swartz, W. F., Cole, T. F., Kuo, K. C., Abeloff, M., Ettinger, D. S., Rosenshein, N. and Young, R. C. (1979). *Journal of Chromatography* **162**, 507.

Gelder, F. B., Reese, C., Moossa, A. R. and Hunter, R. L. (1979). *In* "Immunodiagnosis of Cancer" (R. B. Herberman and K. R. McIntire, Eds), p. 357. Marcel Dekker, Inc. New York.

Gennings, J. N., Leake, B. A. and Bagshawe, K. D. (1979). *In* "Carcino-Embryonic Proteins" (F. G. Lehmann, Ed.), Vol. II, 553. Elsevier/North Holland, Amsterdam.

Gold, P. and Freedman, S. O. (1965a). *Journal of Experimental Medicine* **121**, 439.

Gold, P. and Freedman, S. O. (1965b). *Journal of Experimental Medicine* **122**, 467.

Goldenberg, D. M., DeLand, F., Kim, E., Bennett, S., Primus, F. J., Van Nagell, J. R., Jr, Estes, N., DeSimone, P. and Rayburn, P. (1978). *New England Journal of Medicine* **298**, 1384.

Goslin, R. H., Skarin, A. T., MacIntyre, J. and Zamcheck, N. (1981). *Journal of the American Medical Association* **246**, 2173.

Gropp, C., Havemann, K. and Lehmann, F. G. (1978). *Cancer* **42**, 2802.

Gropp, C., Havemann, K. and Preisser, P. (1979). *In* "Carcino-Embryonic Proteins: Chemistry, Biology, Clinical Applications" (F. G. Lehmann, Ed.), p. 547. Elsevier/North Holland, Amsterdam.

Hallgren, R., Nou, E. and Lundquist, G. (1980). *Cancer* **45**, 780.

Hansen, H. J., Snyder, L. J., Miller, E., Vandervoorde, J. P., Miller, O. N., Hines, L. R. and Burns, J. J. (1974). *Journal of Human Pathology* **5**, 139.

Harris, C. C., Primack, A. and Cohen, M. H. (1974). *Cancer* **34**, 280.

Hartwick, R. A., Krstulovic, A. M. and Brown, P. R. (1979). *Journal of Chromatography* **186**, 659.

Henderson, M. and Kessel, D. (1977). *Cancer* **39**, 1129.

Hazard, J. T. and Drysdale, J. W. (1977). *Nature* **265**, 755.

Hazard, J. T., Yokota, M., Arosio, P. and Drysdale, J. W. (1977). *Blood* **49**, 139.

Hoag, G. N., Franks, C. R. and DeCoteau, W. E. (1978). *Clinical Chemistry* **24**, 1654.

Holyoke, D. and Chu, T. M. (1979). *In* "Immunodiagnosis of Cancer" (R. B. Herberman and K. R. McIntire, Eds), p. 513. Marcel Dekker, Inc. New York.

Hughes, N. R. (1971). *Journal of the National Cancer Institute* **46**, 1015.

Ibrahim, A. N., Rawlins, D., Abdelal, A., Azhar, A., Swammathan, V., Mansour, K. and Nahmias, A. (1980). *Cellular and Molecular Biology* **26**, 327.

Ishitani, K., Niitsu, Y., Watanabe, N., Koseki, J., Oikawa, J., Kadono, Y., Ishii, T., Goto, Y., Onodera, Y. and Urushizaki, I. (1979). *In* "Carcino–Embryonic Proteins" (F. -G. Lehmann, Ed.), Vol. I, 279. Elsevier/North Holland, Amsterdam.

Jordan, T. A., Potter, T. P., Jordan, J. D., Johnston, K. and Lasater, H. A. (1979). *Protides of the Biological Fluids Colloquium* **27**, 95.

Katoh, Y., Stoner, G. D., McIntire, K. R., Hill, T. A., Anthony, R., McDowell, E. M., Trump, B. F. and Harris, C. C. (1979). *Journal of the National Cancer Institute* **62**, 1177.

Kelly, B. S. and Levy, J. G. (1977). *British Journal of Cancer* **35**, 828.

Kelly, B. S. and Levy, J. G. (1980). *British Journal of Cancer* **41**, 388.

Kithier, K., Cejka, J., Belamaric, J., Al–Sarraf, M., Peterson, W. D. Jr, Vaitkevicius, V. K. and Poulik, M. D. (1974). *Clinica Chimica Acta* **52**, 293.

Krant, M. J., Manskopf, G., Brandrup, C. S. and Madoff, M. A. (1968). *Cancer* **21**, 623.

Linder, M. C. (1979a). *In* "Compendium of Assays for Immunodiagnosis of Human Cancer" (R. B. Herberman, Ed.), p. 305. Elsevier/North Holland, New York.

Linder, M. C. (1979b). *In* "Compendium of Assays for Immunodiagnosis of Human Cancer" (R. B. Herberman, Ed.), p. 311. Elsevier/North Holland, New York.

Lipton, A., Harvey, H. A., Delong, S., Allegra, J., White, D., Allegra, M. and Davidson, E. A. (1979). *Cancer* **43**, 1766.

LoGerfo, P. and McLanahan, J. (1976). *Journal of Surgical Research* **20**, 481.

LoGerfo, P., Krupey, J. and Hansen, H. J. (1971). *New England Journal of Medicine* **285**, 481.

Mandel, M. A., Dvorak, K. and DeCosse, J. J. (1973). *Cancer* **31**, 1408.

Manendez–Botet, C. V., Oettgen, H. F., Pinsky, C. M. and Schwartz, M. F. (1978). *Clinical Chemistry* **24**, 868.

Marcus, D. M., Zinberg, N. and Listowsky, I. (1979). *In* "Immunodiagnosis of Cancer" (R. B. Herberman and K. R. McIntire, Eds), p. 473. Marcel Dekker, Inc. New York.

Maxim, P. E., Prather, J. R. and Veltri, R. W. (1980). *Federation Proceedings* **39** (3, part 1), 413.

McGeachin, R. L. and Adams, M. R. (1957). *Cancer* **10**, 497.

Micksche, M. and Kokron, O. (1977). *Oesterreichische Zeitschrift fur Onkologie* **3**, 116.

Nash, D. R. (1979). *Annals of Clinical Research* **11**, 78.

Nash, D. R., McLarty, J. W. and Fortson, N. G. (1980). *Journal of the National Cancer Institute* **64**, 721.

Paris, M., Leclerc, P., Lebeau, B., Rochemaure, J. and Lederc, M. (1980). *Semaine des Hôpitaux de Paris* **56**, 329.

Plesnicar, S. and Rudolf, Z. (1979). *Neoplasma* **26**, 721.

Plow, E. F. and Edgington, T. S. (1979). *In* "Immunodiagnosis of Cancer" (R. B. Herberman and K. R. McIntire, Eds), p. 181. Marcel Dekker, Inc., New York.

Podolsky, D. K., Weiser, M. M., Isselbacher, K. J. and Cohen, A. (1978). *New England Journal of Medicine* **299**, 703.

Potter, T. P., Jr, Jordan, J. D. and Jordan, T. A. (1979). *In* "Compendium of Assays for Immunodiagnosis of Human Cancer" (R. B. Herberman, Ed.), p. 217. Elsevier/North Holland New York.

Reynoso, G., Chu, T. M., Holyoke, D., Chen, E., Nemoto, T., Wang, J. J., Chuang, J., Guinan, P. and Murphy, G. (1972). *Journal of the American Medical Association* **220**, 361.

Rossen, R. D., Reisberg, M. A., Hersh, E. M. and Gutterman, J. U. (1977). *Journal of the National Cancer Institute* **58**, 1205.

Silverman, L. M., Dermer, G. B., Zweig, M. H., Van Steirteghem, A. C. and Tokes, Z. A. (1979). *Clinical Chemistry* **25**, 1432.

Sirsat, A. V., Talavdekar, R. V., Jain, A. K. and Vyas, J. J. (1979). *Indian Journal of Cancer* **16**, 37.

Stolbach, L. L., Krant, J. J. and Fishman, W. H. (1969). *New England Journal of Medicine* **281**, 757.

Theofilopoulos, A. N. (1979). *In* "Compendium of Assays for Immunodiagnosis of Human Cancer" (R. B. Herberman, Ed.), p. 113. Elsevier/North Holland, New York.

Thomson, D. M. P., Krupey, J., Freedman, S. O. and Gold, P. (1969). *Proceedings of the National Academy of Science* **64**, 161.

Tsou, K. C., Lo, K. W., Herberman, R. B., Schutt, A. J. and Go, V. L. (1980). *Journal of Clinical Hematology and Oncology* **10**, 1.

Urushizaki, I., Yoshiro, N. and Ishitani, K. (1979). *In* "Compendium of Assays for Immunodiagnosis of Human Cancer" (R. B. Herberman, Ed.), p. 199. Elsevier/North Holland, New York.

Veltri, R. W., Maxim, P. E. and Boehlecke, J. M. (1980). *British Journal of Cancer* **41**, 705.

Vincent, R. G. and Chu, T. M. (1973). *Journal of Thoracic and Cardiovascular Surgery* **66**, 320.

Vincent, R. G., Chu, T. M., Fergen, T. B. and Ostrander, M. (1975). *Cancer* **36**, 2069.

Vincent, R. G., Chu, T. M., Lane, W. W., Gutierrez, A. C., Stegemann, P. J. and Madajewicz, S. (1979). *In* "Lung Cancer: Progress in Therapeutic Research" (F. Muggia and M. Rozencweig, Eds), p. 191. Raven Press, New York.

Waalkes, T. P., Abeloff, M. D., Woo, K. B., Ettinger, D. S., Ruddon, R. W. and Aldenderfer, P. (1980). *Cancer Research* **40**, 4420.
Waldmann, T. A. and McIntire, K. R. (1974). *Cancer* **34**, 1510.
Weiss, J. F., Mikulski, S. M. and Chretien, P. B. (1979). *In* "Lung Cancer: Progress in Therapeutic Research" (F. M. Muggia and M. Rozenweig, Eds), p. 227. Raven Press, New York.
Wolf, A. (1978). *British Journal of Cancer* **36**, 1046.
Yokoyama, M., Natsuizaka, T., Ishii, Y., Onshima, S., Kasagi, A. and Tateno, S. (1977). *Cancer* **40**, 766.
Zeromski, J., Gorny, M. K., Wruk, M. and Sapula, J. (1975). *International Archives of Allergy and Applied Immunology* **49**, 548.

FERRITIN IN DIAGNOSIS OF LUNG CANCER

I. Urushizaki and Y. Niitsu

*Department of Internal Medicine, Sapporo Medical College,
Sapporo, Japan*

INTRODUCTION

Biochemical abnormalities caused by the release of tumour products in cancer patients can be valuable in assisting tumour detection and staging (Neville and Cooper, 1976). Carcinoembryonic antigen (CEA) has been shown to be of value in this respect in colorectal carcinoma and α-foetoprotein in primary hepato-cellular carcinoma. The situation in lung cancer is less clear and, although workers have attempted to use certain markers to stage this malignancy, the results have not been conclusive (Vincent and Chu, 1978).

Ferritin is an iron storage protein with a molecular weight of approximately 450,000 daltons; it is apparently composed of a number of subunits arranged in the form of a spherical shell around the iron oxide core (Crichton, 1971). Recently, a tumour specific component of ferritin with rapid electrophoretic mobility or an acidic isoelectric point has been reported in various kinds of tumour (Alpert *et al.*, 1973a). In addition, some carcino-foetal proteins in the serum, α_2 H (Buffe *et al.*, 1968) and βFP (Alpert *et al.*, 1973b) were identified as belonging to the ferritin class of proteins. For the detection of circulating ferritin, which, under normal conditions, is present in a very small amounts, a sensitivie immunoradiometric assay has been recently employed (Addison *et al.*, 1972). Elevated levels of ferritin in many tumours and sera of tumour bearing indivi-duals have stimulated interest in ferritin as a potential tumour marker. Elevated serum ferritin levels were described in hepatoma, pancreatic carcinoma, breast

Serono Symposium No. 46, Markers for Diagnosis and Monitoring of Human Cancer, edited by M. I. Colnaghi, G. L. Buraggi and M. Ghione, 1982. Academic Press, London and New York.

cancer and acute leukaemia. So far, there have been few reports on patients with lung cancer (Gropp *et al.*, 1978; Urushizaki *et al.*, 1979).

It is the purpose of this study to define the usefulness of the determination of serum ferritin for the detection of lung cancer. Furthermore, the role of this serum protein for the therapeutic monitoring of lung cancer is discussed.

PATIENTS AND METHODS

Blood samples were drawn from patients with histologically confirmed lung cancer at 3-week intervals. All patients had a measurable lesion on their chest by X-ray examination. Prior to therapy the extent of disease was determined by physical examination, liver chemistries, chest and bone roentgenograms, broncho-graphy and bronchofiberscopy. Roentogenograms, blood and liver chemistries were repeated at intervals during therapy. Normal sera and sera obtained from non-malignant lung diseases, including tuberculosis, bronchitis, sarcoidosis, asthma, bronchiectasis, pneumonia and benign tumours, were used as controls. One-hundred-and-forty-three samples of blind serum, which were sent from the NIH, were also measured to serum ferritin and CEA assays.

Ferritin was isolated from human liver, and an immunoradiometric assay for serum ferritin, using a paper disc as a solid phase material, was performed (Niitsu *et al.*, 1975). The SPAC ferritin kit by radioimmunometric assay was also used (Diichi RI, Tokyo). Assay for CEA was carried out with the CEA Roche kit (Roche, Nutley, USA).

Isolated ferritins from human liver, heart and nude mouse liver were studied by polyacrylamide gel electrophoresis and gel electrofocusing, as described by Urushizaki *et al.* (1973). Antisera against human liver ferritin or mouse liver ferritin were raised in albino rabbit by the method of Marcus and Zinberg (1975). Guinea-pigs were immunized with human heart ferritin by multiple intracutaneous injections of antigen with complete Freund's adjuvant in the back and footpads. Immunoradiometric assays for human and mouse ferritins were carried out according to the method of Watanabe *et al.* (1979). BALB/c nu/nu mice were maintained under SPF conditions inside a vinyl isolator. Specimens of human cancer were resected and two cell lines of oat cell cancer and adenocarcinoma were cultivated and inoculated subcutaneously into nude mice. Nude mice were sacrificed when the tumour grew bigger than the size of the mouse's head and sera were collected for the measurement of ferritin concentration.

RESULTS

Usefulness of the Serum Ferritin Assay in Lung Cancer

Serum Ferritin Concentration in Lung Diseases
The clinical implication of measuring ferritin in the serum has been recently studied by many investigators. An important and well accepted finding is that serum ferritin levels directly reflect the size of mobilizable iron stores in normal subjects as well as in patients with an iron overload or iron deficiency, and,

therefore, its assay provides useful information about the iron status in certain diseases (Walters *et al.*, 1973; Jacobs and Worwood, 1975).

Another possible value of the serum ferritin assay lies in its empirical use for cancer immunodiagnosis (Niitsu *et al.*, 1975; Hazard *et al.*, 1977), despite the fact that the mechanism responsible for the increase in serum ferritin levels in cancer is still uncertain.

Serum ferritin concentration in normal subjects ranged between 10 and approximately 200 ng/ml, with a greater mean concentration in males than in females. In various types of lung diseases elevated levels of serum ferritin were observed in 64.8% (35/54) of patients with lung cancer before any treatment and in 15% of smokers. Serum ferritin levels were almost within the normal range in benign lung diseases including tuberculosis, bronchitis, asthma, bronchiectasis, sarcoidosis, pneumonia and benign tumours (Fig. 1 and Table I).

The importance of serological assay for cancer would be to make a differential diagnosis of malignancies from suspicious benign diseases or to determine the organ site of malignancy by specific markers. Although the determination of

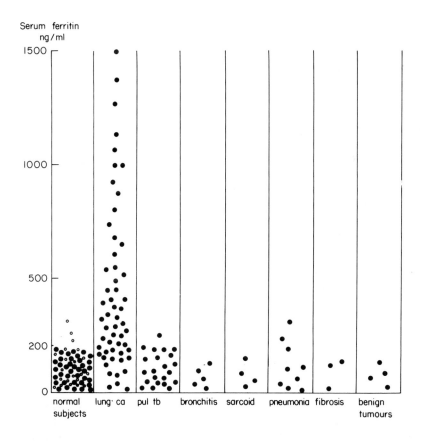

Fig. 1. Serum ferritin concentrations in various lung diseases. (0 = smoker.)

Table I. Usefulness of serum ferritin assay for initial diagnosis of lung cancer.

	No. of individuals	% Elevated (cut-off level 200 ng/ml)
Lung cancer	54	64.8
Benign lung disease[a]	45	4.4
Normal subjects		
Smokers	20	15.0
Non-smokers	38	0

[a] Includes patients with tuberculosis, bronchitis, sarcoidosis, bronchiectasis, pneumonia, fibrosis and benign tumours.

serum ferritin is not specific for the tumour marker of lung cancer, a high incidence of elevated ferritin levels in patients with lung cancer, and a markedly low probability of false positives in other lung diseases, strongly indicate the usefulness of ferritin assay in a differential diagnosis of a suspicious lung lesion.

Usefulness of Serum Ferritin Assay for Initial Staging
The relationship between serum ferritin levels and the stage of lung cancer indicated that there was no apparent correlation between serum ferritin levels and the stage of the disease (Table II). The highest incidence of elevated levels was observed in patients with stage 1. Moreover, in lung cancer the elevation of serum ferritin was neither related to tumour size, as determined by X-ray examination, nor to any particular histological type of tumours.

Table II. Usefulness of serum ferritin assay for initial staging of lung cancer.

Stage	No. of patients	Ferritin concentration[a] Mean + SD (ng/ml)	% Elevated[b] (cut-off level 200 ng/ml)
I	10	645.5 + 524.6	81.0
II	8	472.0 + 463.4	54.0
III	36	487.2 + 532.0	57.1

[a] Time assay performed in relation to pre-treatment.
[b] No significant difference was observed among the various histological types of lung cancer: squamous, adeno, small cell, large cell, alveolar and anaplastic.

The primary purpose in using serodiagnostic tools in cancer is, needless to say, early detection of malignancies. Although, at present, it is not definite that the ferritin assay is of value in detection of early lung cancer, the fact that an elevation of serum ferritin levels occurs in stage 1 lung cancer and that serum ferritin levels of normal subjects never exceed the certain limit (200 ng/ml), suggests that this assay is of some use in detecting lung cancer.

Usefulness of Serum Ferritin Assay for Prognosis
The value of the serum ferritin assay for evaluation of prognosis was examined. The serum ferritin concentration found at the time of diagnosis in patients who

Table III. Usefulness of serum ferritin assay for the prediction of prognosis of lung cancer.

4 months after assay	No. of patients	Ferritin concentration Mean + SD (ng/ml)	% Elevated (cut-off level 200 ng/ml)
Survived	11	433.2 + 561.6	45.4
Dead	24	612.4 + 551.3	65.2

survived for longer than 4 months was slightly lower than in those who died (Table III). However, these small difference do not seem to be indicative of a prediction of prognosis. There was no definitive relationship between serum ferritin concentration and survival time in lung cancer (Table IV).

As for the assessment of prognosis of lung cancer, no promising evidence was observed in our present studies.

Table IV. Relationship between serum ferritin concentration and survival days in lung cancer.

Serum ferritin (ng/ml)	No. of patients	Survival days[a] Mean + SD
0 – 200	5	136.4 + 60.7
200 – 500	10	118.5 + 96.3
500 – 1000	5	109.5 + 91.0
1000 and above	4	111.5 + 96.0

[a] No significant differences.

Serial Determinations of Serum Ferritin

Serial ferritin determinations were performed before and after the treatment. Figure 2 shows serial ferritin determinations in response to operation. Ferritin levels decreased remarkably after operation, but increased at the time of recurrence and tumour progression. Serum ferritin levels appeared to give a good indication of the response to surgical treatment.

Serial ferritin determinations were decreased or unchanged in most patients who responded to radiotherapy, but there were some patients who had a transient ferritin increase during the radiotherapy.

Combination Assay of Serum Ferritin and CEA as a Screening of Lung Cancer

The assessment of ferritin assay for diagnosis of lung cancer is particularly meaningful since complications such as massive bleeding, jaundice, liver damage or iron overload due to repeated transfusions, which can influence serum ferritin levels, are rather rare in lung diseases. The high frequency of elevated ferritin levels at the early stage of lung cancer and the low incidence of false positives in other

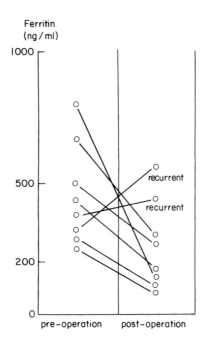

Fig. 2.   Serum ferritin levels in pre- and post-operation of lung cancer.

lung diseases are indicative of the usefulness of the assay in initial diagnosis and in differential diagnosis of a suspicious lung lesion. On the other hand, serum ferritin does not seem to be particularly useful in the prognosis or staging of lung cancer.

It was recently observed that the elevation of CEA in sera of lung cancer is closely related to tumour size, staging and recurrence of lung cancer. The determination of CEA in the serum of lung cancer may be useful as a monitoring method to detect metastases or recurrences and in monitoring the results of the treatment, but not useful for early diagnosis and differential diagnosis because of the high probability of false positivity in non-malignant diseases.

In lung cancer simultaneous determinations of serum ferritin and CEA were performed. There was no definitive relationship between the two markers. In this study we found that the pathological CEA concentration was 52.5% (12/23) of the patients. On the other hand, elevation of serum ferritin was 56.5% (13/23). When both markers were evaluated simultaneously, approximately 80% of patients appeared to have abnormal values in either of these markers (Table V).

Potential for screening of lung cancer was tested in 143 samples of blind serum from the NIH. The sensitivity was somewhat decreased to 43.3% in ferritin assay and 46.7% in CEA assay, but the specificity of both assays was 80%. There was no apparent correlation between serum ferritin and CEA (Table VI). So the use of ferritin assay in combination with CEA might hold promise as a general screen for lung cancer and especially for increasing the specificity of diagnosis.

Table V. Usefulness of combination assay of serum ferritin with serum CEA in lung cancer.

Marker	% Positive[a]
Ferritin	56.5 (13/23)
CEA	52.2 (12/23)
2 markers	30.4 (7/23)
Either one of 2 markers	78.3 (18/23)

[a] Cut-off levels were 5 ng/ml for CEA and 200 ng/ml for ferritin

Table VI. Screening assay of serum ferritin and CEA of blind samples of lung cancer from NIH.[a]

	Ferritin (cut-off level 200 ng/ml)	CEA (cut-off level 5 ng/ml)
Sensitivity	43.3%	46.7%
Specificity	80.0%	83.3%

[a] Blind serum samples were sent from National Institute of Public Health, Bethesda, USA.

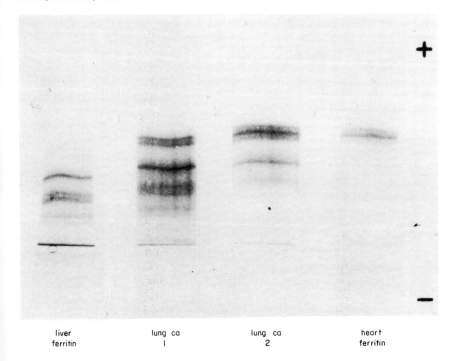

| liver ferritin | lung ca 1 | lung ca 2 | heart ferritin |

Fig. 3. Isoferritin profiles of lung cancers, liver and heart of human beings by gel isoelectric focusing.

Isoferritins in Lung Cancer Tissues

In spite of these apparent clinical implications of serum ferritin in serodiagnosis of lung cancer, the mechanism accounting for the increase in serum ferritin
levels is not fully elucidated. The most plausible and attractive hypothesis is that
the increased ferritin in the circulation conceivably represents secretion or release
from the tumour cells which are synthesizing isoferritin. Recently, more acidic
isoferritin has been found in normal tissues, such as heart, pancreas and kidney,
and, moreover, in cancer tissues and in the serum of cancer patients (Hazard *et al.*,
1977; Hazard and Drysdale, 1977). These isoferritins have more rapid mobility with
an acidic isoelectric point.

We were able to demonstrate an acidic ferritin in lung cancer extract but not
in a normal lung tissue preparation by gel isoelectric focusing (Fig. 3.) This may
indicate that ferritin is synthesized by malignant lung cancer cells.

Ferritinaemia in Nude Mice Bearing Human Lung Cancer

Two histologically different human lung carcinomas, resected by surgical
procedure and cultured *in vitro*, oat cell line and the adenocarcinoma cell line, were
inoculated in nude mice. In order to attain selective measurement of human
ferritin in nude mice sera, an antiserum against human liver was absorbed with
mouse liver ferritin. The resulting antiserum was shown to be non-reactive with
mouse ferritin on radioimmunoassay (Fig. 4.).

Human ferritin could be detected in three sera of four tumour bearing nude
mice using radioimmunoassay specific for human liver ferritin (Table VII). A correlation between tissue ferritin of lung cancer and serum ferritin concentration
of human ferritin was not demonstrated. Using an anti-heart ferritin assay, a
remarkable elevation of the more acidic ferritins in the serum of tumour bearing
nude mice was observed. Serum ferritin increased during tumour growth and
decreased after the removal of the tumour. These results indicate that human
lung cancer bearing nude mice release the ferritin into the circulation.

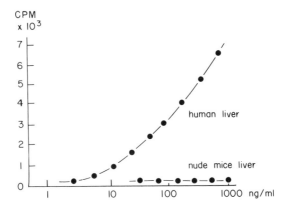

Fig. 4. Immunological reactivity of human liver ferritin and mouse ferritin against anti-
human liver ferritin serum.

Table VII. Serum ferritin concentration in nude mice bearing human lung cancer, measured by RIA using antisera against human liver ferritin and human heart ferritin, and tumour ferritin concentration in corresponding lung cancer.

	Serum ferritin levels (ng/ml)		Tumour ferritin (r/g tissues)
	Anti-liver ferritin assay	Anti-heart ferritin assay	
Lung cancer (Adeno.)	2.5	10.5	38.2
Lung cancer (Squamous)	ND	5.4	22.0
Oat cell line	18.1	30.0	12.4
Adeno. Ca. line	4.0	8.2	–

ND : not detectable; –: not done.

Acidic Ferritin Assay as a New Method to Detect Lung Cancer

Ferritins from tumours generally exhibit more acidic profiles on isoelectric focusing than their normal tissue counterparts (Urushizaki *et al.*, 1973). However, this acidic profile is not unique to malignant tissue since certain normal tissues, such as heart or pancreas, also have isoferritins with more acidic isoelectric points than normal liver ferritin (Arosio *et al.*, 1976). These acidic isoferritins differ immunologically from normal liver ferritin (Fig. 5). A radioimmunoassay based on the more acidic heart ferritin showed a higher elevation of serum ferritin in tumour bearing nude mice, when compared with the conventional measurement of liver ferritin assay. As this is the case in human serum, ferritin assay presently used may probably be underestimating the ferritin levels in lung cancer sera because ferritin from tumour tissue is generally more acidic and is

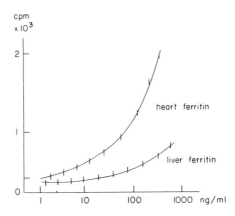

Fig. 5. Immunological reactivity of human liver ferritin and heart ferritin by heart ferritin assay.

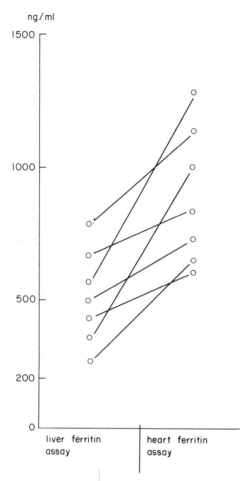

Fig. 6. Comparison of serum ferritin values in lung cancer by simultaneous measurements using liver ferritin and heart ferritin assays.

immunologically less reactive to antiserum against normal liver ferritin. Therefore, we made an acidic ferritin assay which used antisera against heart ferritin. Preliminary results showed a remarkable elevation of ferritin levels in the serum of lung cancer compared to the basic ferritin assay (Fig. 6). The evaluation of acidic isoferritin assay for cancer diagnosis is considered to be an important area for future research.

SUMMARY

The clinical significance of serum ferritin was studied for its possible use in serodiagnosis of lung cancer. Using immunoradiometric assay, elevated levels of serum ferritin were observed in 64% of patients with lung cancer and 15% of smokers. In benign lung diseases, including tuberculosis, bronchitis, asthma, sarcoidosis, bronchiectasis, pneumonia and benign tumours, serum ferritin levels were almost within the normal range. In lung cancer, the elevation of serum ferritin neither related to the tumour size as determined by X-ray examination, nor to any particular histological type of tumour. There was no apparent correlation between serum ferritin and CEA levels in lung cancer. In some instances, serial ferritin levels proved useful in monitoring the efficacy of treatment or in differential diagnosis but not of any use in the estimation of prognosis or staging. Its potential for screening lung cancer, in general, was tested in 143 blind serum samples from the NIH. The sensitivity was somewhat decreased to 52% but the specificity was high in both assays of serum ferritin and CEA. As there was no apparent correlation between serum ferritin and CEA levels in lung cancer, the combination of ferritin assay and CEA might be useful as a general screen for lung cancer and especially for increasing the specificity of diagnosis.

Tumour tissues of lung contained a moderate amount of acidic isoferritin. In addition to this, it was clearly demonstrated that serum ferritin of patients with lung cancer could be directly derived from the tumour tissues, by using nude mice inoculated with human lung cancer.

The acidic isoferritin assay of heart ferritin appears to be very valuable for the diagnosis of lung cancer.

REFERENCES

Addison, G. M., Beamish, M. R., Hales, C. N., Hodgkins, M. and Jacobs, A. (1972). *Journal of Clinical Pathology* 25, 326.

Alpert, E., Coston, R. L. and Drysdale, J. W. (1973a). *Nature* 242, 194.

Alpert, E., Isselbacher, K. J. and Drysdale, J. M. (1973b). *Lancet* 1, 43.

Arosio, P., Yokota, M. and Drysdale, J. W. (1976). *Cancer Research* 36, 1735.

Buffe, D., Rimbaut, C. and Burtin, P. (1968). *International Journal of Cancer* 3, 850.

Crichton, R. R. (1971). *New England Journal of Medicine* 284, 1413.

Gropp, C., Havemann, K. and Lehmann, F. -G. (1978). *Cancer* 42, 2802.

Hazard, J. G. and Drysdale, J. W. (1977). *Nature* 265, 755.

Hazard, J. G., Yokota, M. and Drysdale, J. W. (1977). *Blood* 49, 139.

Jacobs, A. and Worwood, M. (1975). *New England Journal of Medicine* 292, 951.

Marcus, D. M. and Zinberg, N. (1975). *Journal of National Cancer Institute* 55, 791.

Neville, A. M. and Cooper, E. H. (1976). *Annals of Clinical Biochemistry* 13, 283.

Niitsu, Y., Kohgo, Y., Yokota, M. and Urushizaki, I. (1975). *Annals of New York Academy of Science* 259, 450.

Urushizaki, I., Ishitani, K., Natori, H., Yokota, M., Kitago, M. and Niitsu, Y. (1973). *Gann* 64, 237.

Urushizaki, I., Niitsu, Y. and Ishitani, K. (1979). *In* "Compendium of Assays for Immunodiagnosis of Human Cancer" (R. Herberman, Ed.), pp. 199–204. Elsevier North-Holland, Amsterdam

Vincent, R. G. and Chu, T. M. (1978). *In* "Workshop on Immunodiagnosis of Human Cancer" (R. Herberman Ed.), p. 239. NCI. USA.

Walters, G. O., Miller, F. M. and Worwood, M. (1973). *Journal of Clinical Pathology* 26, 770.

Watanabe, N., Niitsu, Y., Koseki, J., Oikawa, J., Kadono, Y., Ishii, T., Goto, Y., Onodera, Y. and Urushizaki, I. (1979). *In* "Carcino-Embryonic Proteins" (F.-G. Lehmann, Ed.), Vol. 1, 273–278. Elsevier North-Holland, Amsterdam.

TUMOR MARKERS RELATED TO LUNG CANCER:
A DISCUSSION

R. B. Herberman

*Laboratory of Immunodiagnosis, National Cancer Institute,
National Institutes of Health, Bethesda, Maryland, USA*

There are some particularly favorable aspects regarding the application of
markers to problems with diagnosis or management of lung cancer. In regard to
screening, there are known, very high risk groups that can be focused upon for
detailed studies. These include heavy smokers and particularly those who also
have industrial exposure to co-carcinogenic agents like asbestos or uranium. In
such groups, one can anticipate annual incidence rates of greater than 1:1000 as
opposed to a considerably lower incidence in the general population. With this
disease, there is also at least the potential for obtaining tumor cells directly in the
sputum, for cytological examination. Lung cancer would also appear to be an
advantageous tumor site for tumor localisation studies since it is relatively easy to
visualise most parts of the lungs by X-rays and by computerised tomographic CT
scans. Prognostic assessment in lung cancer also has some definite advantages. By
careful lymph node examination, it is possible to get detailed information at the
time of surgery regarding the stage of disease; such information has been shown
to have a correlation with the prognosis of the patients. Lung cancer is an
aggressive type of tumor in which, despite removal of most tumor by surgery or
the reduction of small cell carcinoma to low levels by chemotherapy, there is
still a high rate of recurrence of progressive disease within 1–2 years. Therefore,
it is relatively easy to design trials to evaluate the importance of markers for
prognosis, as an aid in determining therapy, or for following patients for early
detection of recurrent disease.

Serono Symposium No. 46, Markers for Diagnosis and Monitoring of Human Cancer, edited
by M. I. Colnaghi, G. L. Buraggi and M. Ghione, 1982. Academic Press, London and New
York.

In regard to the available markers and those that may be developed in the foreseeable future, it is important to consider what are the approaches and the prospects for the valuable utilisation of markers for practical clinical purposes in lung cancer.

Firstly, let us consider the possible value of tumor markers for screening, especially of high risk groups. With tumor markers, one is faced with the combined problems of limited sensitivity and specificity of most of the available tests. It was of interest that circulating levels of serum ferritin were detected with rather high frequency in patients with stage I lung cancer. It will be important to evaluate this marker in the earliest stages of lung cancer, including *in situ* lung cancer. It should also be noted that, despite the relatively low incidence of elevated levels of pro-ACTH in the studies of Dr Ratcliffe, similar studies by Wolfsen and Odell (1979) have indicated that this marker may be useful in the early detection of lung cancer in patients with chronic pulmonary disease. The reasons for the major discrepancies between the studies are not obvious, but it would seem important to examine this issue further and determine whether the procedures used by Wolfsen and Odell can be reproduced. An alternative approach to the application of tumor markers to screening would be the detection of tumor markers on cells in the sputum. For the past several years, the National Cancer Institute in the USA has supported an early lung cancer detection project, based on careful examination of sputum cytology. Using standard cytological techniques, it has been possible to detect a number of patients with *in situ* carcinoma of the lung and Dr McIntire has told me that those patients detected on the basis of positive cytology alone have had a high rate of apparently curative surgical removal of their tumors. Fluorescence or immunohistochemical staining of such cytology specimens by antibodies to selective lung tumor markers may aid early detection of cancer. One would require an antigen that is not on normal lung epithelial cells and is not a differentiation antigen but rather one which would be expressed on most or all lung cancer cells. The use of such a reagent with the fluorescence activated cell sorter might allow screening of large numbers of cells to detect positive cells at a low frequency. Among the markers discussed at this meeting, one might consider the value of the lung tumor associated antigen of Braatz and McIntire and possibly some of the other lung tumor associated antigens that were described by Dr McIntire (this volume, p. 95). In addition, Dr John Minna's group and several other groups have been preparing monoclonal antibodies to lung tumor associated antigens and perhaps one or more these will be sufficiently discriminatory for such an application.

Another potential approach to early diagnosis of lung cancer might be to look for immune responses to tumor associated antigens. One might be able to detect antibodies or cellular immune responses to such antigens at an early stage in the development of lung cancer. However, none of the available procedures are sufficiently well standardised and reproducible to be used for large-scale clinical studies.

It should be noted that the ideal would be to find positive results with a tumor marker without clear evidence of cancer by classical cytology, X-ray examination or other accepted diagnostic techniques. This then would lead to a vigorous search for tumor. Such findings in a screening study would also require careful follow-up of the screened population to determine who subsequently develops cancer. It would be necessary to follow the individuals who were both positive and negative for the particular marker, to determine whether the incidence of subsequent cancer would be higher in the marker positive group. It should be noted that in such studies, even if a marker was not sufficiently discriminatory to allow early diagnosis in a particular patient, if the marker would only be elevated or positive in the subpopulation of individuals at highest risk of developing cancer, such information could be quite useful for focusing the follow-up and for epidemiological evaluation. In all screening studies, the ultimate criterion for success would be whether the early detection of cancer would lead to improved survival of the patients beyond that which is associated with the standard diagnosis of lung cancer.

In regard to initial diagnosis, the problem is to discriminate reliably between patients with cancer and those with benign lung lesions or with background pulmonary problems related to smoking and/or chronic obstructive pulmonary disease. In regard to circulating markers, one would need a marker that is elevated in a relatively high percentage of patients with localised cancer and which is low in most patients with benign lung disease and in smokers. As pointed out earlier, the assays for ferritin or possibly for pro-ACTH may be helpful in this area. In a study reported by Wolfsen and Odell (1979) on 100 consecutive patients with abnormal chest X-rays, 77% of those subsequently diagnosed as having cancer were found to have elevated ACTH or another hormone, whereas all individuals found to have benign disease were negative for these hormones. Cytological examination of the sputum or of bronchial washings or of pleural effusions for the expression of tumor markers on the cells may be quite useful and perhaps more discriminatory than the circulating markers. One can also envision the usefulness of radioimmunodetection for discrimination between benign and malignant lesions in the lungs. One might particularly hope that monoclonal antibodies to lung cancer antigens would be helpful in this regard. It should be noted that antibodies to a lung cancer antigen which does not enter the circulation might be particularly useful since circulating antigen might interfere with adequate localisation. Such an approach might also help to identify lesions which would not be easily visible on X-rays or CT scans.

In regard to the application of tumor markers to prognosis in lung cancer, the real question is whether the markers could add to the staging information that is obtained at surgery. It would be very helpful if it were possible to classify patients better in regard to responsiveness to therapy. This might be done pre-operatively, to help to identify patients with unresectable disease. There have been some indications for the value of CEA in this regard, with circulating levels above about 3 ng/ml indicating high likelihood for unresectable disease. Immunological approaches might also be helpful to identify cancer in metastatic sites. In addition to radioimmunodetection, one could envision the use of cytological approaches for detection of small numbers of malignant cells in bone marrow or possibly even in the peripheral blood. Markers associated with metastatic lung cancer might be expected to be most useful in this regard. At the time of surgery, the challenge would be to determine whether a tumor marker could subdivide patients within a particular TNM stage of disease. Examination of removed lymph nodes for small numbers of tumor cells might improve the staging considerably. After surgery, one would like to be able to utilise tumor markers to detect residual disease, which might lead to further surgery or to more aggressive chemotherapy or radiotherapy. For this, some of the circulating markers might be helpful, including ferritin, CEA, and some of the hormones. Identification of patients with continued elevation of markers might be expected to help in assigning patients to adjuvant chemotherapy studies.

In regard to the monitoring of patients after primary therapy, again one could envision several possible valuable applications of tumor markers. Firstly, following marker levels during chemotherapy or radiotherapy might help to provide early indications of response to treatment. Such testing might also be expected to be very useful to predict responsiveness to new chemotherapeutic agents, and thereby identify a wider array of potentially useful drugs for this disease. In fact, another major application of the markers for monitoring, the earlier detection of recurrence, would only be expected to be useful if we had better chemotherapeutic agents to then treat patients with detected recurrent tumor. In regard to detection of recurrent disease, the important question is whether a particular marker would reliably provide positive results prior to clinical detection of recurrence, Furthermore, it would be important to determine whether this earlier detection was actually clinically useful, particularly leading to improved survival of the patients. For these approaches, CEA, ferritin, hormones and, possibly, other lung tumor associated markers might be useful.

I would now like to briefly comment further on some of the particular markers that were mentioned during this session. The study of Kelly and Levy that was mentioned by Dr McIntire initially seemed quite promising. However, in a recent evaluation of their tests with coded serum specimens provided from the NCI Mayo Clinic Serum Bank, the test was unable to discriminate significantly between the cancer specimens and the benign disease controls. In contrast, it is noteworthy that in a similar evaluation of the tissue polypeptide antigen in conjunction with CEA, it was possible to demonstrate that a discriminant could be used to distinguish most of the cancer specimens from the control specimens; therefore, although these tests are not highly tumor specific, they might still be quite useful for various problems of management of lung cancer. In regard to the presentation on ferritin by Dr Urushizaki (Urushizaki and Nitsu, this volume, p. 111), I now provide some additional information concerning the specimens that he tested from the NCI Mayo Clinic Serum Bank. He detected that about 15% of the smokers and some of the benign disease patients had elevated ferritin levels and, rightly, raised the question as to whether this might represent earlier detection of occult malignancy in some of those individuals. However, I have just checked on the follow-up of most of these patients in the study and during the subsequent 2.5–3 years since the specimens were collected, there has been no detection of cancer among any of the control individuals. Therefore, it does appear that the radioimmunoassay for at least the common variety of ferritin has some definite problems with false positive results.

It is clear from the presentations at this meeting and from the above discussion that we still do not have entirely satisfactory markers for any of the important clinical applications related to lung cancer. I hope that, in the coming years, better markers will be developed and demonstrated to be particularly valuable for one or more of the important clinical applications. The advent of monoclonal antibodies has led to more optimism in this regard. One would hope that some of these antibodies would be sufficiently specific to allow reliable detection of lung cancer cells and perhaps might help to detect circulating tumor markers. One might also envision the use of this technology to attempt development of new antibodies against the "pro" pieces of the ectopic hormones like ACTH that may be produced by lung tumor cells and, thereby, develop assays which would be much more discriminatory than those which are currently available.

REFERENCE

Wolfsen, A. R. and Odell, W. D. (1979). *In* "Compendium of Assays for Immuno-diagnosis of Human Cancer (R. B. Herberman, Ed.), p. 293, Elsevier North Holland, Amsterdam.

NEW DEFINITIONS IN THE MARKER APPROACH FOR DIAGNOSIS AND MONITORING OF HUMAN CANCER: A DISCUSSION

B. Serrou, D. Cupissol, F. Favier and C. Favier

Laboratoire d'Immunopharmacologie des Tumeurs, INSERM U–236, ERA–CNRS N. 844, Centre Paul Lamarque, Montpellier, France

Despite formidable, international research, markers for diagnosis and monitoring of human cancer are, in our opinion, still inadequately defined. Our impression, based on the discussions presented on leukaemia, breast and lung cancer, is that there is no clear-cut proof for the existence of the so-called tumour specific antigen. Indeed, stronger and stronger arguements favour the concept of "differentiation antigens", a term which we propose to characterize antigens expressed on and by human cells. The time has come to reconsider our overall approach to cancer which has probably suffered as a result of a comparison with the transplantation approach and the "transplantation antigens". Cancer can be viewed as the expression of the autologous dysregulation. Therefore, progress can only come about by comprehensive consideration of cell function and interaction. Until now, the immunological system has been looked upon as a means of destroying foreign aggressors and not a regulatory system for cell growth, proliferation and differentiation. Reconsideration of these aspects should, by definition, yield new insights and strongly stimulate new avenues of research as well as point to the necessity of close collaboration between the basic scientist and clinician.

Following these general considerations, we would like to focus to some key points which are: (1) tumour specificity; (2) non-specific tumour markers; (3) other immunological markers; and (4) the definition of clinical phases for evaluating new markers.

Serono Symposium No. 46, Markers for Diagnosis and Monitoring of Human Cancer, edited by M. I. Colnaghi, G. L. Buraggi and M. Ghione, 1982. Academic Press, London and New York.

TUMOUR SPECIFICITY*

For many years now, systematic attempts have failed to provide proof of
tumour specific antigens, both *in vivo*, using living or modified cells, and *in vitro*
by trying to purify and characterize the possible molecules involved. Even after
a study of human models and research devoted to the CALL antigen, I am aware
of any clear evidence supporting antigens expressed either on the membrane
or the cytoplasm of tumour cells. This could be related to the fact that tumour
cells take their origin from normal autologous cells and under different influences
give rise to only weak, if any, tumour specific antigen. Our own impression is
that we are dealing with differentiation antigens which could be expressed differently either quantitatively or qualitatively at the cell level, thereby explaining
the difficulties in demonstrating small antigenic differences between autochthonous tumour and normal cells. In addition, differences in the cell cycle (cells at
different phases) could also, at least partly, explain some inconsistent and non-
reproducible results which have appeared in the literature. It therefore seems
reasonable to us to support a well organized international research team such as
the one formed a few years ago for HLA typing. This would include an exchange
of reagents and antibodies, leading to the creation of a panel of antibodies obtained
from tissue culture and freshly explanted cells. The monoclonal antibody approach
further supports this kind of proposal. This approach deals with monoclonal
antibodies directed against specific lymphocyte characteristics. Recent developments of this technique are resulting in a large panel of antibodies capable of
characterizing very precise antigenic determinants at different stages of differentiation and different phases of the cell cycle. The use of the fluorescent cell sorter
(FACS) could prove to be very helpful in this approach by allowing the detection
of a very small number of cells expressing a given tumour marker. These considerations, in themselves, emphasize the complexity and difficulty of the tumour
specificity approach. However, the capability of detecting the difference between
normal and tumour cells could suffice to: (1) furnish proof for the existence of
a persistent small tumour cell burden in the patient, and (2) give rise to the
use of monoclonal antibodies to treat cancer patients, either injected directly as
such, or as drug vectors.

NON-SPECIFIC TUMOUR MARKERS

Concerning non-specific markers, there are few positive points and many
negative ones. A few markers, like HCG for trophoblastic tumours, are altogether
appropriate for diagnostic purposes, follow-up and adapting treatment. However,
in our opinion, this is not the case for the majority of markers evaluated up to
now, particularly CEA as evaluated by McIntire (this volume, p. 95) (Tables I
and II). High cost vs effectiveness must be reviewed. It seems unreasonable to
us to witness and read about so many uncontrolled and unevaluable studies.
In terms of the present economical situation, this becomes even more unacceptable.
How many studies have been carried out and how many CEA tests have been

*Saunders *et al.* (1981).

Table I. Relationship between the survival and the CEA baseline.

CEA baseline	Patients total no.	Dead	Alive
$\geq$ 20 ng/ml	42	27	15
$<$ 20 ng/ml	68	15	53
TOTAL	110	42	68

$P = 0.001$.

Table II. CEA level and survival time (percentage).

	Months				
	2	4	6	8	10
(1) CEA $\geq$ 20 ng/ml	25	20	5	5	5
(2) CEA $<$ 20 ng/ml	80	75	60	50	50

1 vs 2 = $P < 0.01$.

Table III. Ferritin in patients bearing lung cancer with liver metastases.

Groups	Number of patients	Ferritin (μg/ml)
Healthy donors	34	75 ± 39
Lung cancer patients with liver metastases	10	400 ± 10

$P < 0.05$.

and are still performed every day without any clear indication for them? After so many years, it is indeed surprising that it is still not possible to benefit from more conclusive evidence concerning the CEA evaluation in cancer patients, particularly since this is the result of well executed clinical evaluations. I shall return to this point later. Ferritin, as suggested by Urushizaki and Niitsu (this volume, p. 111) and also based on our results (Table III), would be a good candidate for such trials. Another possible approach would be to apply the techniques employed to evaluate new drugs or treatments to specific markers such as CEA for breast or gastrointestinal tumours. This kind of project has already begun for the evaluation of some recent chemotherapeutic drugs and new biological response modifiers. However, this particular area, as already seen for hormonal markers of, for example, lung cancer (Ratcliffe, this volume, p. 85), has yet to be adequately developed. This is also true of antigenic expression of the different stages of normal and tumour cell differentiation. But, in our opinion, the clinical evaluation of these markers has to be completely re-analysed.

Table IV. Circulating immune complexes (CIC) levels in lung cancer patients.

Groups	IgG (UI/ml)	IgM (UI/ml)	IgA (UI/ml)
(1) Healthy donors	1.25 ± 0.4	10.60 ± 3	1.80 ± 0.3
(2) Lung cancer patients in complete remission	1.57 ± 0.8	8.55 ± 7	1.85 ± 0.8
(3) Lung cancer patients in relapse	2.10 ± 1.4	14.0 ± 10	2.25 ± 1.2

IgG and IgM = 1 and 2 vs 3 = $P < 0.05$.

OTHER IMMUNOLOGICAL MARKERS

As developed during this meeting, immunological markers would appear to be useful for the classification of leukaemias and lymphomas, but we do not want to focus on this particular aspect.

The outcome of research on circulating immune complexes has been rather disappointing as a whole, owing, in part, to technical problems and also to the fact that we do not know the exact nature of these complexes—whether they are actually related to tumour, or if they contain antigen and if so, what kind? Moreover, their biological significance and role are unknown (Gauci *et al.*, 1981; Serrou and Rosenfeld, 1981a). We must consider the possibility that the presence of circulating immune complexes could be the expression of either a satisfactory immune response or an overloaded and partially blocked immune system. There is some evidence suggesting that immune complexes could induce regulatory or suppressor cells known to exist in cancer patients. A better characterization of these complexes (which most often reflect tumour burden), improved detection techniques and well conducted randomized clinical studies are a few simple suggestions to reinforce research in this promising field (Table IV).

When considering the regulatory role of the immune system, it must be under-

Table V. BCG antibodies in lung cancer patients.

	Low titre	Medium titre	High titre
Patients in complete remission	30%[a]	29%	41%
	$P < 0.05$		$P < 0.05$
Patients in progression	55%	45%	0%

[a]Percentage of patients.

stood that all, even small, modifications of this system may correlate with a given stage of tumour evolution and the expression of a new equilibrium in the host tumour relationship (Serrou *et al.,* 1980; Serrou and Rosenfeld, 1981b). Along these lines, the recent availability of monoclonal antibodies directed against functional lymphocyte subsets may help detect relapse in the preclinical stage to facilitate follow-up of the patient and adapt treatment. This might prove particularly useful if linked with the evolving therapeutic concept of biological response modifiers or employed in the detection of high risk groups. This type of detection is an often evoked goal. Evaluation of NK cell activity may be a goal candidate for this particular use (Serrou *et al.,* 1980, 1981; Serrou and Rosenfeld, 1980). We do not wish to pursue this subject any further except to mention antidrug antibodies used to monitor patient treatment, establish a prognosis and adjust patient therapy (Table V) (Serrou and Rosenfeld, 1981c).

A WELL DEFINED APPROACH FOR EVALUATING NEW TUMOUR MARKERS

As we have previously pointed out, the clinical evaluation of new tumour markers seems to be poorly adapted from a scientific and economic viewpoint. For this reason, we propose the same scheme of evaluation for tumour markers as that used for drug evaluation. Phase 1 studies would be devoted to evaluation of the feasibility of a given assay and the technical adjustments required after the preclinical stage; phase 2 would determine the type of tumour for which the test is appropriate and phase 3 would deal with the introduction of the new marker into clinical randomized studies to evaluate new therapeutic approaches. This would be accompanied by and compared with the most reliable currently employed test for the type of tumour studied. This kind of project obviously requires close collaboration between the basic scientist and clinician, not only at the local level, but at national and international levels as well. This would be facilitated by already existing cooperative efforts. A cooperative project would be able to evaluate new tumour markers better and more quickly, avoiding loss of time and money. This should not only serve the interests of the patient and treatment department, but the community as well. In conclusion, I would like to say that we now know "where" we want to go, we are beginning to know "how" to get there, but precisely "how" has yet to be resolved.

REFERENCES

Gauci, L., Caraux, J. and Serrou, B. (1981). *In* "Human Cancer Immunology" (B. Serrou and C. Rosenfeld, Eds), Vol. 1, 37–98. Elsevier North-Holland, Amsterdam.

Saunders, J. P., Daniels, J. C., Serrou, B., Rosenfeld, C. and Denney (Eds). (1981). *In* "Fundamental Mechanism in Human Cancer Immunology". Elsevier North-Holland, Amsterdam, New York.

Serrou, B. and Rosenfeld, C. (Eds) (1980). *In* "New Trends in Human Immunology and Cancer Immunotherapy". Doin Publ., Paris.

Serrou, B. and Rosenfeld, C. (Eds) (1981a). *In* "Human Cancer Immunology", Vol. 1. Elsevier North-Holland, Amsterdam.
Serrou, B. and Rosenfeld, C. (Eds) (1981b). *In* "Human Cancer Immunology", Vol. 2. Elsevier North-Holland, Amsterdam. (In press.)
Serrou, B. and Rosenfeld, C. (Eds). (1981c). *In* "Human Cancer Immunology", Vol. 3. Elsevier North-Holland, Amsterdam. (In press.)
Serrou, B., Gauci, L., Caraux, J., Cupissol, D., Thierry, C. and Estève, C. (1980). *In* "Recent Results in Cancer Research" (G. Mathe and F. Muggia, Eds), Vol. 75, 41–46. Springer–Verlag, Heidelberg, New York.
Serrou, B., Herberman, R. and Rosenfeld, C. (Eds) (1981). *In* "Human Cancer Immunology", Vol. 4. Elsevier North-Holland, Amsterdam. (In press.)

MARKERS OF PANCREATIC CANCER

R. Hunter[1], F. Gelder[2], T. Ming Chu[3] and A. R. Moossa[4]

Emory University, Atlanta, Georgia[1],
Louisiana State University, Shreveport, Louisiana[2],
Roswell Park Memorial Institute, Buffalo, New York[3]
and the University of Chicago, Chicago, Illinois[4], *USA*

INTRODUCTION

Several candidate pancreatic tumor antigens have been reported since Banwo *et al.* (1974) reported an oncofetal antigen associated with fetal pancreas and adult pancreatic tumors. Some have been studied very little and others were demonstrated to be known materials such as α-fetoprotein (reviewed by Shimano *et al.*, 1981). This report reviews the work on the most extensively studied antigen: pancreatic oncofetal antigen (POA). It was originally described by Gelder *et al.* (1978a, b) who purified the material and studied its distribution among tissues and in the sera of several hundred patients with diverse benign and malignant conditions. Working independently, Shimano *et al.* (1981) isolated a pancreatic cancer associated antigen (PCAA) which had similar biochemical properties and was found in a similar distribution in the sera of patients. We have recently found that PCAA and POA produce a line of complete immunological identity in Ouchterlony immunodiffusion analysis, confirming the suggestion that POA and PCAA are the same material. The purpose of this communication is to review the biochemical, biological and clinical data from both groups.

Serono Symposium No. 46, Markers for Diagnosis and Monitoring of Human Cancer, edited by M. I. Colnaghi, G. L. Buraggi and M. Ghione, 1982. Academic Press, London and New York.

PURIFICATION OF ANTIGEN AND PREPARATION OF ANTISERA

The first antisera against POA were prepared by immunising rabbits with saline extracts of human fetal pancreas obtained following second trimester prostaglandin induced abortions. The antisera contained many specificites to normal pancreas and serum proteins. Those to adult pancreas were removed by adsorption with gluteraldehyde insolubilised normal human pancreas and adult serum. The resultant antisera reacted strongly with α-fetoprotein and weakly with another material, later called POA. It did not react with extracts of adult pancreas, other adult tumors or serum proteins. POA also showed patterns of immunological non-identity with carcinoembryonic antigen (CEA), ferritin and several other known tumor associated antigens.

Double immunodiffusion analyses were performed on 110 serum samples from patients with various diagnoses. POA was demonstrated in the sera of 20 of 26 patients with carcinoma of the pancreas. It was isolated from the plasma of a patient who had approximately 150 μg/ml. A large amount of plasma was obtained from this individual and was used as a reference standard for further studies. POA was purified by ammonium sulfate precipitation, cryoprecipitation, ultracentrifugation, and chromatography on a Sepharose 6B column. The product formed a single band on polyacrylamide gel electrophoresis. It was a glycoprotein with molecular weight of approximately 800,000 which had an α2 mobility on electrophoresis. It was highly sensitive to trypsin and perchloric acid, but was resistant to RNase and DNase. It contained no detectable lipid. Subsequent isolates from other patients had similar properties except for a variation in electrophoretic mobility from the α2 to the β region and a variation in molecular weight between 800,000 and a little over 1,000,000.

Purified adult POA was used to prepare antisera for the development of a quantitative rocket immunoelectrophoresis assay. The specificity of the antisera was established by comparison with our standards, other antisera and POA from several sources. On Oucterlony analysis, lines of complete immunological identity were formed between several preparations of adult and fetal POA using antisera against either preparation.

Antisera against PCAA were prepared by different procedures. Normal plasma proteins were removed from ascitic fluid from a patient with pancreas cancer by means of an immunoabsorbent column. The non-binding material was concentrated and used to immunise rabbits. The resulting antisera was adsorbed with gluteraldehyde insolubilised normal plasma and was used to monitor the purification of PCAA from ascitic fluid. The purification utilised ultracentrifugation, ammonium sulfate precipitation and Sepharose 6B chromatography, and DEAE sephacell ion exchange chromatography. The purified material migrated as a single protein band on polyacrylamide gel electrophoresis. An enzyme immunoassay using horse-radish peroxidase conjugated antisera was developed. This assay was more sensitive than the rocket assay used for POA. It measured levels down to 0.1 μg/ml as opposed to 1 μg/ml for POA. However, the coefficient of variation of the two assays are similar: 3–5%. The biochemical properties of PCAA are similar to those of POA except that molecular weights as high as 1,200,000 were found. PCAA consisted of 20% carbohydrate and 80% peptide with an isoelectric point of 4.7 and migration in the α2 β region of electrophoresis.

DISTRIBUTION OF THE ANTIGEN IN TISSUES

Using double immunodiffusion analysis, POA was demonstrated in ten of 13 fetal pancreas extracts and in fetal small bowel extracts but not in other fetal tissues. It was not detected in multiple adult tissue extracts except for trace amounts in one of six colon extracts and two of six small bowel extracts. Since POA is highly sensitive to proteolytic enzymes, these analyses were carried out in the presence of enzyme inhibitors. Results with assays for PCAA in tissue using the enzyme immunoassay technique were similar if one allows for the increased sensitivity of this technique. PCAA was found in concentrations of > 0.3 $\mu g/mg$ of protein in three of six pancreas tumor extracts, both of two colon tumor extracts, two of six breast tumor extracts, and all of three normal color extracts. None was detected in three lung tumors or 23 normal tissue extracts.

The distrubution of the antigens in tissue was also studied by fluorescence microscopy. Both POA and PCAA were found in the cytoplasm of ductal cells of malignant pancreas tissue. The antigen was also present in signet ring cells of stomach cancer as well as in goblet cells of normal gastrointestinal tissue. The ductal cells of fetal pancreas and fetal gastric epithelial cells also demonstrated the antigen by immunofluorescence. It was not demonstrated in other fetal or adult tissues.

Table I. Serum levels of POA in various conditions.

Patient condition[a]	POA[b]		PCAA[c]	
	% Positive	No. tested	% Positive	No. tested
Pancreatic cancer	62	143	67	43
Biliary tract cancer	59	17	–	–
Hepatocellular cancer	33	18	–	–
Lung cancer	20	90	36	30
Colorectal cancer	16	129	27	37
Breast cancer	8	147	16	36
Gastric cancer	20	50	–	–
Duodenum, small intestine	0	5		
Pancreatitis	17	91		
Biliary stone, cirrhosis, cholecystitis	12	91		
Pregnancy	10	109		
Normal	3	233	5	40

[a]Patient samples were collected at several institutions before therapy. [b]POA was measured by a rocket immunoelectrophoresis assay. Positive values were greater than 14 standard units which is about 18–20 $\mu g/ml$. [c]PCAA was measured by an enzyme immunoassay. Positive values are greater than 16 $\mu g/ml$ which is 2 standard deviations above the mean for normal people.

STUDIES WITH PATIENT SERA

The results of tests for POA and PCAA in the sera of several groups of patients are shown in Table I. The sera were obtained from several sources including the University of Chicago, the Roswell Park Memorial Institute, the Mayo NCI Serum Plasma Bank and the Louisiana State University Medical Center. The sera from patients with adenocarcinoma of the pancreas had elevated levels of POA more frequently than those from any other group. Most of the patients with elevated levels had moderate to well differentiated carcinomas while many with levels in the normal range had poorly differentiated tumors. The levels tended to rise with increasing size of the tumor but elevated levels were found in approximately one-third of patients with resectable pancreas cancer. Elevated levels of POA were found in a similar proportion of patients with biliary tract cancer although the numbers studied are smaller. A smaller proportion of patients with other malignancies also had elevated levels of the antigen in their sera. Immunofluorescence studies have recently been carried out on a number of patients with elevated POA levels in breast cancer. The tumors were all negative. The patients with elevated serum levels of POA all had liver metastases, suggesting that the elevated levels were associated with the effects of the tumor on the liver rather than a product of the tumor cells themselves. Consequently, it appears that POA is produced by malignant cells in pancreatic and probably biliary tract cancers, but is also produced by reactive cells in other conditions.

FACTORS AFFECTING SERUM ASSAYS

Serum samples from patients with various levels of POA were drawn with a variety of anticoagulants and stored under various conditions in an effort to identify factors which would affect the antigen. POA levels were not detectably affected by any of the anticoagulants, freezing, thawing, or refrigerator storage for a period of at least several weeks. They remained unchanged at $-70°$ for more than 2 years. In the initial studies of POA, care was taken to obtain samples only prior to treatment. Consequently, the elevated levels could not be attributed to the activity of drugs.

Extensive studies were carried out searching for antigenic isotypes of POA. Ouchterlony double immunodiffusion assays were carried out with each positive specimen and serum sample. Lines of complete immunological identity were found in almost all cases. However, occasional patient sera demonstrated lines of partial immunological identity indicating that isotypes of POA do exist. They have not yet been characterised. The variation in electrophoretic mobility and molecular weight among POA and PCAA samples isolated from different patients was usually not paralleled by a change in antigenic determinants detectable on immunodiffusion analysis. This suggests that the isolates differ in carbohydrate content but have similar or identical peptide components.

USE OF SERUM ASSAYS IN DIAGNOSIS OF PANCREAS CANCER

The early detection of pancreatic cancer is seldom possible. In the absence of jaundice, early symptoms are generally vague and non-specific. Consequently, approximately 85% of people have regional or distant metastases at the time of diagnosis. Even among symptomatic patients, the diagnosis is frequently difficult. Several years ago, three institutions (Mayo Foundation, Memorial Sloan Kettering Cancer Center and the University of Chicago) carried out a prospective study to compare and evaluate the diagnostic accuracy of available procedures among patients who were suspected of having pancreatic cancer. Three-hundred-and-sixty-eight patients with unexplained gastrointestinal symptoms which were suggestive of pancreatic cancer were studied: 36% of them did have pancreatic cancer, 11% had other cancers, 11% pancreatitis, 30% biliary tract disease and 12% had abdominal pain of indeterminate cause.

Not every patient was tested with every procedure available, but the results were generally concordant and could be summarised as follows. A battery of potential serological markers which included gastrin, parathyroid hormone, calcitonin, glucagon, insulin, C-peptide, human chorionic gonadotrophin, RNase, glucose, alkaline phosphatase, POA and CEA were measured. The most useful assay of this battery in the diagnosis or exclusion of pancreatic cancer was POA. It had a positive predictive value of 80% and a negative predictive value of 73% (Mackie *et al.*, 1979a, 1980). CEA was elevated in 83% of the patients with pancreatic cancer but also in 65% of patients with other cancers and 45% of those with benign diseases. A highly elevated CEA (greater than 9 mg/ml) was indicative of metastatic or unresectable pancreatic cancer and did not differentiate it from other advanced intraabdominal tumors. In this study, the prevalence of pancreatic cancer was 32%. The value of POA in identifying pancreatic cancer in populations with lower prevalence, i.e. in those not clinically suspected of having the disease, is much less.

This multi-institutional study was also designed to evaluate the effectiveness of combinations of tests in addition to that of individual tests. Ultrasonography achieved the highest rate of correct diagnoses (97% of patients diagnosed with 84% accuracy) (Mackie *et al.*, 1979b). The most accurate test was endoscopic retrograde cholangiopancreatography (ERCP) with duodenal drainage and cytology. The results suggested that ultrasonography was the best non-invasive test and that a combination of ERCP, pancreatic juice assay and cytology in a single procedure was the best discriminating investigation. Studies were carried out to determine if assays for POA and CEA could improve the diagnostic accuracy of ultrasonography (Mackie *et al.*, 1979b). In a series of 134 examinations in patients suspected of having pancreatic cancer, 34 had a positive ultrasonographic diagnosis, 66 had a negative study or other diagnosis, and 20 had a doubtful result. At the completion of the diagnostic work-up, the sensitivity and specificity of ultrasonography for pancreatic cancer varied according to whether the 20 doubtful results were considered normal or abnormal. If they were normal, the tests had a sensitivity of 76% and a specificity of 91%. If they were called abnormal, the sensitivity rose to 87% but the specificity fell to 74%. The addition of assays of POA and CEA to this group of patients with doubtful ultrasound examinations increased the sensitivity to 85% and the specificity to 90% which was a significant increase at the $P < 0.01$ level. Neither the CEA nor POA were able to identify the false results in the groups of patients confidently diagnosed by ultrasound. Chronic pancreatitis is a frequent source of false ultrasound reports in pancreatic cancer. This problem besets most, if not all, pancreatic investigations. Elevations of CEA are found in as many as 68% of patients with chronic pancreatitis. Elevated levels of POA are found in a smaller proportion and the levels are generally lower than those found in pancreatic cancer. In summary, serum assays for POA appeared to be neither sensitive nor specific enough to be used as stand alone procedures, but they can significantly improve the overall diagnostic accuracy when used in appropriate combinations with other tests. Much more work in this area is needed.

POA assays were performed serially in patients with pancreatic cancer in an effort to monitor the course of therapy. If a patient had a high level before treatment, it invariably fell within a few weeks following resection and then rose with development of clinical metastases in a fashion analogous to that which has been reported with CEA (Gelder, 1978a; Hunter, 1979 and unpublished observations). Patients who did not have elevated levels of POA at the time of initial diagnosis generally did not develop them with recurrence. However, one patient with a normal level before operation developed a rapidly rising level of POA with recurrence of disease. Consequently, it appears that serial determinations of POA can be of value in monitoring the course of therapy of pancreatic cancer. The clinical value of this monitoring depends upon the nature of available therapy.

REFERENCES

Banwo, O., Versey, J. and Hobbs, J. R. (1974). *Lancet* 1, 643.
Gelder, F. B., Reese, C. J., Moossa, A. R., Hall, T. and Hunter, R. (1978a). *Cancer Research* 38, 313.
Gelder, F., Reese, C., Moossa, A. R. and Hunter, R. (1978b). *Cancer* 42, 1635.
Hunter, R., Gelder, F. and Moossa, A. R. (1979). *In* "Compendium of Assays for Immunodiagnosis of Human Cancer" (R. Herberman, Ed.), pp. 247–250, Elsevier North Holland, New York.
Mackie, C. R., Cooper, M. J., Lewis, M. H. and Moossa, A. R. (1979a). *Annals of Surgery* 189, 480.
Mackie, C. R., Bowie, J., Cooper, M. J., Lewis, M. H. and Moossa, A. R. (1979b). *Archives of Surgery* 114, 889.
Mackie, C. R., Moossa, A. R., Go, V. L. W., Nobel, G., Sizemore, G., Cooper, M. J., Wood, R. A. B., Hall, A. W., Waldman, T., Gelder, T. and Rubenstein, A. W. (1980). *Digestive Diseases and Sciences* 25, 161.
Shimano, T., Loor, R. M., Papsidero, L. D., Kuriyama, M., Vincent, R. G., Nemoto, T., Holyoke, E. D., Berjian, R., Douglass, H. O. and Chu, T. M. (1981). *Cancer* 47, 152.

CEA AND CSAp MARKERS IN THE DETECTION AND MONITORING OF COLORECTAL CANCER

D. M. Goldenberg

*Division of Experimental Pathology, Department of Pathology,
University of Kentucky Medical Center, Lexington, Kentucky, USA*

GASTROINTESTINAL CANCER MARKERS

Beginning perhaps with the identification of α-fetoprotein (AFP) by Abelev *et al.* (1963) and of carcinoembryonic antigen (CEA) by Gold and Freedman (1965), the gastrointestinal system has been the focus of much attention in our efforts to define tumor and organ distinct markers. A list of the principal markers of current interest in gastrointestinal tissues and tumors is presented in Table I. Only a few have retained organ or cell specific properties, while none has yet attained the rank of a cancer specific marker. Those six antigens represented as cell specific, such as IMG, CMA, CSAs, SGA, GOA, and CSAp, are glycoproteins selectively distributed in goblet cells and in signet ring tumor cells (Kawasaki *et al.*, 1971; Gold and Miller, 1974; Goldenberg *et al.*, 1976a; Bara *et al.*, 1978; Rapp *et al.*, 1979; Gold, 1979; Gold and Goldenberg, 1980; Pant *et al.*, 1977, 1978; Pant and Goldenberg, 1979).

Table II summarises some clinical findings of the elevation of some of these markers in patients with gastrointestinal tumors. The best discrimination between malignant and benign diseases appears to be for GT-II, which is elevated in a high percentage of all four tumor types listed. It is further apparent, among gastrointestinal tumors, that none of these markers is strictly tumor type specific. Nevertheless, the markers of most interest in the case of colorectal cancers are CEA, GT-II, TennaGen, and CSAp.

*Supported in part by NIH grants CA-25584, CA-17742 and CA-15799

Serono Symposium No. 46, Markers for Diagnosis and Monitoring of Human Cancer, edited by M. I. Colnaghi, G. L. Buraggi and M. Ghione, 1982. Academic Press, London and New York.

Table I. Tumor associated markers in gastrointestinal cancer.[a]

Antigen	Investigator	Year	Organ specific	Cancer specific
(1) AFP, α-fetoprotein	Abelev *et al.*	(1963)	No	No
(2) CEA, carcinoembryonic antigen	Gold and Freedman	(1965)	No	No
(3) FSA, fetal sulfoglyco-protein	Häkkinen *et al.*	(1968)	Perhaps	No
(4) IMG, intestinal mucosa specific glycoprotein	Kawasaki *et al.*	(1971)	Cell specific	No
(5) CMA, colonic muco-protein antigen	Gold and Miller	(1974)	Cell specific	No
(6) CSAs, colon specific antigens	Goldenberg *et al.*	(1976a)	Cell specific	No
(7) SGA, sulfated glyco-peptidic antigen	Bara *et al.*	(1978)	Cell specific	No
(8) GOA, goblet cell antigen	Rapp *et al.*	(1979)	Cell specific	No
(9) ZGM, zinc glycinate marker	Pusztaszeri *et al.*	(1976)	No	No
(10) CSAp, colon specific antigen p	Pant *et al.*	(1977)	Cell specific	No
(11) BFP, basic fetoprotein	Ishii	(1979)	No	No
(12) GT–II, galactosyltrans-ferase isoenzyme	Podolsky *et al.*	(1978)	No	No
(13) POA, pancreatic oncofetal antigen	Gelder *et al.*	(1978)	No	No
(14) TennaGen	Potter *et al.*	(1979)	No	No

[a]From Goldenberg (1981).

Table II.   Selected blood markers for gastrointestinal cancer.[a]

	% Elevated						
Diagnosis	AFP	CEA	GT 11	POA	BFP	TnGn	CSAp
Stomach ca.	18	61	75	25	31	74	0
Colorectal ca.	5	72	73	14	26	89	52
Pancreas ca.	23	91	83	48	NA[b]	92	20
Primary liver ca.	70	NA	100	0	NA	NA	NA
Benign GI disease	35[c]	37	0	18	3	36	10
Normals	1	11	0	3	0	7	8

[a]From Goldenberg (1981). [b]NA, not available. [c]Hepatitis for AFP cases.

CEA levels are raised in a high percentage of patients with colorectal cancer, ranging from 72 to 82% for all stages, with the more advanced clinical stages showing the highest frequency of plasma CEA elevation (Table III). Unfortunately, the relatively high percentage of patients with benign gastrointestinal diseases showing CEA elevations precludes its use, alone, for diagnosis (Goldenberg, 1979). Pre-operative CEA values appear to have some prognostic significance in colorectal cancer, where high levels indicate a greater probability of more advanced disease (Herrera et al., 1976; Wanebo et al., 1978). The CEA test is most generally accepted for monitoring disease activity in colorectal cancer patients (Holyoke et al., 1975; Mayer et al., 1978; Mach et al., 1978; Sugarbaker et al., 1976). Recently, prospective studies of CEA used alone as an indication for second-look surgery have indicated that a high rate of localised tumor can be detected (Martin et al., 1979), and it appears that this 65% rate of localised tumor found at second-look surgery is much higher than the results published for this procedure prior to the advent of the CEA test (Gilbertsen and Wangensteen, 1962). It should be pointed out, however, that single CEA values are not as reliable as frequent monitoring of circulating CEA for assessing clinical status in a colorectal cancer patient.

Galactosyltransferase isoenzyme-II, or GT-II, is an interesting recent marker which appears to be more specifically associated with malignancy than most other substances available (Table IV). Although normal individuals who were tested did not appear to have elevated GT-II, abnormal serum values were found in patients with celiac disease and with alcoholic hepatitis (Podolsky et al., 1978). As is also the case for CEA, GT-II titers increase with advanced stage of disease in colorectal cancer (Podolsky et al., 1978).

Although the substance described as TennaGen, or Tennessee antigen, is present in a number of cancer types, it appears to have the highest incidence of elevation in adenocarcinomas of the gastrointestinal tract (Potter et al., 1978). However, it is also elevated in patients with benign gastrointestinal and benign pulmonary disease (Table V), thus limiting its value as a diagnostic marker. However, in contrast to almost all of the other markers discussed, TennaGen seems to be elevated in a large number of patients with early colorectal cancer, showing levels

Table III.   Circulating CEA levels in various conditions.[a]

Clinical status	% Elevated CEA
Malignant diseases	
Colorectum, all stages	72–81
Dukes' A	38–44
Dukes' B	60–76
Dukes' C	60–75
Metastasised	80–89
Stomach	61
Pancreas	91
Breast	47
Lung	76
Prostate	40
Bladder	42
Gynecological	65
Lymphomas	35
Acute and chronic leukemias	37
Non-malignant diseases	
Alcoholic cirrhosis of liver	70
Alcohol addiction	65
Pulmonary emphysema	57
Kidney transplant	56
Pancreatitis	53
Granulomatous colitis	47
Pneumonia	46
Gastric ulcer	45
Ulcerative colitis	31
Normals	
Healthy, unselected	11
Healthy, non-smokers	3
Healthy, smokers	19
Healthy, pregnant	3

[a]From Goldenberg (1981).

of over 90% positivity in patients with Dukes' A and B lesions (Potter *et al.*, 1978). Furthermore, changes in the titer of the antigen in the serum appears to correspond to disease activity following therapy (Potter *et al.*, 1978).

During the search for organ specific markers of the colon (Goldenberg *et al.*, 1976a), we identified a glycoprotein antigen in a xenografted human colonic carcinoma, GW-39 (Goldenberg *et al.*, 1966), which was water soluble and destroyed in immunoreactivity by such mucoprotein extraction agents as perchloric acid and phenol, thus being distinct from the other colorectal glyco-proteins described previously (Goldenberg *et al.*, 1976b; Pant *et al.*, 1977, 1978; Pant and Goldenberg, 1979; Shochat *et al.*, 1981). Initial tissue studies revealed that this antigen, called colon specific antigen p, or CSAp, is present in colorectal

Table IV. Results of serum galactosyltransferase isoenzyme (GT–II) tests.[a]

Diagnosis	No. positive/total	% Positive
Colorectal ca.	85/117	73
Inflammatory bowel	0/20	0
Pancreas ca.	15/18	83
Pancreatitis	0/15	0
Stomach ca.	12/16	75
Esophageal (squamous) ca.	4/9	44
Gall bladder and biliary ca.	2/4	50
Cholelithiasis and biliary cirrhosis	0/6	0
Hepatoma	2/2	100
Alcoholic hepatitis	3/15	20
Celiac disease	18/20	90
Breast ca.	18/23	78
Bronchogenic ca.	13/20	65
Prostatic ca.	4/4	100
Renal ca.	1/2	50
Hodgkin's lymphoma	4/8	50
Chronic lymphocytic leukemia	2/2	100
Melanoma	0/2	0
Osteosarcoma	0/1	0
Unknown primary	3/4	75
Normals	0/85	0

[a]Adapted from Podolsky *et al.* (1978); reproduced from Goldenberg (1981).

Table V. Results of TennaGen test.[a]

Diagnosis	No. positive/total	% Positive
Colorectal ca.	170/192	89
Benign G.I. disease	197/548	36
Stomach ca.	28/38	74
Pancreas ca.	23/25	92
Lung ca.	68/86	79
Benign lung disease	46/139	33
Breast ca.	60/133	45
Other malignant tumors	100/183	55
Normals: smokers	41/590	7
Normals: non-smokers	19/282	7

[a]Adapted from Potter *et al.* (1979), reproduced from Goldenberg (1981).

D. M. Goldenberg

tissues, including normal, benign disease, and malignant, as well as in some mucinous cystadenocarcinomas of the ovary (Pant *et al.*, 1977). After developing a solid phase radioassay for CSAp, we have found, in our initial analysis of patient sera, that CSAp was elevated in 52% of advanced colorectal cancer patients, 20% of patients with pancreatic cancer and in 10% of individuals with non-neoplastic, benign gastrointestinal diseases (Table VI) (Goldenberg, 1981; Pant *et al.*, 1981). Other tumor types investigated to date have not shown CSAp serum elevations in more cases than was true for normal individuals. Thus, CSAp appears to be

Table VI. CSAp radioassay results.[a]

Diagnosis	No. positive/total	% Positive
Gastric ca.	0/10	0
Colorectal	16/31	52
Pancreatic ca.	3/15	20
Ovarian ca.	0/24	0
Bronchogenic ca.	2/29	7
Cervical ca.	1/19	5
Benign GI disease	1/10	10
Normals	2/25	8

[a]From Goldenberg (1981).

restricted to gastrointestinal lesions, particularly colorectal cancer. Unfortunately, however, with the current radiometric assay for CSAp, it appears that this marker has little value in the initial diagnosis of colorectal cancer, except that a positive result is highly indicative of a colorectal neoplasm or possibly a pancreatic carcinoma. Because of this high specificity for colorectal cancer, we postulated that the CSAp assay would be more predictive of colorectal cancer when combined with the CEA test. Figure 1 presents a comparative analysis of plasma CEA and serum CSAp elevations in 31 colorectal cancer patients, using cut-offs of 5 ng/ml

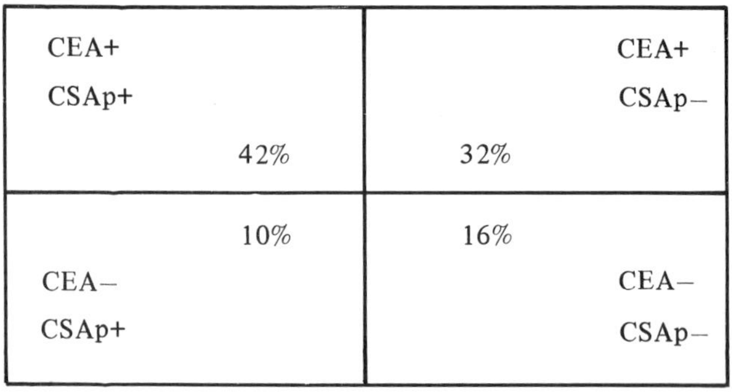

CEA+ CSAp+ 42%	CEA+ CSAp− 32%
10% CEA− CSAp+	16% CEA− CSAp−

Fig. 1. Comparative analysis of plasma CEA and serum CSAp elevations in 31 colorectal cancer patients, using cut-offs of 5.0 ng/ml and 10.0 U for CEA and CSAp, respectively. (From Goldenberg, 1981.)

and 10 U for CEA and CSAp, respectively. A 10% increase over CEA positivity could be achieved with the CSAp assay, and either test was positive in 84% of the cases. However, in reviewing the different disease states and tumor types showing CEA elevations (Table III), it would appear that performing the CSAp assay in a patient with an elevated CEA titer with an as yet undiagnosed primary tumor may be of some diagnostic value if the CSAp titer is elevated. More work is required, however, to test this supposition and to possibly improve the sensitivity of our assay.

RADIOIMMUNODETECTION OF CANCER

The previous discussion has been concerned with tumor markers present in the blood and being used as an indication of tumor burden. The presence or absence of increased quantities of such markers in the blood depends on a number of factors, including synthesis and release or shedding for some, degradation and metabolism once released, cell death and turnover, etc. However, it is reasonable to expect that the immediate tumor milieu would have sufficient amounts of these tumor markers to provide a gradient between tumor and other tissues, and that this gradient may serve to differentiate such tumors from non-neoplastic tissues and even benign disease states. If the markers at the tumor site can be used as targets for specific, antigen binding antibodies, then these same antibodies may serve as carriers for diagnostic or therapeutic molecules. If a diagnostic dose of a radionuclide is employed, then its emissions may serve to reveal sites of antigen-antibody binding, and in turn tumor, by using appropriate sensors of the radio-activity. This is the principle of radioimmunodetection of cancer (Goldenberg, 1978; Goldenberg *et al.*, 1978). Our initial clinical studies with cancer radio-immunodetection were undertaken with CEA radioantibodies, and to date we have studied more than 300 patients by this method. We have recently summarised our results in 142 patients receiving radioactive CEA antibodies (Goldenberg *et al.*, 1980a). This and previous publications (Goldenberg *et al.*, 1978; DeLand *et al.*, 1980) describe the technology in detail. In brief, purified CEA is used to immunise goats, and the resulting serum is purified by an automated affinity chromatography system in which CEA cross-reactive antigens are removed and the antibody is adsorbed onto a CEA affinity column. This brings the antibody from a 30% to an over 70% immunoreactivity with CEA (Goldenberg *et al.*, 1979). Thereafter, the antibody IgG is isolated and labeled by the chloramine-T procedure with I-131. After the prospective subject has been shown to be negative for hypersensitivity by skin testing and KI has been administered orally to reduce thyroid uptake of radioiodine, the radioactive antibody is injected i.v. at a dose of 2-3 μg antibody IgG/kg body wt, amounting to 1-2 mCi of I-131 per patient. We have found that injection of the radioactive antibody IgG by itself proves difficult to discriminate between target (tumor) and non-target and blood pool radioactivity. Therefore, we found it necessary to devise a method to compensate for circulating and interstitial non-specific radioactivity, consisting of the computer assisted sub-traction of technetium components (99m-Tc labeled human serum albumin and 99m-Tc pertechnetate) injected shortly before each imaging session (Goldenberg *et al.*, 1978). The I-131 and Tc-99m images are stored in a computer, which then permits the subtraction of the 140 keV of Tc from the 364 keV image of I-131, resulting in a tumor associated radioscintiscan. This procedure has been shown to enhance the target/non-target ratios by an average of about 2.5 (Goldenberg *et al.*, 1980a).

Our radioimmunodetection results in the first 157 patients studied with radioactive CEA antibodies are summarised in Table VII. When analysing various body regions in which no evidence of tumor could be obtained by other clinical methods, a true negative rate (specificity) for radioimmunodetection was found between 83 and 100% for the various tumor types included in the study. The true positive rate, or sensitivity, varied from 50% in a small series of pancreatic cancer patients to 90% in cervical and other uterine cancers.

Table VII. CEA radioimmunodetection results according to tumor sites.

Primary diagnosis	No. of pts.	Sensitivity (true positive rate)			
		Primary site	Secondary site	TOTAL	%
Colorectal cancer	52	10/12	41/45	51/57	89
Ovarian cancer	19	10/10	11/14	21/24	88
Lung cancer	13	8/12	4/5	12/17	71
Mammary cancer	6	2/5	7/9	9/14	64
Pancreatic cancer	6	3/6	1/2	4/8	50
Cervical cancer	15	6/8	13/13	19/21	90
Other uterine cancers	5	3/3	6/7	9/10	90
Gastric cancer	4	2/3	3/3	5/6	83
Unknown origin	9	NA[a]	8/9	8/9	89
Miscellaneous cancers	26	9/21	8/9	17/30	57
Lymphoma	2	0/2	0/2	0/4	0

[a]NA, not applicable.

A detailed analysis of our radioimmunodetection results in 51 patients with a confirmed history of colorectal cancer is given in Table VIII. These patients had a total of 54 confirmed tumor sites, of which 47 could be demonstrated by radioimmunodetection. Two of the six missed by radioimmunodetection were lung lesions less than 2 cm in diameter (as measured on the chest roentgenogram), in patients nos 92 and 250. Of the two primary tumors missed, one involved an incomplete study (no. 262), while we are unable to explain our failure in the second case (no. 261). In a liver metastasis not seen by radioimmunodetection (patient no. 349), the corresponding liver radionuclide scan also failed to show any abnormality. It is interesting that a number of patients with normal plasma CEA titers had primary or metastatic tumors demonstrable by radioimmunodetection, while the very high blood titers in other patients did not appear to hinder successful antibody localisation. Particularly worthy of note is that in 11 of these patients (marked with asterisks in Table VIII) correct tumor radioimmunodetection results were obtained when other diagnostic measures were negative, including such methods as i.v. pyelography, abdominal computed tomography, liver scanning and ultrasonography. In one case (patient no. 193), the pelvic tumor superior and posterior to the urinary bladder was revealed by radioimmuno-detection while the pelvic computed tomograms and i.v. pyelograms were negative at the time of study. Twenty-eight weeks later, a repeat CT scan revealed a lesion consistent with a growing neoplasm. At the time of the radiolocalisation study, the CT scan could not differentiate between a presumed enlarged prostate and a neoplasm. Similar findings were obtained in the other ten studies showing true positive radioimmunodetection results prior to other clinical evidence of similar sites of tumor. A report of the practical value of CEA radioimmunodetection in one of these patients (no. 327) has appeared recently (DeLand *et al.*, 1981). Thus, although CEA radioimmunodetection is still in an early phase of development, some practical and useful results in the management of colorectal cancer have been obtained in 11 of the first 51 patients with this tumor studied to date. A similar experience has been made with a more limited number of patients receiving radioactive antibodies to human chorionic gonadotropin, where sites of tumor were detected which were negative in a number of other clinical tests (Goldenberg *et al.*, 1980b; Javadpour *et al.*, 1981).

Evidence for the tumor specificity of radioimmunodetection has been derived from several sources. In our original clinical study of radioimmunodetection (Goldenberg *et al.*, 1978), evidence supporting authentic radioantibody interaction with CEA was derived by showing I–131 radioactivity associated with CEA at a molecular size range above that which is appropriate for either IgG or CEA alone, when a colonic cancer extract obtained at surgery 5 days after administration of radioactive antibody was analyzed immunochemically; this result suggested the formation of a radioantibody-antigen complex in the tumor. In this case, tumor radioactivity exceeded that in adjacent normal colonic tissue by a factor of 2.5. In another analysis of radioimmunodetection (Goldenberg *et al.*, 1980a), injection of radioactive antibody into cancer patients having benign non-neoplastic lesions resulted in only a non-specific localisation of less than 2%. Furthermore, normal goat IgG administered to a group of cancer patients resulted in a 13% non-specific tumor localisation rate, and it appeared that this was related to the large size of the tumors localised (Goldenberg *et al.*, 1980a).

To conclude, our studies to date suggest that radioimmunodetection will have a role in the pre- and post-operative evaluation and monitoring of cancer patients whose tumors contain markers which can serve as targets for localising antibodies. We have been able to identify tumors which were not revealed by conventional detection methods, even when an elevated or rising plasma CEA titer was recorded (DeLand *et al.*, 1981; Goldenberg *et al.*, 1978; Goldenberg *et al.*, 1980a; van Nagell *et al.*, 1980; Table VIII). Similar examples have been found with hCG radioimmunodetection (Goldenberg *et al.*, 1980b; Javadpour *et al.*, 1981). Nevertheless, we appreciate that many opportunities remain for improving the sensitivity and specificity of the technique, particularly by improving on the immunological reagents, the choice of radionuclide, and the scanning devices. Further advances in radioimmunodetection may also come from the simultaneous application of antitumor antibody mixtures, as we have recently described in our colonic cancer model with radioactive CEA and CSAp antibody combinations (Gaffar *et al.*, 1981).

Table VIII. Plasma CEA and radioimmunodetection results in 5 colorectal cancer patients.

| Patient | Plasma CEA (ng/ml)[a] | Radioimmunodetection results | |
		Primary site	Secondary sites
108	2210.0	0[b]	+, abdomen (1)[c]; +, liver (1); ?+ mediastinum (1)
92	16.4	0	−, lung ($<$ 2 cm)
136/58/269*	2.8	0	N
86	2.1	0	+, abdomen (1)
90/112	1190.0	0	+, liver (1)
152*	3150.0	0	+, abdomen (1); +, liver (1)
5/8	10.7	+ (1)	N
73	2.5	+ (1)	N
81/201	80.0	0	N
84	48.0	0	N
40/88	116.0	0	N
24	2.1	0	N
21	116.0	0	+, liver (1)
189	612.0	0	N
206	1.4	0	N
42	3.3	0	N
57	10.3	+ (1)	+, abdomen (1); +, liver (1)
64/78	0.8	+ (1)	N
195*	12.2	0	+, liver (1); +, abdomen (1)
191*	9.0	0	+, abdomen
126	62.0	0	N
244	2.1	0	+, abdomen
250	0.0	0	−, lung ($<$ 2 cm)
203	188.0	0	+, abdomen (1); +, lung (1)
150	40.0	+ (1)	+, liver (1); +, lung (1)
128	16.1	+ (1)	+, lung (1)
87	154.0	0	+, lung (1)
96	152.0	0	+, abdomen (1)
26*	0.9	+ (1)	N
38	68.0	+ (1)	N
60*	5600.0	+ (1)	+, liver (1)
83	5.4	0	+, abdomen (1); +, submandible (1)
85	9.0	0	N
20	11.7	0	+, liver (1)
255*	17.5	0	+, abdomen (1)
6	0.3	0	+, abdomen (2)
262	212.0	− (1)[e]	+, liver (1)
297	48.0	0	+, sacral (1)
292/270*	172.0	0	+, abdomen (1)
209	9.9	0	+, liver (1)
261	16.5	−	+, liver (1)
181	1.3	0	+, abdomen (1); +, kidney (1)
193*	46.0	0	+, liver; +, pelvis (1)

Table VIII cont.

| Patient | Plasma CEA (ng/ml)[a] | Radioimmunodetection results | |
		Primary site	Secondary sites
218	4.7	0	+, liver
283	9.0	0	N
322	185.0	0	+, liver (1); −, abdomen (1); +/−, lung
310	112.0	0	+, liver (1); +/−, abdomen (1)
309	13.0	0	+/−, liver (1)
327*	72.0	0	+, liver (1); +, abdomen (1)
349	44.0	+ (1)	−, liver (1); ʄ+, lumbar (1)
347*	96.0	0	+, abdomen

*Cases positive for tumor by radioimmunodetection prior to other detection methods.
[a]A value above 2.5 ng/ml is considered to be abnormal. [b]+, tumor identified; −, tumor missed; 0, tumor excised; N, no tumor identified or missed; ?+, positive scan with or without confirmatory clinical data available; +/−. questionable scan with or without correlative data. [c]Number in parentheses, number of tumor sites imaged. [d]Patients with two or more numbers underwent a repeat radioimmunodetection study. [e]Incomplete study, since lateral view not scanned. [f]Liver radionuclide scan also unrevealing.

SUMMARY

This paper first reviews the current status of gastrointestinal tumor markers. In colorectal cancer, the principal markers of immediate clinical interest are carcinoembryonic antigen (CEA), galactosyltransferase isoenzyme-II (GT-II), Tennessee antigen (TennaGen), and colon specific antigen p (CSAp). Review of the available clinical results with these four markers reveals that they are neither cancer specific nor diagnostic of colorectal cancer. A combined study of blood titers of CEA and CSAp shows that either marker was increased in 84% of 31 patients with colorectal cancer, suggesting a possible value in testing both markers in prospective colorectal cancer patients. Most of these tumor markers present in the blood serve as indicators of tumor burden.

The use of radioactive antitumor antibodies for the external scintigraphic detection of cancer, called radioimmunodetection, is reviewed in terms of our clinical experience with CEA tumor radioimmunodetection. Among a series of 52 patients with a history of colorectal cancer, 83% of primary and 91% of metastatic tumor sites could be detected, thus yielding an overall true positive detection rate (sensitivity) of 89%. A number of patients with normal plasma CEA titers had primary and metastatic tumors demonstrable by radioimmunodetection, while very high blood titers in other patients did not hinder successful antibody localisation. In 11 of 51 patients studied, true positive radioimmunodetection results were obtained when other diagnostic measures were unrevealing, thus indicating the clinical utility of this new approach despite its early history and level of development. It is suggested that improvement in antibody reagents, in choice of radionuclides, and in the scanning devices used, together with the application of multimarker antibody mixtures, may advance radioimmunodetection to achieve improved sensitivity and specificity for early, small tumor lesions.

ACKNOWLEDGEMENTS

I am indebted to Dr Frank H. DeLand, Dr E. Edmund Kim, Dr Sidney J. Bennett, Mr Jimmy R. Salyer and Ms Usha Shah for their collaboration in the clinical radioimmunodetection studies, and to Dr Keshab D. Pant, Dr Dan Shochat and Mr Howard L. Dahlman for their contributions in the study and development of CSAp.

REFERENCES

Abelev, G. I., Perova, S. D., Khramkova, N. I., Postnikova, Z. A. and Irlin, I. S. (1963). *Transplantation* **1**, 174.
Bara, J., Paul-Bardais, A., Loisillier, F. and Burtin, P. (1978). *International Journal of Cancer* **21**, 133.
DeLand, F. H., Kim, E. E., Simmons, G. and Goldenberg, D. M. (1980). *Cancer Research* **40**, 3046.
DeLand, F. H., Kim, E. E., Casper, S., Corgan, R. L., Dine, M. E. and Goldenberg, D. M. (1981). *American Journal of Roentgenology*. (In press.)
Gaffar, S. A., Pant, K. D., Shochat, D., Bennett, S. J. and Goldenberg, D. M. (1981). *International Journal of Cancer* **27**, 101.
Gelder, F. B., Reese, C. J., Moossa, A. R., Hall, T. and Hunter, R. (1978). *Cancer Research* **38**, 313.
Gilbertsen, V. A. and Wangensteen, O. H. (1962). *Surgery, Gynaecology and Obstetrics* **114**, 438.
Gold, D. V. (1979). *In* "Compendium of Assays for Immunodiagnosis of Human Cancer" (R. B. Herberman, Ed.), pp. 231–236. Elsevier North-Holland, New York.
Gold, D. V. and Goldenberg, D. M. (1980). *In* "Cancer Markers. Diagnostic and Developmental Significance" (S. Sell, Ed.), pp. 329–369. Humana Press, Clifton, N.Y.
Gold, D. V. and Miller, F. (1974). *Immunochemistry* **11**, 369.
Gold, P. and Freedman, S. O. (1965). *Journal of Experimental Medicine* **122**, 467.
Goldenberg, D. M. (1978). *Cancer Bulletin* **30**, 213.
Goldenberg, D. M. (1979). *Acta Hepato-Gastroenterologica* **26**, 1.
Goldenberg, D. M. (1981). *In* "Gastrointestinal Cancer". Raven Press, New York. (In press.)
Goldenberg, D. M., Witte, S. and Elster, K. (1966). *Transplantation* **4**, 760.
Goldenberg, D. M., Pant, K. D. and Dahlman, H. L. (1976a). *Cancer Research* **36**, 3455.
Goldenberg, D. M., Pant, K. D. and Dahlman, H. L. (1976b). *Proceedings of the American Association for Cancer Research* **17**, 155.
Goldenberg, D. M., DeLand, F. H., Kim, E., Bennett, S., Primus, F. J., van Nagell, J. R., Jr, Estes, N., DeSimone, P. and Rayburn, P. (1978). *New England Journal of Medicine* **298**, 1384.
Goldenberg, D. M., DeLand, F. and Primus, F. J. (1979). *In* "Immunodiagnosis of Cancer, Part 1" (R. B. Herberman and K. R. McIntire, Eds), pp. 265–304. Marcel Dekker Inc., New York.
Goldenberg, D. M., Kim, E. E., DeLand, F. H., Bennett, S. and Primus, F. J. (1980a). *Cancer Research* **40**, 2984.
Goldenberg, D. M., Kim, E. E., DeLand, F. H., van Nagell, J. R., Jr and Javadpour, N. (1980b). *Science (Wash. D. C.)* **208**, 1284.

Häkkinen, I. P. T., Jarvi, O. and Gironross, J. (1968). *International Journal of Cancer* **3**, 572.
Podolsky, D. K., Weiser, M. M., Isselbacher, K. J. and Cohen, A. M. (1978). *New England Journal of Medicine* **299**, 703.
Herrera, M. A., Chu, T. M. and Holyoke, E. D. (1976). *Annals of Surgery* **183**, 5.
Holyoke, E. D., Chu, T. M. and Murphy, G. P. (1975). *Cancer* **25**, 830.
Ishii, M. (1979). *In* "Compendium of Assays for Immunodiagnosis of Human Cancer" (R. B. Herberman, Ed.), pp. 45–50. Elsevier North-Holland, New York.
Javadpour, N., Kim, E. E., DeLand, F. H., Salyer, J. R., Shah, U. and Goldenberg, D. M. (1981). *Journal of the American Medical Association.* (In press.)
Kawasaki, H., Imasato, K. and Kimoto, E. (1971). *Gann* **62**, 171.
Mach, J. -P., Vienny, H., Jaeger, P., Haldemann, B., Egely, R. and Pettavel, J. (1978). *Cancer* **42**, 1439.
Martin, E. W., Jr, Cooperman, M. and Minton, J. P. (1979). *In* "Compendium of Assays for Immunodiagnosis of Human Cancer" (R. B. Herberman, Ed.), p. 215. Elsevier North-Holland, New York.
Mayer, R. J., Garnick, M. B., Steele, G. D., Jr and Zamcheck, N. (1978). *Cancer* **42**, 1428.
Pant, K. D. and Goldenberg, D. M. (1979). *In* "Compendium of Assays for Immunodiagnosis of Human Cancer" (R. B. Herberman, Ed.), pp. 225–229. Elsevier North-Holland, New York.
Pant, K. D., Dahlman, H. L. and Goldenberg, D. M. (1977). *Immunological Communications* **6**, 411.
Pant, K. D., Shochat, D., Nelson, M. O. and Goldenberg, D. M. (1981). *Proceedings of American Association of Cancer Research* **22**. (In press.)
Potter, T. P., Jr, Jordan, T., Jordan, J. D. and Lasater, H. (1978). *In* "Prevention and Detection of Cancer, Part II, Detection, High Risk Markers, Detection Methods and Management" (H. E. Nieburgs, Ed.), pp. 467–490. Marcel Dekker, New York.
Potter, T. P., Jr, Jordan, J. D. and Jordan, T. A. (1979). *In* "Compendium of Assays for Immunodiagnosis of Human Cancer" (R. B. Herberman, Ed.), pp. 217–224. Elsevier North-Holland, New York.
Pusztaszeri, G., Saravis, C. A. and Zamcheck, N. (1976). *Journal of the National Cancer Institute* **56**, 275.
Rapp, W., Windisch, M., Peschke, P. and Wurster, K. (1979). *Virchows Archiv, A Pathologie, Anatomie und Histologie* **382**, 163.
Shochat, D., Archey, R. L., Pant, K. D., Dahlman, H. L., Gold, D. V. and Goldenberg, D. M. (1981). *Journal of Immunology* **126**, 2284.
Sugarbaker, P. H., Bloomer, W. D., Corbett, E. D. and Chaffey, J. T. (1976). *American Journal of Roentgenology* **127**, 641.
van Nagell, J. R., Jr, Kim, E. E., Casper, S., Primus, F. J., Bennett, S., DeLand, F. H. and Goldenberg, D. M. (1980). *Cancer Research* **40**, 502.
Wanebo, H. J., Bhaskar, R., Pinsky, C. M., Hoffman, R. G., Stearns, M., Schwartz, M. J. and Oettgen, H. F. (1978). *New England Journal of Medicine* **299**, 448.

A NON-CEA MARKER IN COLORECTAL CANCER

D. M. P. Thomson

The Montreal General Hospital, Montreal, Quebec, Canada

INTRODUCTION

Historically, the search for constituents that are unique to tumor tissue began over 100 years ago. With the introduction of inbred strains of mice, Foley (1953) produced the first evidence for antigenicity of experimentally induced tumors.

Many human tumor antigen systems have been described in recent years. Some of the molecules that have the properties of tumor markers may, in fact, be normal tissue constituents produced in increased quantities as a result of malignant transformation. Tumor cells, as a result of the failure to differentiate, synthesise tissue constituents that are normally expressed during human fetal and embryonic life. These oncofetal molecules may represent developmental enzymes or substances of unknown functions such as carcinoembryonic antigen and α1-fetoprotein. Many of the substances have been termed tumor antigens, largely because they are measured by immunological methods, but in actual fact may not be immunogeneic in man.

The ability of the host to mount a specific antitumor immune response indicates the presence of specific tumor antigens. Evidence has accumulated during the past 15 years that human cancers express neoantigens. Moreover, many studies with a variety of *in vitro* methods suggest that the commonest neoantigens are organ specific. But most *in vitro* assays used to detect the host's immune response to the neoantigens are hampered by complexity and disclaimed for irreproducibility. Halliday and Miller (1972), however, described a most promising *in vitro* assay of antitumor immunity which is based on the phenomenon that

Serono Symposium No. 46, Markers for Diagnosis and Monitoring of Human Cancer, edited by M. I. Colnaghi, G. L. Buraggi and M. Ghione, 1982. Academic Press, London and New York.

leukocytes from patients with cancer, after being incubated with extracts of cancer of the same organ and histogenesis, lose their former ability to adhere to glass surfaces. A modified assay (Holan *et al.*, 1974), called tube LAI (Leukocyte Adherence Inhibition) by Grosser and Thomson (1975), was adopted and it was automated by computer driven image analysis (Tataryn *et al.*, 1978).

For years it has been customary to believe that the tumor associated phenotypes could be exploited in immunological assays to identify patients with cancer. Phenotypic tumor markers, such as carcinoembryonic antigen, α1-fetoprotein, acid phosphatase, and chorionic gonadotropin, have been clinically useful in discovering and monitoring patients with advanced cancers. But because they are metabolised, diluted in the body fluids and excreted, they are usually detectable only when most of the cancers are large. As a result they have not proved useful for diagnosing early and curable cancer. The organ specific neoantigens, unlike the other tumor phenotypes, are immmunogenic in humans; even small quantities of shed tumor antigens stimulate the host's immune system. The immune response becomes amplified, so that antitumor immunity can be detected when many cancers are small, even *in situ* and curable.

In this review of LAI in colorectal cancer, we will describe some of the features of the LAI response, which we have studied, the evidence for the diagnostic ability of the assay, and the characteristics of putative antigens expressed by colorectal cancers.

TUBE LAI ASSAY

The assay has been described previously (Grosser and Thomson, 1975). Buffy coat peripheral blood leukocytes, admixed with crude extracts from solid tumor and in medium without fetal calf serum, are incubated in glass tubes placed horizontally to allow the cells to adhere to the glass surface. Later nonadherent cells are counted automatically by a computer linked image analyzer. The computer expresses the difference on nonadherent cells as a nonadherence index (NAI):

$$NAI = \frac{A - B}{B} \times 100$$

where A equals a sample of the nonadherent cells incubated with specific cancer, and B equals a sample of the nonadherent cells incubated with the other unrelated, control cancer extract. NAIs $\geqslant$ 30 are accepted as positive because less than 5% of hospitalised patients with benign diseases or cancer of organs unrelated to the specific cancer extracts have NAIs $\geqslant$ 30 (Grosser and Thomson, 1975; Marti and Thomson, 1976; Flores *et al.*, 1977; Lopez *et al.*, 1978; O'Connor *et al.*, 1978; Tataryn *et al.*, 1979; Ayeni *et al.*, 1980).

Of critical importance is that the leukocytes' recognition of tumor antigen is determined by their difference in nonadherence when incubated with the specific and non-specific cancer extracts at the same time. By always examining the leukocytes' reactivity to two tumor extracts in a criss-cross fashion, it is possible to be certain that the changes in their glass adherence properties under differing experimental conditions represents a specific physiological change. Failure to test the leukocytes response against two differing cancer extracts accounts for many of the reported failures to find tumor specific reactivity (Hellstrom *et al.*, 1976, 1977; Ballard and Dickinson, 1980; Dusheiko *et al.*, 1979).

In the studies reported in this review, colon and other cancer specimens, obtained at necropsy from metastatic deposits in the liver, were homogenised in phosphate buffered saline. A principle drawback of the assay is the dependance on surgical or necropsy specimens which can be expected to vary in their antigenic content because of events which befall the tissues before their preservation by freezing. So recently, we have been examining cancer cells that are able to grow in nude mice or tissue culture. Four differing human tumors grown in nude mice were supplied to us coded. Four of four transplanted human cancers—colon, pancreas, lung and breast –were found to express their organ specific neoantigens, but less well than cancers metastatic in the liver.

We have found, as have others, that tissue cultured cancer cells also express organ specific neoantigens as assayed by LAI (Khosravi *et al.*, 1981; Sanner *et al.*, 1980). We have used a bladder cancer cell line for 8 months as a source of antigen for LAI. It seems to express a higher and better content of tumor antigen than primary or metastatic bladder cancer. The cost, however, of growing enough cells for each different type of cancer is prohibitive for us. Besides, metastatic colon specimens have usually expressed reasonable tumor antigen activity. Nonetheless, tissue cultured cancer cells may prove to be a reliable antigen source that would allow different laboratories to work with standardised cancer extracts.

SPECIFICITY OF ANTITUMOR IMMUNITY

Most serological assays are controlled internally by using standards which give positive and negative results. Cell mediated assays like LAI, on the other hand, depend upon fresh leukocytes as one of the reactants. Ideally, the LAI assay is standardised daily with fresh leukocytes from different patients; some of which react positively, and others negatively, to the specific cancer extracts. A negative control can easily be included in the assay daily by testing leukocytes from a variety of hospitalised patients without the specific cancer.

Figure 1 show a histogram for the NAI distribution of 653 patients without cancer or benign diseases of the colorectum whose leukocytes were tested against extracts of colon and lung cancer. The NAI is almost normally distributed about the zero value. And less than 5% have had an NAI $\geq$ 30 to the colon cancer extract.

As leukocytes from hospitalised patients suspected of having colon cancer become available, they too are tested to assess whether they exhibit a greater response than the control subjects to the colon cancer extract. Figure 1 shows a histogram for the NAI distribution of 101 patients with stage A and B colorectal cancer. Unlike the controls, patients with early colon cancer have NAIs whose frequency distribution is markedly skewed to the right and is significantly different ($P < 0.001$) from the control patients. Sixty-six per cent, in fact, have an NAI $\geq$ 30. Figure 1 shows the NAI distribution of 163 patients with advanced cancer; only about 20% respond positively. But if patients with stage IV cancer are divided on the basis of their clinically apparent tumor burden, those with

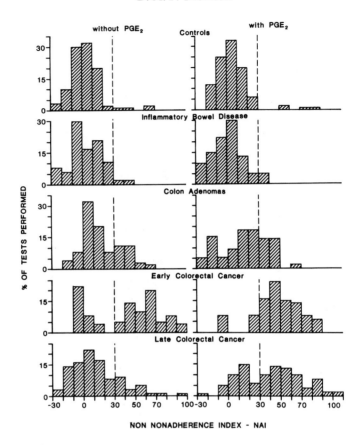

Fig. 1. Distribution of NAIs. Colon cancer is the specific extract, and lung cancer is the non-specific, control extract. Controls were hospital patients without colorectal disease or lung cancer.

solitary lesions often react (87%), while those with multiple metastatic foci seldom react (17%).

The specificity of the response is further evaluated by testing the LAI response of patients with colon polyps and inflammatory bowel disease. Less than 5% of patients with inflammatory bowel disease have an LAI$^+$ response (Fig. 1). Patients with colon adenomas, on the other hand, often react in the tube LAI assay to the colon cancer extract (Fig. 1).

Organ Specific Neoantigen of Human Cancer

Human cancers, arising in an organ and of similar histogenesis, express a cell surface molecule with a common antigenic epitope to which only patients with a like cancer react; the organ specific neoantigens are recognised by allogeneic or autochthonous leukocytes from patients with the same cancers. Leukocytes from patients with cancer other than colorectum react positively with colorectal cancer extracts so seldom that, when it does occur, we are never certain whether it represents an example of more than one neoantigen being expressed by the principal cancer or an antigenic stimulus from a dysplastic lesion or early cancer of the colorectum. Figure 2 shows that patients with colon cancer respond only to colon cancer neoantigens. Other cancers arising in nearby or even distant organs express organ specific neoantigens which have antigenic determinants that do not cross react. So we find that cancers of the stomach, pancreas and colon exhibit no cross-reactivity amongst themselves. For that matter, even cancers of the small intestine express an organ specific neoantigen that is distinct from the colorectal cancer neoantigen.

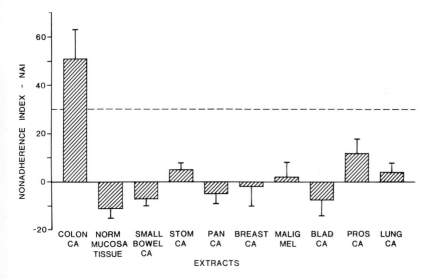

Fig. 2. The NAI of leukocytes from LAI[+] colon cancer patients to different extracts, tested in a paired fashion. Colon cancer extract was paired with a lung cancer extract as was the normal colon mucosa extract.

Expression of Organ Specific Neoantigens by Pre-malignant Lesions

In most tissues the development of a neoplasm is a gradual process involving a series of sequential alterations during pre-neoplastic and pre-malignant phases (Foulds, 1975). The ultimate cancer phenotype is associated with the loss of some specialised functions and with the appearance of proteins which are usually present either at an earlier stage in development or in a different tissue (Potter, 1978). Consequently, many types of human and experimental malignant neoplasms are associated with phenotypic characteristics of embryonal, fetal or regenerating cells or tissues (Weinhouse and Ono, 1972). Some markers, in fact, appear early in the cancer process and long before the appearance of overt cancer (Farber et al., 1979; Ogawa et al., 1979). Indeed, the phenotypic cancer markers are often considered to be the result of altered gene control and expression, and they seem to be intimately associated with the malignant behavior (Holliday, 1979).

Potter (1978) makes the point that a fetal organ consists of a cell population that participates in an organised series of changes resulting in a functional organ. A clonal neoplasm, to the contrary, will not recall the total program although it may have much of the phenotypic variation seen in a population of normal cells from the same organ. The neoplastic cells, unlike the normal, have a block in their differentiation; called either "blocked ontogeny" or "partially blocked ontogeny" (Potter, 1978).

Stem cells of an organ, presumably at some point during their differentiation, express organ specific neoantigens, but the final adult cells of the organ do not. And yet, when cells become dysplastic or cancerous, they express, once again, the organ specific neoantigen; their differentiation is blocked, so it seems, at the point where the organ specific neoantigens are expressed. Even though the organ specific neoantigens are yet another cancer phenotype, the unique characteristic of these antigens is their immunogenicity in humans, for none of the other phenotypic cancer markers, described so far, share this feature.

Yet some investigators—on the basis of their results with *in vitro* assays—have concluded that cancer patients are sensitised to normal tissue antigens of the organ. But as far as we can tell, leukocytes of most cancer patients are not sensitised to normal tissue antigens: first, leukocytes from LAI^+ patients do not react to extracts of the normal organ (Fig. 2); second, patients with severe inflammatory organ disease, as a rule, are not LAI^+ (Fig. 1). And yet there are patients without cancer but with dysplastic lesions who do react specifically to the cancer extracts (Fig. 1) (Flores *et al.*, 1977; O'Connor *et al.*, 1978; Tataryn *et al.*, 1979).

The LAI^+ responses of patients with colon adenomas were shown not to be directed against normal tissue antigens in extracts prepared from the normal organ (Thomson *et al.*, 1979a; Tataryn *et al.*, 1979). Their response, tested against the partially purified organ specific neoantigen, was similar to the patient with cancer of the same organ (Thomson *et al.*, 1979a). Furthermore, when the benign lesion or the cancer was excised, the positive response disappeared about 3 months later, indicating that the excised lesion was responsible for stimulating the antitumor immune response (Tataryn *et al.*, 1979). Apparently, some adenomas express organ specific neoantigen like cancers arising from the same organ.

Others have accumulated evidence to suggest that colon adenomas have malignant potential, and the histogenesis of the polyp cancer sequence has been documented repeatedly (Morson, 1974; Enterline, 1976; Fenoglio *et al.*, 1977). Figure 1 shows how the NAIs of 110 patients with adenomas, unlike the controls, are distributed biphasically and skewed to the right; 24% of this group react to the colon cancer extract. The LAI^+ patients with adenomas, of course, do not react against extracts of normal colon mucosa.

Adenomas, they approach but do not attain the final adult state, are a case of "partially" blocked ontogeny. As part of the block in their differentiation, some express a phenotypic marker of cancer, the immunogenic organ specific neoantigen. So far there is no evidence to suggest that adenomas expressing organ specific neoantigens are less differentiated so more prone to become cancers than the adenomas not expressing organ specific neoantigens. Needless to say, the assay would be of considerable value if it did distinguish adenomas likely to become a cancer shortly.

MECHANISM MEDIATING LAI PHENOMENON

LAI Reactive Cell and Arming

Maluish and Halliday (1975) found that the LAI reactive cell, when it bound the sensitising tumor antigen, released mediators causing other leukocytes to be nonadherent, the leukocytes that released the mediators were reported to be T cells. Other investigators have confirmed their findings, and we too have observed that armed macrophages are able to release mediators. Originally, however, we failed to detect mediators in the tube LAI assay (Grosser and Thomson, 1975; Marti *et al.,* 1976).

To define the cell mediating the LAI phenomenon, subpopulation of PBL, deleted and/or enriched, were put into the tube LAI assay. Only leukocytes enriched for monocytes reacted (Grosser *et al.,* 1976). If, as our experiments indicated, the monocyte reacts directly with the tumor antigen, then the mechanism by which the tumor antigen was recognised had to be demonstrated, for we had not excluded the possibility that products from small numbers of lymphocytes contaminating the monocyte cell population produced mediators to alter the monocytes' adhesiveness, When serum, or the IgG fraction, from LAI$^+$ patients was preincubated with normal PBL, the "armed" cells reacted in an immunologically specific manner (Marti *et al.,* 1976). Whenever LAI$^+$ leukocytes were detected, the serum of these patients were found to contain arming antitumor antibody.

Other investigators have confirmed that serum from LAI$^+$ patients can arm normal PBL to react specifically (Bhatti *et al.,* 1979; Goldrosen *et al.,* 1979). In this regard, it is especially interesting that Sanner *et al.* (1980) using the hemocytometer assay, has been able to arm normal leukocytes with serum from LAI$^+$ patients.

Cross-linking of Cell Surface IgG

The interaction of antigen with antigen sensitive cells is required to initiate the programmed cell functions. Cross-linking of cell bound IgG molecules with secondary bridging of IgG–Fc receptors initiates a complex series of events in the plasma membrane, and a signal is delivered to antigen sensitive cells as a consequence. This leads to biochemical reactions that culminate in physiological responses, producing the phenomenon of LAI. Human IgGs, heat aggregated for 15 and 30 min, and the same quantity of natural IgG, were added separately to normal leukocytes. The leukocytes incubated with heat aggregated IgG exhibited enhanced nonadherence from the glass; cross-linked IgG, in the form of heat aggregated IgG, binding to leukocytes mediates LAI. In a second experiment, cell surface γ-globulins of normal leukocytes were cross-linked with similar amounts of anti-human IgG, and IgA, and IgM. The anti-human IgG, but not anti-human IgA and IgM, enhanced leukocyte nonadherence; the leukocyte nonadherence simulated a positive LAI response.

Calcium Ion Fluxes

Calcium ion influx is a critical link between a specific stimulus and the physiological response. When a cell is stimulated one of the first events triggered is a transient, but marked, increase in free intracellular calcium concentrations. The increase plays an important role as a signal to produce the appropriate responses in many biological processes.

Calcium ionophore increases the permeability of cell membranes to calcium, and calcium thus flows down a concentration gradient. Leukocytes incubated with the ionophore exhibited enhanced nonadherence (Fig. 3). Not unexpectedly, when LAI$^+$ leukocytes were preincubated with 2×10^{-6} M ionophore, their reactivity to the sensitising tumor antigen was negated.

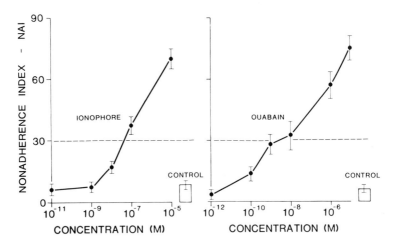

Fig. 3. Concentration effect curves for calcium ionophore or Ouabain on normal leukocyte adherence inhibition. Extract A containing the drug is the specific antigen and extract B containing a similar amount of protein but no drug being the control antigen. The control bar is the nonadherence of leukocytes to extracts A and B not containing any drug.

In a second experiment, Ouabain was used to increase intracellular calcium. Inhibiting sodium potassium ATPase, Ouabain's overall effect is to increase the net intracellular calcium concentration. Normal leukocytes responded to the admixture of extract and Ouabain as though the cell were sensitised to the Ouabain (Fig. 3). Then as expected, LAI$^+$ leukocytes preincubated with 2×10^{-6} M Ouabain had their response nullified.

The two preceding experiments indicated that increasing the intracellular concentration of Ca^{2+} triggers a response which is manifested by the loss of the leukocytes' glass adherence properties. Experiments where calcium ion fluxes were prevented were then undertaken with Intal$^{®}$ (Na cromoglycate), lidocaine, and the inorganic and organic Ca^{2+} channel antagonists, La^{3+} and nifedipine, respectively. At the appropriate concentrations, they had no effect on the glass adherence properties of normal leukocytes. But when LAI$^+$ leukocytes were preincubated with them, the leukocytes' subsequent reactivity to the sensitising tumor antigen was inhibited, indicating the importance of calcium ion fluxes and the calcium channel in triggering the leukocytes' response after binding tumor antigens.

Prostaglandins

Leukocytes from LAI^+ patients, for 1-2 weeks after surgery, cease to react (Grosser and Thomson, 1975; Marti and Thomson, 1976). In studying the possible mechanism(s) of the immunosuppression, corticosteroids were implicated as being important: corticosteroid levels rose during surgery and remained elevated for some days (Flores *et al.*, 1976); corticosteroids added *in vitro* to the assay inhibited LAI activity (Flores *et al.*, 1976; Grosser *et al.*, 1980) and LAI^+ leukocytes were inhibited from reacting when the patients had received corticosteroids shortly before (Grosser *et al.*, 1980).

A key step in the synthesis of prostaglandins is the freeing of arachidonate from membrane phospholipids. Steroidal anti-inflammatory drugs, preventing phospholipase A_2 activation, inhibit the removal of arachidonic acid from membrane phospholipids, and this blocks the synthesis of products from it. Accordingly, what effect PGE_2 had when added to the leukocytes after surgery was examined. PGE_2 reversed the surgical immunosuppression of LAI activity (Fig. 4). Figure 5 shows that only a narrow concentration range of PGE_2 converts the response to positive. For PGE_2, effects were undetected below 10^{-6} M, were nearly maximal between 10^{-6} and 10^{-5} M, and declined above 10^{-5} M; at 10^{-4} M PGE_2 induced minimal or no response.

Leukocytes from advanced cancer patients seldom react in the assay because excess circulating tumor antigen desensitises their reactivity (Grosser and Thomson, 1976); we hypothesised that this was induced by antigen coating all binding sites of the reactive cells (Grosser and Thomson, 1976). In fact, LAI^- cells from advanced cancer patients were converted to positive by exposing them to a

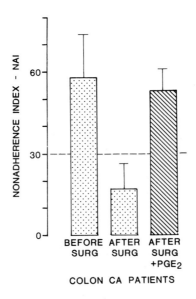

Fig. 4. The effect of PGE_2 stimulation on LAI^+ leukocytes after surgery. Before surgery the leukocytes of the patients with colon cancer were LAI^+. Five days after surgery the leukocytes' response was negative, but if the leukocytes were incubated with 10^{-6} M PGE_2 for 5 min, the response reverted to positive.

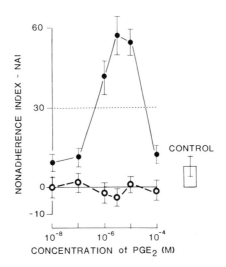

Fig. 5. The effects of PGE_2 concentrations on the NAI. After surgery, leukocytes from now LAI^- early cancer patients (● ———●), and control patients (○ - - - -○) were stimulated with different concentrations of PGE_2 for 5 min and then plated in the assay, and the difference to the specific and non-specific cancer extracts determined. The control bar represents the NAI of LAI^- early cancer patients after surgery in the absence of PGE_2 stimulation.

critical concentration of trypsin (Grosser and Thomson, 1976; Thomson *et al.*, 1979b). Previously, we suggested that trypsin acted by digesting the tumor antigen from the leukocytes' cell surface (Grosser and Thomson, 1976; Thomson *et al.*, 1979b). But proteolytic enzymes, particularly trypsin, activate cell surface adenylate cyclase, increasing intracellular cyclic AMP (Parker, 1974). So it seemed appropriate to determine whether PGE_2 stimulated leukocytes from advanced cancer patients could be rendered reactive.

PGE_2 converted the negative response of advanced cancer patients to positive (Kaneti *et al.*, 1981). The change was affected swiftly, but there was only a narrow dose-response range. Figure 1 shows the distribution of the NAI values of patients with differing stages of colon cancer without and with PGE_2 stimulation. The LAI responses of patients with Dukes' A and B colorectal cancer, was largely unaffected by PGE_2 stimulation (Fig. 1). But many more leukocytes from advanced colon cancer patients responded to the colon cancer extract if preincubated for 5 min with 5×10^{-6} M PGE_2 (Fig. 1). The change in LAI activity is immunologically specific, for leukocytes from patients with cancers other than colon cancer showed no change in their reactivity to the colon cancer or the control, non-specific antigen (Fig. 1).

PGE_2, it is known, stimulates adenylate cyclase to raise intracellular levels of cyclic AMP. In fact, the leukocytes' intracellular cyclic AMP was elevated four- to five-fold immediately after incubation with PGE_2. Other substances that elevate intracellular cyclic AMP or inhibit its degradation heightened the LAI response, too.

To show how tumor antigen can negate the LAI^+ response and how PGE_2 can convert it back, LAI^+ leukocytes from patients with early colon cancer were preincubated with serum from advanced cancer patients, colon and breast

(Fig. 6). LAI[+] leukocytes from colon cancer patients, preincubated with serum from colon cancer or breast cancer patients, had their response blocked in an immunologically specific manner only by serum from advanced colon cancer patients (Fig. 6). The same cells, after preincubation with the colon cancer patients' serum, washed once, and then incubated briefly with PGE_2 before plating in the assay, had their specific LAI reactivity restored (Fig. 5).

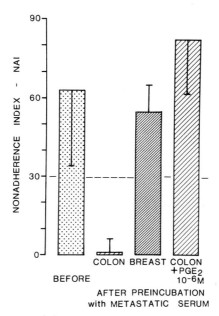

Fig. 6. Specific inhibition of LAI[+] response by colon cancer tumor antigen and restoration of LAI response by PGE_2 stimulation.

Effect of Arachidonic Acid Metabolism on LAI Response

By stimulating the synthesis of intracellular nucleotides, prostaglandins seem to modulate the LAI response of sensitised leukocytes. To evaluate whether prostaglandin metabolites were essential for the reactivity of primed LAI[+] leukocytes, we examined the effect of indomethacin, a competitive inhibitor of the cyclo-oxygenase pathway of arachidonic acid metabolism. Over a range of concentrations maintained throughout the 2 h assay, indomethacin, if anything, enhanced the LAI responses; possibly by inhibiting the cyclo-oxygenase pathway for arachidonic metabolism, more arachidonic acid was being diverted to the lipoxygenase pathway.

Mepacrine (Blackwell *et al.*, 1978; Burka and Paterson, 1980) and BPB (Roberts *et al.*, 1977), like corticosteroids, exert much of their inflammatory action by inhibiting phospholipase A_2, limiting free endogenous arachidonic acid which serves as a substrate for cyclo-oxygenase and lipoxygenase metabolic pathways (Flower and Blackwell, 1976). Mepacrine and BPB inhibited LAI activity in a dose-response fashion (Fig. 7). Since the experiments with indomethacin indi-

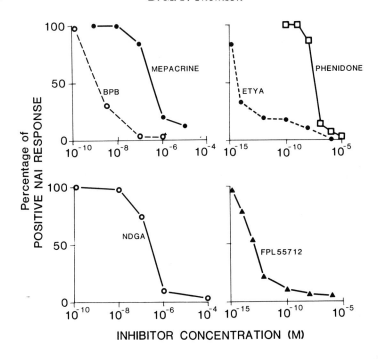

Fig. 7. Effects of BPB, mepacrine ETYA, phenidone, NDGA, and FPL 57712 on LAI$^+$ response. The results are expressed as percentages of the activity found for untreated LAI$^+$ cells.

cated that primed leukocytes do not require metabolites of the cyclo-oxygenase pathway for them to respond upon initial exposure to the sensitising tumor antigen, other arachidonic acid metabolic pathways must be more critical in mediating the phenomenon of LAI. For this reason we assessed whether lipoxygenase inhibitors negated the expression of LAI activity. ETYA (Hamberg and Samuelsson, 1974) or phenidone (Blackwell and Flower, 1978), lipoxygenase/ cyclo-oxygenase inhibitors, nullified the LAI$^+$ response to tumor antigen (Fig. 7); the failure of arachidonic acid to be metabolised by the lipoxygenase pathway, so it seems, is responsible for inhibiting LAI.

Nordihydroguaiaretic acid (NDGA), an anti-oxidant, has been reported to be a specific inhibitor of the lipoxygenase pathway and methyltransferase-like enzymes (Naccache *et al.*, 1979; Hamberg, 1976), though it is also considered by some to inhibit thromboxane synthesis. When LAI$^+$ leukocytes were briefly incubated with NDGA, their response was negated in a dose-dependant fashion (Fig. 7). LAI$^-$ leukocytes from advanced cancer patients, converted to positive with PGE$_2$ or aminophylline stimulation, also had their LAI response inhibited by being incubated with NDGA, mepacrine, BPB, ETYA or phenidone.

Slow reacting substance of anaphylaxis (SRS-A) is a product of the lipoxygenation pathway; leukotriene C and D (LTC$_4$ and LTD$_4$) seem to be the functionally critical components of SRS-A (Parker *et al.*, 1979; Goetzl, 1980). FPL 55712 is reported to be a specific antagonist of SRS-A (Augstein *et al.*, 1973).

When LAI$^+$ leukocytes, either with or without PGE$_2$ stimulation, were preincubated with FPL 55712, a dose-dependent inhibition is obtained between 10^{-13} to 10^{-6} M (Fig. 7). Varying degrees of inhibition are found, however, at concentrations as low as 10^{-14} M.

Modulation of the Expression of Human Antitumor Immunity

The leukocytes' adherence properties to glass reflect its physiological status. Stimulation of leukocytes by an antigen receptor reaction triggers biochemical reactions and physiological responses, altering the leukocytes' adherence properties. But if a drug blocks a critical biochemical reaction the leukocytes' glass adherence properties remain unaltered because, we believe, physiological responses do not attain full development. Seemingly there is a close relationship between the complete expression of the leukocytes' programmed cell function and changes in glass adherence properties.

For the expression of the effector arm of human antitumor immunity *in vitro,* the interplay of calcium fluxes, intracellular cyclic nucleotides, and metabolites of arachidonic acid are critically important. The movement of Ca^{2++} ions into the cell, by either calcium ionophore or Ouabain, triggers changes that alter the glass adherence properties of the leukocytes which initiate the phenomenon of antigen induced LAI. Prostaglandins modulate the expression of antitumor immunity by affecting intracellular nucleotides. Lipoxygenase products of arachidonic acid seem to be essential if the cells after binding tumor antigen and delivering a signal are to express their programmed function. Inhibitors of ATP synthesis, microfilament and microtubular function do not alter the adherence properties of the resting cell but do prevent the changes that normally follow binding of tumor antigen (Thomson *et al.,* 1981).

When the cancer is not advanced, the host bearing the tumor reacts briskly against the tumor *in vitro* and *in vivo.* Having encountered repeatedly tumor antigen *in vivo,* leukocytes from patients with advanced cancer have already undergone a series of biochemical and physiological response which has desensitised the cells, explaining why they fail to respond in the LAI assay.

A variety of substances that affected intracellular nucleotides, including dibutyryl cyclic AMP and dibutyryl cyclic GMP, reversed the deactivated state of leukocytes from advanced cancer patients. Cyclic AMP and cyclic GMP are thought to regulate many opposing functions of leukocytes and other cells (Hadden *et al.,* 1975), and we had expected to find that the refractory state of leukocytes could be reversed only by substances that stimulated the intracellular production of either cyclic AMP or cyclic GMP. However, it has been speculated that changes in the ratio of intracellular nucleotides may be more important for regulating cellular activities than are their absolute concentrations (Watson *et al.,* 1973).

The results of our studies indicate clearly that leukocytes obtained from patients after surgery or with advanced cancer lacked sufficient intracellular nucleotides to reverse the cellular re-arrangements signalled by either stress hormones or free tumor antigen binding to cell surface receptors. In both situations the production of prostaglandins, it seems, was wanting. Likewise, in mice bearing B-16 melanomas immune responses were profoundly suppressed

(Favelli *et al.,* 1980). Favelli *et al.* (1980) showed that these responses were significantly augmented by treating the mice with a long acting analog of PGE_2. Indomethacin only impaired the responses further (Favelli *et al.,* 1980). Others have suggested that overproduction of PGE_2 by macrophages, the prinicpal source of leukocytes PGE_2 (Ferraris *et al.,* 1974), may be responsible for depressed immune responses (Goodwin *et al.,* 1977; Stenson and Parker, 1980: Strom *et al.,* 1977; Fulton and Levy, 1980).

Leukocytes seem unable to respond repeatedly to tumor antigen unless after each encounter intracellular nucleotide production is activated, reaching a sufficient level to reverse the deactivated state. Prostaglandins synthesised during the immune effector response may, in fact, be an important feed-back mechanism by which the cells maintain an antigen responsive state. Corticosteroids, and presumably indomethacin, over a longer period have an inhibitory effect on LAI activity, immune responses and inflammation by preventing prostaglandin synthesis and/or enhancing prostaglandin breakdown (Moore and Hoult, 1980a, b).

Prostaglandins, so it seems, prime the cell and reverse the refractory state of leukocytes triggered by binding antigen. Our studies show, conclusively, that leukocytes from patients bearing advanced cancers are not primed to react to tumor antigen; presumably this is because monocyte derived prostaglandins have not been able to maintain adequate intracellular nucleotide synthesis in the face of continual encounters with tumor antigen *in vivo* and not because prostaglandins are acting as physiological inhibitors of the immune effect or response (Goodwin *et al.,* 1980; Plescia *et al.,* 1975).

Calcium is the second messenger that mediated the cell's response to bound tumor antigen. Cyclic nucleotides, raised by a variety of mechanisms, seem to be the physiological agents which control the biochemical reactions activated by calcium entry and mediate cell recovery (Adelstein and Hathaway, 1979). Cyclic AMP levels were higher in cells stimulated with tumor antigen. The site(s) of action of cyclic nucleotides that enables them to execute these effects is as yet obscure. They nevertheless produce many and perhaps all of their effects by stimulating the phosphorylation of certain cell proteins by activating a protein kinase; high levels could inactivate calcium channels and stimulate the calcium extrusion pump ATPase; equally important, other proteins may be phosphory-lated, to reverse the biochemical reactions and physicological changes, and in this way the cells are reprimed to be triggered once again by antigens.

DIAGNOSTIC VALUE OF LAI

The tube LAI assay detects early neoplastic growth, consistently and accurately. All the same, the diagnostic potential of the assay had not been compared with other routine and acceptable investigational procedures used for the discovery of cancer. That was why we compared the LAI assay, barium enema and colono-scopy with regard to ability to detect colon cancer in patients with gastrointestinal complaints and no definite diagnosis, attending a colonoscopy clinic (Ayeni *et al.,* 1981).

Table I. Diagnosis and leukocytes adherence inhibition results of patients who had a colonoscopy.

Diagnosis of Leukocyte donor	No.[c] tested	No. LAI positive
Colorectal cancer		
In situ	1	1
Dukes' A	3	2
Dukes' B	4	3
Dukes' C	2	1
Dukes' D	7	3
Other abdominal cancers	3	0
Polyps		
Hyperplastic	2	0
Adenoma		
Tubular	7	1
Villotubular	14	6
Villous	1	1
Recurrent polyps[a]	2	2[b]
Undefined (no biopsy)	23	2
Other colon abnormalities		
Inflammation	16	0
Diverticulosis	14	0
Hemorrhoids	2	0
None	42	0

[a]Recurrent polyps by history. [b]One patient had no lesion demonstrated by either barium enema or colonoscopy. [c]None were tested with PGE_2 stimulation.

Table I lists the final diagnosis and LAI results of 142 patients who attended the colonoscopy clinic of the Montreal General Hospital with gastrointestinal complaints. Six of eight (75%) patients with *in situ*, stage A or B colorectal cancer were LAI[+]. When the colorectal cancer was Dukes' C or D, four of nine (44%) patients were LAI[+].

Colorectal adenomas were removed from 22 patients, eight of whom (36%) were LAI[+] (Table I). In another 23 patients, polyps were observed only; two of these patients had an LAI[+] response which remained the same when retested 3 months later. Another two patients with a history of recurrent adenomas were LAI[+] though only one of them had a polyp visualised.

No patients with hyperplastic polyps, inflammatory disease or diverticulosis of the colorectum, and none of the remaining patients, who had no specific colon abnormality, were LAI positive (Table I).

D. M. P. Thomson

Comparison of Results of LAI, Colonoscopy and Barium Enema

Cancer Patients

Ten patients with colon cancer were LAI^+; colonoscopy detected seven and barium enema detected eight of the lesions (Table II). One patient, not diagnosed by barium enema or colonoscopy, had long standing ulcerative colitis and a concomitant stage C cancer of the ascending colon. Not surprisingly, both barium enema and colonoscopy missed diagnosing another patient with a solitary brain metastasis from a previous primary. Another patient was not diagnosed by colonoscopy because of difficulty in advancing the colonoscope to the lesion, on the right side (Table III). In two other instances, barium enema and colonoscopy detected colon abnormalities that were not characterised exactly.

Seven patients were LAI^-: one each with Dukes' A, B, and C, and four with Dukes' D colon adenocarcinomas. The colon lesions of all seven of them were diagnosed by barium enema and in six of them by colonoscopy (Table II).

The LAI^- patient with Dukes' A cancer was again tested before and 1 month after surgery, and all results were negative. The patient with stage C colorectal cancer who had an NAI of 29 was reported as LAI^-, though we indicated that if cancer was suspected clinically, then the NAI value strongly suggested the existence of a more advanced cancer.

LAI, colonoscopy and barium enema detected 59% (10 of 17), 76% (13 of 17) and 88% (15 of 17), respectively, of patients with colorectal cancer, attending a colonoscopy clinic. None of these patients was tested with PGE_2 stimulation.

Polyp Patients

Twenty-two patients attending the colonoscopy clinic had colorectal adenomas excised and examined by pathology (Table I), and eight of these patients were LAI^+. Most of the adenomas that were removed were diagnosed by barium enema and/or colonoscopy.

Two patients with a history of recurrent adenomas were LAI^+ (Table I). One of the patients had undergone four previous polypectomies for eight adenomas, still the colonoscopy and barium enema findings were normal although the LAI response of his leukocytes has remained steadfastly positive for 12 months. The other patient, with a history of villotubular adenoma 3 years before and positive NAIs for 5 months, had a new polyp in the transverse colon observed by barium enema that was not removed because of certain difficulties.

Colorectal polyps in 23 patients remain undefined because they were not visualised or removed by endoscopy.

Evaluation of Diagnostic Value of LAI

For LAI to be of diagnostic value, sensitivity and specificity must be ≥ 1.0. In the evaluation of the diagnostic value of the assay for colorectal cancer, we compared the results of the 17 patients who proved to have cancer with 78 patients who had neither cancer nor polyps: 74 patients with other colon abnormal-

Table II. Diagnosis of LAI positive and negative patients and results of barium enema and colonoscopy.

Diagnosis of patients	LAI positive			LAI negative		
	No.	No. diagnosed by barium enema	colonoscopy	No.	No. diagnosed by barium enema	colonoscopy
Colorectal cancer						
In situ	1	1	1	—	—	—
Dukes' A	2	2	2	1	1	1
Dukes' B	3	3	3	1	1	1
Dukes' C	1	0	0	1	1	1
Dukes' D	3	2	1	4	4	3
Other abdominal cancers	—	—	—	3	2	2
Polyps inflammatory	—	—	—	1	1	1
Hyperplastic	—	—	—	2	2	2
Adenomas						
Tubular	1	1	1	6	4	6
Villotubular	6	4	6	8	7	6
Villous	1	0	1	—	—	—
Recurrent polyps	2[a]	1	0	—	—	—
Undefined	2	2	0	21	21	0
Other colon abnormalities						
Inflammation	—	—	—	16	13	15
Diverticulosis	—	—	—	14	14	3
Hemorrhoids	—	—	—	2	0	2
None	—	—	—	42	—	—

[a]One of the LAI positive patients had no polyp shown by either barium enema or colonoscopy.

Table III. Outcome of diagnostic procedure[a].

Disease	Procedure	Sensitivity[a]	Specificity[b]	Sum[c]
All Colorectal Cancer	Tube LAI	0.58	0.99	1.57
	Barium enema	0.93	1.0	1.93
	Endoscopy	0.76	1.0	1.76
Dukes' A and B	Tube LAI	0.75	0.99	1.74
	Barium enema	1.0	1.0	2.0
	Endoscopy	1.0	1.0	2.0
Dukes' C and D	Tube LAI	0.44	0.99	1.42
	Barium enema	0.77	1.0	1.77
	Endoscopy	0.55	1.0	1.55

[a]Sensitivity is the proportion of true positive among diseased. [b]Specificity is the proportion of true negative among non-diseased. [c]Sum is sensitivity and specificity, and it must be > 1.0 for a procedure to be of diagnostic value; if this sum is 2.0, the test is ideal.[d] A statistical test for validity of the procedure is performed in each as the usual χ^2 test for 2×2 tables. All procedures were highly significant ($P < 0.005$).

ities, three patients with other abdominal cancer, and one LAI$^+$ patient with a history of recurrent adenomas but without any lesion found by barium enema or endoscopy (Tables I and II). The results of this comparison are shown in Table III. In testing the null hypothesis that the proportion of positives is equal for patients with or without colorectal cancer, there is evidence to reject it for all procedures in diagnosing colorectal cancer, as well as early and late colorectal cancer. Hence, all three diagnostic procedures can be characterised as valid (Table III).

The sensitivity and specificity of a test do not alone determine its ability to predict the presence or absence of a disease in a population (Watson and Tang, 1980). The positive and negative predictive values (Table IV) are dependent not only on sensitivity and specificity of the test but also on the prevalence of the disease in the population to which the test will be applied. Given data on test sensitivity, specificity and prevalence, the probability that a patient with a positive or negative test does or does not have cancer can be estimated. In the colonoscopy clinic, where the prevalence of cancer was almost 18%, under the given sensitivity and specificity, patients with a positive LAI results would have a 92% probability of cancer. A patient with a negative result would have a 92% probability of no cancer. We would anticipate that for every 108 patients with a positive test result, 100 have cancer.

However, if the prevalence of colorectal cancer was 50 per 100,000 (0.05%), under these conditions there is a positive predictive value of 2.8%; that is, a patient selected at random who has a positive test result has only one chance in 36 (100/2.8) of colorectal cancer. Or only one out of every 36 subjects with a positive test would, in probability, have colorectal cancer. It is clear that the LAI assay will have a useful role in populations that have a high prevalance of colorectal cancer.

The LAI assay in colorectal cancer, we believe, approaches the lower limits of sensitivity necessary for a diagnostic assay for cancer. (Halliday *et al.*, 1977; Shani *et al.*, 1978; Tataryn *et al.*, 1979). Clearly, antitumor immunity *echoes* the early growth of a neoplasm; yet it remains true that the antitumor immune response can be dampened by a number of factors: cancer bulk (Grosser and Thomson, 1975), surgical stress (Flores *et al.*, 1976; Marti and Thomson, 1976) and corticosteroids (Flores *et al.*, 1976; Grosser *et al.*, 1980). More than once, technical problems with the assay have yielded what we call both false positive and negative results: that is, assays which when repeated give a different answer (O'Connor *et al.*, 1978).

Some of the false results will never be entirely eliminated because the assay involves a moderately complex series of manipulations and, even in the most skilled hands, errors can be made, though not more frequently than in 3% of tests (Ayeni *et al.*, 1980; Grosser and Thomson, 1975; O'Connor *et al.*, 1978; Tataryn *et al.*, 1979). Once the skill has been acquired to perform the assay—the principal factor limiting its success—another serious problem is a constant source of putative tumor antigen guaranteed to have and to retain its activity, since, in our (O'Connor *et al.*, 1978) and others' (Shani *et al.*, 1978) experience, extracts from autopsy specimen can both lose or lack strong putative antigen activity. Unexpected changes in tumor antigen activity have resulted in early colorectal patients not reacting when they should. Consequently, important technical variables inherent in the tube LAI assay still must be solved if the method is ever to be routinely adopted.

Table IV. A comparison of positive and negative predictive values of the tube LAI assay, barium enema and colonoscopy for colorectal cancer.

Disease	Procedure	Predictive value[a]		% Efficiency[b]
		+ve	−ve	
All Colorectal Cancer	Tube LAI	92	92	92
	Barium enema	100	99	98
	Endoscopy	100	81	96
Dukes A and B	Tube LAI	88	80	97
	Barium enema	100	100	100
	Endoscopy	100	100	100
Dukes C and D	Tube LAI	84	94	93
	Barium enema	100	97	98
	Endoscopy	100	95	96

$$^{a}PV \text{ pos} = 100 \times \frac{(Se)(P)}{(Se)(P) + (1 - Sp)(1 - P)}$$

$$PV \text{ neg} = 100 \times \frac{(1 - P) \times Sp}{(1 - P) Sp + P(1 - Se)}$$

$$P = \text{Prevalence} = \frac{17}{95} = 0.1789$$

Se = sensitivity; Sp = specificity.
[b]Efficiency was considered as the percentage of patients who were correctly classified, and was determined according to the formula $[P Se + (1 - P)Sp] \times 100$.

Monitoring LAI Reactivity After Surgery

Immediately after surgery the LAI⁺ response is lost for about 2 weeks unless the leukocytes are stimulated with PGE_2. The response becomes positive about 2 weeks after surgery and remains positive for another 2-3 months (Flores *et al.*, 1977; Lopez *et al.*, 1978). Then it becomes undetectable unless the patient has a sizeable amount of residual cancer that apparently acts as a stimulus to maintain the immune reactivity. Patients who are free of cancer remain LAI⁻ We have observed, in a few instances, patients apparently free of cancer who have had a positive test, confirmed by a repeat test, more than 6 months after surgery that was transient in nature; that is, it persisted for only 1 or 2 months (Ayeni *et al.*, 1980). The biological significance of this brief reactivity is unknown. Leukocytes from patients who harbour micrometastasis remain LAI⁻ even with PGE_2 stimulation until the cancer reaches a sufficient size to once again stimulate the host's antitumor immune response. When carefully monitored, the LAI response of most patients turns positive before there is clinical evidence of recurrent cancer (Flores *et al.*, 1977). The LAI response has been observed to be positive up to 1 year before recurrence of cancer. In other instances, the LAI response seems to turn positive only shortly before the recurrent cancer is discovered.

As the cancer mass increases, tumor antigen shed from the tumor nullifies the LAI response. So that it is possible to predict the tumor burden by determining the LAI response with and without PGE_2 stimulation. When leukocytes are LAI⁺ with and without PGE_2 stimulation, patients usually have a small tumor burden. In contrast, when leukocytes are LAI⁺ only with PGE_2 stimulation, patients usually have a large tumor burden.

PGE_2 stimulation of leukocytes now allows the tube LAI assay to detect and distinguish patients with more advanced cancers. Not all patients with colorectal cancer, of course, are LAI⁺ even with PGE_2 stimulation of their leukocytes. Patients with Dukes' B colorectal cancer that has invaded through the colon wall and into adjacent tissues, in fact, are often LAI⁻ even after PGE_2 stimulation of their leukocytes. We have collected nine patients with this type of colorectal cancer and LAI⁻ pattern of reactivity. With and without PGE_2 stimulation, their mean NAI was 2 and 13, respectively. So far four have returned 1 month after surgery and with PGE_2 stimulation there was still no improvement of their LAI reactivity. The explanation for this failure to respond is unknown.

ISOLATION AND CHARACTERISATION OF THE OSN OF COLORECTAL CANCER

Isolation from Solid Tumor

The putative tumor antigen in a crude PBS extract elutes in the void volume of Sepharose 4B molecular sieve column because it is part of the cell membrane. KBr ultracentrifugal flotation has been used to separate melanoma associated antigen (MAA) and HLA antigens (McCabe *et al.*, 1978). HLA antigens, associated with high density lipoproteins, are found in the upper fraction. LAI active material,

in additon, is recovered in the upper fraction. As described in more detail elsewhere by Khosravi *et al.* (1981) they supplied us with coded samples of KBr
separated tumor materials from malignant melanoma and colon cancer cells
grown in tissue culture. Specificity of the LAI blocking was shown in criss-cross
experiments; for both cancers, the LAI active material was in the upper fraction,
enriched for HLA antigens and β_2-microglobulin.

Histocompatibility antigens of normal tissues and TSAs of many chemically
induced animal tumors are an integral part of the cell membrane. Their isolation
depends on making them water soluble. Limited papain digestion of purified
cell membranes was the method originally used to isolate HLA antigens; it also
was chosen to solubilise human cancer antigens. Besides, this was the approach
used for solubilising TSAs of chemically induced tumors (Baldwin and Glaves,
1972; Thomson and Alexander, 1973). The papain solubilised tumor antigens
eluted in all molecular weight ranges assayed, but the principal activity was consistently found at a molecular weight of 100,000 daltons or so. This material,
analyzed by sodium dodecyl sulfate gel electrophoresis, was composed of smaller
subunits, and outstanding was a band at 12,00 molecular weight. This suggested
that the material might contain β_2-microglobulin.

Intrigued by the possibility that the neoantigens of human tumors might
be similar to histocompatibility antigens in structure and linkage to β_2-micro-
globulin, we passed the human material with putative tumor antigen activity
through an affinity column of horse anti-human β_2-microglobulin. Retained by
the affinity column, the putative tumor antigen was eluted with a chaotropic
agent, KSCN (Thomson *et al.*, 1976). The tumor antigen seems to bind
to the affinity column specifically; the putative tumor antigen does not bind
to an immunoadsorbent column of normal IgG (Thomson *et al.*, 1978); nor
does the putative antigen bind to an affinity column of antisera raised to the
material that had not bound to the anti-β_2-microglobulin affinity column (Thomson
et al., 1980). Doubtlessly, the putative tumor antigen co-purifies with β_2-micro-
globulin. Carcinoembryonic did not bind to the anti-β_2-microglobulin affinity
column (Thomson *et al.*, 1979a). Confirming our studies, Malley *et al.* (1979)
reported that the malignant melanoma tumor antigen, as assayed by LAI, co-
purifies with β_2-microglobulin. Using antisera raised in monkeys to melanoma
associated antigens, Khrosavi *et al.* (1980) found that both MAA and HLA activity
were enriched in the upper KBr fraction. Moreover, they applied shed material
from melanoma cultures to a Sepharose 4B rabbit anti-human β_2-microglobulin
IgG affinity column, eluted the bound material with 3 M KSCN, and found
that β_2-microglobulin, HLA and MAA had bound to the affinity column. These
findings lend further support to our original report on the association of β_2-micro-
globulin with one type of MAA.

The colon tumor antigens, isolated from the anti-β_2-microglobulin affinity
column, have three principal bands when analyzed by SDS gel electrophoresis:
molecular weights of about 12,000, 25,000–30,000 and 40,000 daltons (Thomson
et al., 1976; Thomson *et al.*, 1978). Nonetheless, the molecular weight of the
polypeptide chain carrying the organ specific neoantigen determinant is, as yet,
unknown.

Originally, the HLA large component and no other membrane components
were reported to be bound to β_2-microglobulin (Robb *et al.*, 1976; Nakamuro

et al., 1977). Recent studies indicate that β_2-microglobulin does bind certain membrane components that are the same in molecular size as the HLA large components but are different antigenically from the HLA large components (Tada *et al.*, 1978). For that matter, the T/a and Qa-2 antigens in the mouse, it is reported, are linked to β_2-microglobulin (Ostberg *et al.*, 1975; Michailson *et al.*, 1977). Besides, the male specific antigen (H-Y) is associated with β_2-microglobulin, though coded for by the Y chromosome (Fellous *et al.* 1978). Membrane proteins, associated with β_2-microglobulin, may possibly have a regulatory role during cell differentiation; so the expression of a β_2-microglobulin linked cell surface protein with organ specificity would be in keeping with the concept that β_2-microglobulin associates with cell surface proteins that, somehow, play a role in cell differentiation.

Because the organ specific neoantigen co-isolates with β_2-microglobulin and, when analyzed on SDS gel electrophoresis, resembles the pattern of histocompatibility antigens, we suggested that the organ specific neoantigen may well be part of an "altered-self" histocompatibility antigen (Thomson *et al.*, 1976). Other possibilities include: HLA molecules acting as adaptors that combine with the antigenic molecule to form hybrid antigens, containing elements of self and non-self; or the organ specific neoantigens could be expressed separately on the cell surface, but share many of the structural and antigenic features of the HLA antigens (Thomson *et al.*, 1978).

The HLA complex consists of a set of genes on chromosome 6 that controls polymorphic cell surface antigens which provoke graft rejection. The known loci span sufficient DNA to code for about 2,000 average proteins, but at present much of the DNA has no defined function. So yet another possibility is that the organ specific neoantigens are like embryonic analogs of the adult HLA antigens, each system operating as mediator of cell–cell recognition, the former functioning only in the embryo and the latter both in the fetus and in the adult. But why the organ specific neoantigens should be immunogenic in the adult host if they are coded for by a normal gene locus is not yet understood.

Isolation from Serum

As the tumor grows, tumor antigen is shed from the cell surface membranes into the local milieu, and, eventually, when the tumor mass has grown larger, antigen escapes into the systemic circulation. Some of the organ specific neoantigens are eliminated by kidney filtration after being degraded from their high molecular weight form (Lopez and Thomson, 1977).

On a molecular sieve column of Sephadex G-150, the putative colon cancer antigens present in the serum elutes in the molecular weight range of 80,000 to $\geqslant$ 150,000 (Lopez and Thomson, 1977; Thomson *et al.*, 1980); like HLA antigens it is precipitated by polyanions and co-isolates with the HDL fraction of serum (Allison *et al.*, 1977; Lopez and Thomson, 1977). CEA in serum is not precipitated by the polyanions (Thomson *et al.*, 1980). The HDL fraction of serum elutes in a broad peak in the excluded and included volumes of a Sephadex G-150 column; tumor antigen activity is found in this peak. Also a small protein peak which has antigen activity is often observed at a molecular weight of about 48,000.

Isolation from Urine

The tumor antigens from urine of patients with metastatic colon cancer were partially purified by a combination of physicochemical methods and affinity chromatography using IgG from the sera of patients who were LAI$^+$ to the appropriate cancer antigen (Thomson *et al.,* 1980). The final material, containing the putative colon cancer tumor antigen, was greatly enriched and revealed an unique band on SDS gels about 38,000–40,000 molecular weight and residual fine bands at about 25,000–30,000 molecular weight. But when we tried to expand the scale of isolation by affinity chromatography with γ-globulin from LAI$^+$ patients, the quantity of contaminates, presumably light chain bleeding from the affinity columns, became a serious drawback for this method; consequently, we turned to using physicochemical separation methods.

The first problem in isolating a sufficient quantity of tumor antigen from urine is that large volumes of fluid have to be concentrated. The 2 l Amicon$^{\circledR}$ stirred cell works well in concentrating 50–200 l of urine. DEAE ion exchange chromatography, using a shallow, step-wise salt gradient separates rapidly tumor antigen from most urinary protein. Blue Sepharose CL-6B$^{\circledR}$ affinity chromatography removes albumin. And an anti-human light chain affinity column is essential to remove the abundant light chains which because of their heterogeneous charge and dimerisation are difficult to separate completely from the tumor antigens. Steric exclusion chromatography, Sephadex G-75$^{\circledR}$ superfine, separate low and high molecular weight contaminates from the tumor antigen. Still other contaminates are removed by hydroxyapatite chromatography. This approach to purifying the colon tumor antigen yields about 3 mg of material from 100 l of urine which is enriched 10,000-fold for LAI activity. On SDS gels the LAI active material resembles the papain solubilised tumor antigen.

Recent Progress in Purification of Organ
Specific Neoantigens

The slow progress in purifying the OSNs has been largely the fault of the LAI assay. Initially, tumor isolates were substituted for the PBS cancer extracts, consuming considerable quantities of the scarce, isolated materials in the titration process and leaving not enough material to continue (Thomson *et al.,* 1976). When the blocking LAI assay was introduced (Thomson *et al.,* 1978), excessive consumption of materials was no longer a problem, and enrichment of antigen activity could be calculated because the blocking assay was not affected by the protein concentration of the isolates. Then, the limiting factor became an adequate supply of LAI$^+$ leukocytes, for these came from patients with small cancers before surgery. Obviously, these patients were not plentiful. Supplies of LAI$^+$ leukocytes became ample with the discovery that PGE$_2$ stimulated leukocytes from advanced cancer patients now responded positively (Kaneti *et al.,* 1981). Now, the greater availability of reactive cells means that new approaches can be tried, and more fractions can be prepared and tested from each isolation step. By pooling only those fractions with LAI activity more impurities can be eliminated at each isolation step. So, recently, we have turned our attention to examining what additional steps could be used to yield a pure tumor antigen.

The principal problem associated with using the anti-β_2-microglobulin affinity column step is that light and heavy chains of γ-globulin bleed from the column and contaminate the bound and eluted isolate. To separate the putative tumor antigen isolated from the anti-β_2-microglobulin affinity column from the contaminants, preparative isoelectric focusing in flat beds was undertaken. The LAI active material was recovered from the pI range of 5.5–6.0. On steric exclusion HPL chromatography this material showed a discrete protein peak which was LAI active (Fig. 8). On SDS gels the pattern of the LAI active material is similar to that previously described (Fig. 9). Presumably the higher molecular weight forms of the molecule, often noted when the antigen was isolated first by molecular sieve chromatography (Thomson *et al.*, 1976), represent dimerised polypeptide chains that are disrupted by eluting the antigens from the affinity column with 3 M KSCN.

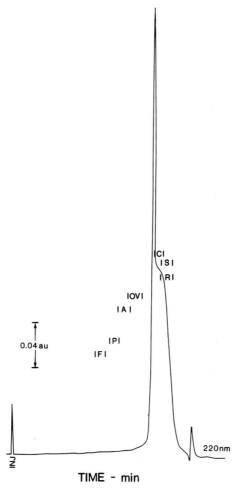

TIME - min

Fig. 8. Elution curve of LAI active papain soluble colon cancer material. Column: TSK 3000 SW. Solvent: 0.3 M NaCl 0.1 M phosphate buffer pH 7.0. Flow rate: 1.0 ml/min. Sample volume: 7 μl. Elution position of protein standards: F, ferritin; P, phosphorylase B; A, albumin; O, ovalbumin; C, carbonic anhydrase; S, soybean anhydrase; R, ribonuclease.

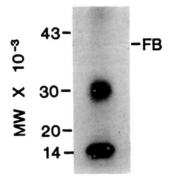

Fig. 9. SDS gel pattern of ^{125}I-labeled colon cancer from the peak of the chromatographic profile shown in Fig. 8. FB = faint band seen on autoradiograph.

Characteristics

We believe that the organ specific neoantigen exhibited by colon cancer is physicochemically similar to other neoantigens expressed by cancers arising in other organs. Nonetheless, subtle differences exist in the organ specific neoantigens, for those of each organ are recognised separately by the tumor bearing host's immune response. The difference in the organ specific neoantigens from one organ to another is probably no greater than are the allotypes of HLA antigens from each other. No doubt, the antigenic determinant on the polypeptide chain that is responsible for organ specificity will reside in a small number of amino acid residues located on the surface of the molecule and will probably depend on the conformation of the negative molecule. It might be expected that all organ specific neoantigens will have a similar framework structure or common portion, which may even be identical to proteins expressed on fully differentiated cells of the same organ, and it will be a hypervariable region that bestows organ specificity.

The significance of the organ specific neoantigens in ontogeny is unknown, but clearly each cancer cell, no matter how undifferentiated it appears morphologically, expresses this cell surface protein. Seemingly, the organ specific neoantigen is coded for by the cell genome, and so it is not a new, unique antigen like tumor specific transplantation antigens of chemically induced animal tumors. If this is a molecule that is normally expressed by stem cells, it is indeed curious how this antigen has not induced tolerance during fetal development. With a purified antigen it should prove possible to develop new, simple immunodiagnostic assays. By knowing the structure of the tumor antigen, then possibly its relationship to other cell surface proteins and its biological significance in the neoplastic process might be better understood.

ACKNOWLEDGEMENTS

I thank Mary Sutherland, Paula Friedlander, Sylvia van den Hurk and Kerry Phelan for their expert technical assistance. McGill Biomedical Engineering developed the computer programs that allowed the storage and analysis of the

demographic and test data on the patients described in this review.
I thank Mrs Mary Bergin for typing the manuscript.
This work was supported by grants from the Medical Research Council of
Canada, the National Cancer Institute of Canada and the Cancer Research Society
Inc. of Montreal.

REFERENCES

Adelstein, R. S. and Hathaway, D. R. (1979). *American Journal of Cardiology*
44, 783.
Allison, J. P., Pellegrino, M. A., Ferrone, S., Callahan, G. N. and Reisfeld, R. A.
(1977). *Journal of Immunology* **118**, 1004.
Augstein, J., Farmer, J. B., Lee, T. B., Sheard, P. and Tattersall, M. L. (1973).
Nature New Biology **245**, 215.
Ayeni, R. O., Tataryn, D. N., MacFarlane, J. K. and Thomson, D. M. P. (1980).
Surgery **87**, 380.
Ayeni, R. O., Thomson, D. M. P., MacFarlane, J. K. and Daly, D. (1981). *Cancer*
(In press.)
Baldwin, R. W. and Glaves, D. (1972). *Clinical and Experimental Immunology*
11, 51.
Ballard, C. M. and Dickinson, J. P. (1980). *Clinical and Experimental Immunology*
40, 383.
Bhatti, R. A., Ablin, R. J., Condoulis, W. and Guinan, P. D. (1979). *Cancer
Research* **39**, 3328.
Blackwell, G. J. and Flower, R. J. (1978). *Prostaglandins* **16**, 417.
Blackwell, G. J., Flower, R. J., Ni jkamp, F. P. and Vane, J. R. (1978). *British
Journal of Pharmacology* **62**, 79.
Burka, J. F. and Peterson, N. A. M. (1980). *Prostaglandins* **19**, 499.
Dusheiko, G. M., Kew, M. C. and Rabson, A. R. (1979). *British Journal of Cancer*
40, 397.
Enterline, H. T. (1976). *Current Topics in Pathology* **63**, 95.
Farber, E., Cameron, R. G. and Laishes, B. A. (1979). *In* "Carcinogens: Identi-
fication and Mechanisms of Action", p. 319. Raven Press, New York.
Favalli, C., Garaci, E., Etheredge, E., Santoro, M. G. and Jaffe, B. M. (1980).
Journal of Immunology **125**, 897.
Fellous, M., Gunther, E., Kemler, R., Wiels, J., Berger, R., Guenet, J. L., Jacob,
H. and Jacob, F. (1978). *Journal of Experimental Medicine* **148**, 58.
Fenoglio, C. M., Kaye, G. I., Pascal, R. R. and Lane, N. (1977). *Pathology Annual*
12, 87.
Ferraris, V. A., DeRubertis, F. R. C., Hudson, R. H. and Wolfe, L. (1974). *Journal
of Clinical Investigation* **54**, 378.
Flores, M., Thomson, D. M. P. and MacFarlane, J. K. (1976). *Surgical Forum*
XXVII, 91.
Flores, M., Marti, J. H., Grosser, N., MacFarlane, J. K. and Thomson, D. M. P.
(1977). *Cancer* **39**, 494.
Flower, R. J. and Blackwell, G. J. (1976). *Biochemical Pharmacology* **25**, 285.
Foley, E. J. (1953). *Cancer Research* **13**, 835.
Foulds, L. (1975). *In* "Neoplastic Development", Vol. 2, 549–636. Academic
Press, New York.
Fulton, A. M. and Levy, J. G. (1980). *International Journal of Cancer* **26**, 669.
Goetzl, E. J. (1980). *New England Journal of Medicine* **303**, 822.
Goldrosen, M. H., Russo, A. J., Howell, J. H., Leveson, S. H. and Holyoke, E. D.
(1979). *Cancer Research* **39**, 587.

Goodwin, J. S., Messner, R. P., Bankhurst, A. D., Peake, G. T., Saiki, J. H. and Williams, R. G., Jr (1977). *New England Journal of Medicine* **297**, 963.

Goodwin, J. S., Husby, G. and Williams, R. C., Jr (1980). *Cancer Immunology and Immunotherapy* **8**, 3.

Grosser, N. and Thomson, D. M. P. (1975). *Cancer Research* **35**, 2571.

Grosser, N. and Thomson, D. M. P. (1976). *International Journal of Cancer* **18**, 58.

Grosser, N., Marti, J. H., Proctor, J. W. and Thomson, D. M. P. (1976). *International Journal of Cancer* **18**, 39.

Grosser, N., Thomson, D. M. P., Flores, M. and MacFarlane, J. K. (1980). *Cancer Immunology and Immunotherapy* **7**, 263.

Hadden, J. W., Hadden, E. M., Johnson, L. D. and Johnson, E. M. (1975). *In* "Lymphocytes and Their Interactions" (R. C. Williams, Ed.), p. 27. Raven Press, New York.

Halliday, W. J., Maluish, A. E., Stephenson, P. M. and Davis, N. C. (1977). *Cancer Research* **37**, 1962.

Halliday, W. J. and Miller, S. (1972). *International Journal of Cancer* **9**, 477.

Hamberg, M. and Samuelsson, B. (1974). *Proceedings of the National Academy of Sciences of USA* **71**, 3400.

Hamberg, M. (1976). *Biochimica et Biophysica Acta* **431**, 651.

Hellstrom, I., Hellstrom, K. E. and Shantz, G. (1976). *International Journal of Cancer* **18**, 354.

Hellstrom, I., Hellstrom, K. E. and van Belle, G. (1977). *American Journal of Clinical Pathology* **68**, 706.

Holan, V., Hasek, M., Bubenik, J. and Chutna, J. (1974). *Cellular Immunology* **13**, 107.

Holliday, R. (1979). *British Journal of Cancer* **40**, 513.

Kaneti, J., Thomson, D. M. P. and Reid, E. C. (1981). *Journal of Urology*. (In press.)

Khosravi, M., Liao, S. K. and Dent, P. B. (1980). "XIth International Pigment Cell Conference, Japan." (In press.)

Khosravi, M., Liao, S. K., Thomson, D. M. P. and Dent, P. B. (1981). (Submitted for publication.)

Lopez, M. J. and Thomson, D. M. P. (1977). *Nature* **251**, 547.

Lopez, M., O'Connor, R., MacFarlane, J. K. and Thomson, D. M. P. (1978). *British Journal of Cancer* **38**, 660.

Malley, A., Burger, D. R., Vandenbark, A. A., Frikke, M., Finke, P., Begley, D., Acott, K., Black, J. and Vetto, R. M. (1979). *Cancer Research* **39**, 619.

Maluish, A. E. and Halliday, W. J. (1975). *Cellular Immunology* **17**, 131.

Marti, J. and Thomson, D. M. P. (1976). *British Journal of Cancer* **34**, 116.

Marti, J. H., Grosser, N. and Thomson, D. M. P. (1976). *International Journal of Cancer* **18**, 48.

McCabe, A., Ferrone, S., Pellegrino, M. A., Kern, D. H., Holmes, E. C. and Reisfeld, R. A. (1978). *Journal of the National Cancer Institute* **60**, 773.

Michailson, J., Flaherty, L., Vitetta, E. and Poulik, M. D. (1977). *Journal of Experimental Medicine* **145**, 1066.

Moore, P. K. and Hoult, J. R. S. (1980a). *Nature* **288**, 269.

Moore, P. K. and Hoult, J. R. S. (1980b). *Nature* **288**, 271.

Morson, B. (1974). *Proceedings of the Royal Society of Medicine* **67**, 451.

Naccache, P. H., Showell, H. J., Becker, E. L. and Sha'afi, R. I. (1979). *Biochemical and Biophysical Research Communications* **89**, 1224.

Nakamuro, K., Tanigaki, N. and Pressman, D. (1977). *Immunology* **32**, 139.

O'Connor, R., MacFarlane, J. K., Murray, D. and Thomson, D. M. P. (1978). *British Journal of Cancer* **38**, 674.

Ogawa, K., Medline, A. and Farber, E. (1979). *British Journal of Cancer* **40**, 782.
Ostberg, L., Rask, L., Wigzell, H. and Peterson, P. A. (1975). *Nature* **253**, 735.
Parker, C. W. (1974). *Biochemical and Biophysical Research Communications* **61**, 1180.
Parker, C. W., Huber, M. M., Hoffman, M. K. and Falkenhein, S. F. (1979). *Prostaglandins* **18**, 673.
Plescia, O. J., Smith, A. H and Grinwich, K. (1975). *Proceedings of the National Academy of Sciences of USA* **72**, 1848.
Potter, V. R. (1978). *British Journal of Cancer* **38**, 1.
Robb, R. J., Strominger, J. L. and Mann, D. L. (1976). *Journal of Biological Chemistry* **251**, 5427.
Roberts, M. F., Deemer, R. A., Mincey, T. C. and Dennis, E. A. (1977). *Journal of Biological Chemistry* **252**, 2405.
Sanner, T., Kotlar, H. K. R. and Eker, P. (1980). *Cancer Letters* **8**, 283.
Shani, A., Ritts, R. E., Jr, Thynne, G. S., Weiland, L. H., Silvers, A. and Moertel, C. G. (1978). *International Journal of Cancer* **22**, 113.
Stenson, W. F. and Parker, C. W. (1980). *Journal of Immunology* **125**, 1.
Strom. T. B., Carpenter, C. B., Cragoe, E. J., Jr, Norris, S., Devlin, R. and Perper, R. J. (1977). *Transplantation Proceedings* **9**, 1075.
Tada, N., Tanigaki, N. and Pressman, D. (1978). *Journal of Immunology* **120**, 513.
Tataryn, D. N., MacFarlane, J. K., Murray, D. and Thomson, D. M. P. (1979). *Cancer* **43**, 898.
Tataryn, D. N., MacFarlane, J. K. and Thomson, D. M. P. (1978). *Lancet* **1**, 1020.
Thomson, D. M. P. and Alexander, P. (1973). *British Journal of Cancer* **27**, 35.
Thomson, D. M. P., Gold, P., Freedman, S. O. and Shuster, J. (1976). *Cancer Research* **36**, 3518.
Thomson, D. M. P., Rauch, J. E., Weatherhead, J. C., Friedlander, P., O'Connor, R., Grosser, N., Shuster, J. and Gold, P. (1978). *British Journal of Cancer* **37**, 753.
Thomson, D. M. P., Tataryn, D. N., O'Connor, R., Rauch, J., Friedlander, P., Gold, P. and Shuster, J. (1979a). *Cancer Research* **39**, 604.
Thomson, D. M. P., Tataryn, D. N., Schwartz, R. and MacFarlane, J. K. (1979b). *European Journal of Cancer* **15**, 1095.
Thomson, D. M. P., Tataryn, D. N., Weatherhead, J. C., Friedlander, P., Rauch, J., Schwartz, R., Gold, P. and Shuster, J. (1980). *European Journal of Cancer* **16**, 539.
Thomson, D. M. P., Phelan, K., Scanzano, R. and Fink, A. (1981). (Submitted for publication.)
Watson, R. A. and Tang, D. B. (1980). *New England Journal of Medicine* **303**, 497.
Watson, J., Epstein, R. and Cohn, M. (1973). *Nature* **246**, 405.
Weinhouse, S. and Ono, T. (1972). *In* "Isozymes and Enzyme Regulation in Cancer". University Park Press, Baltimore.

MARKERS OF GI TRACT TUMOURS: A DISCUSSION

P. Burtin

Institut de Recherches Scientifique sur le Cancer, Villejuif, France

Dr Burtin:

As an immunochemist, I am always interested by new tumour associated antigens. The results presented in this session are very rewarding in this respect. I would like first to have a discussion on Dr Hunter's paper, then on that of Dr Thomson.

To a question of Dr Mach, Dr Hunter answers on the relationship between his POA and that described by Dr Hobbs: he explains that Dr Hobbs' group published two subsequent papers on this topic. The antigen described in the first one was not available for comparison. The antiserum described in the second article was sent to Dr Hunter: it contained two antibodies, one of them identical to Hunter's anti-POA.

Dr Burtin asks several questions:

Dr Hunter, you described POA as present in foetal pancreas of less than 18 weeks. Does it mean that you did not study pancreas of older foetuses, or that you did not find POA in these pancreas?

Dr Hunter:

We studied a few older pancreas. They became negative after 18 weeks of gestation.

Serono Symposium No. 46, Markers for Diagnosis and Monitoring of Human Cancer, edited by M. I. Colnaghi, G. L. Buraggi and M. Ghione, 1982. Academic Press, London and New York.

Dr Burtin:

You described the presence of relatively high amounts of POA in normal sera. Where does it come from, as you find it in only a few goblet cells of the intestine? Furthermore, antigens of the goblet cells are generally destined to be excreted in the intestinal lumen. Hence, why are these relatively high levels present in normal sera?

Dr Hunter:

I don't know.

Dr Burtin:

You mentioned that your new antisera showed spurs between precipitin lines obtained with various pancreatic cancer sera; you considered these patterns as due to heterogeneity of POA. Could they be explained also by a discrete proteolysis?

Dr Hunter:

That could be.

Dr Herberman:

May I remind you of the problems experienced by Dr McIntyre and Dr Braatz with their lung tumour associated antigen. A strong cross-reaction was seen between this antigen and the chymotrypsin inhibitor present in normal serum.

Dr Franchimont:

Is the POA present in the serum identical to that of tissues, or only a fragment of it?

Dr Hunter:

Probably identical.

Dr Burtin:

Is the elevation of POA in serum seen in cases of biliary obstruction, whatever their cause?

Dr Hunter:

I have no answer to this question.

Then the discussion turns to Dr Thomson's paper.

Dr Burtin:

Many groups in the world studied the reactivity of patients' lymphocytes to tumour extracts by LMI or LAI methods. Very often they obtained less clear results than you have. For instance, in my laboratory, by using LMI, we found about 50% of positive results with leucocytes of colorectal cancer patients (65% in non-invasive carcinomas, 40% in the advanced ones). But 65% of patients with an inflammatory intestinal disease (ulcerous colitis, Crohn's disease, etc.) also gave positive results. Hence, your data are much better. Maybe it is because you explored B lymphocytes' reactivity, whereas other groups studied T cell reactivity. Let me now ask you several questions. First of all, do you know if this organ specific antigen is of foetal (or embryonic) origin?

Dr Thomson:

We never tested that point.

Dr Burtin:

Did you try to immunize animals with your purified antigen, and to set up a radioimmunoassay?

Dr Thomson:

I am afraid of the risk of producing hetero antibodies that would reveal only the common part of these organ specific antigens, and not their specific part. The same was observed with hetero antisera against HLA antigens.

Dr Burtin:

Let us imagine a hetero antiserum reacting with the common part of all these organ specific tumour associated antigens. It would be an especially interesting reagent.

Dr Koldovsky:

I agree with Dr Burtin's idea that your antigen could be of embryonic origin. That would not exclude its antigenicity in adults. Let me remind you that in Simonen's experiments immunological tolerance was not obtained in young chicken embryos, but only after 12 days of gestation. Furthermore, immunological tolerance acquired to foetal antigens does not last the whole lifetime.

Dr Burtin:

Could I mention here the results obtained by Bansal and Sjögren? Both groups demonstrated that immunization with foetal extracts allowed some degree of protection against intestinal tumours in mice and rats. From another point of view, Zöller *et al.* showed that leucocytes of colorectal cancer patients had reactivity to human foetal extracts by the LMI method.

Dr Franchimont:

I would like to comment on the mechanism of the reaction you are dealing with: you have production of monokines, not of lymphokines, don't you?

Dr Thomson:

It is possible to arm monocytes of normal subjects with the serum of cancer patients. But it is very difficult to perform it.

Dr Herberman:

It would be very interesting to have a reaction between your purified antigen and patients' serum immunoglobulins, such as a binding assay. Positive reactions would validate your previous data.

USE AND LIMITATIONS OF MONOCLONAL ANTI CEA
ANTIBODIES IN IMMUNOASSAYS AND IN TUMOUR
LOCALIZATION BY IMMUNOSCINTIGRAPHY: A DISCUSSION

J.-P. Mach, F. Buchegger, C. Girardet, M. Forni, J. Ritschard, R. S. Accolla
and S. Carrel

*Ludwig Institute for Cancer Research, Lausanne Branch, and
Institute of Biochemistry, University of Lausanne, Epalinges, Lausanne, and
Clinique Médicale and Division de Médecine Nucléaire, Department of Medicine,
University Hospital of Geneva, Geneva, Switzerland*

INTRODUCTION

Carcinoembryonic antigen (CEA) (Gold and Freedman, 1965) is a well
characterized tumour marker associated with the most common human carcinoma.
Recently, using the method of Köhler and Milstein (1975), we produced monoclonal antibodies (Mab) reacting specifically with CEA (Accolla *et al.*, 1979,
1980). The specificity of these antibodies for CEA molecules was demonstrated in
an inhibition radioimmunoassay performed in low molarity buffer (0.02 M Tris-
HCl, pH 7.4). It was shown that one thousand times more crude perchloric acid
extract of normal colon or normal lung was necessary to give the same inhibition
as purified colon carcinoma CEA. Furthermore, a purified preparation of the
known antigen cross-reacting with CEA called NGP or NCA (Mach and Pusztaszeri,
1972; von Kleist *et al.*, 1972) gave almost no inhibition in this RIA using either
one of two different Mab anti CEA described (Accolla *et al.*, 1980). Further
evidence of the CEA specificity of these Mab was provided by the fact that they
recognized precisely the CEA present on frozen sections of colon carcinoma using

Serono Symposium No. 46, Markers for Diagnosis and Monitoring of Human Cancer, edited
by M. I. Colnaghi, G. L. Buraggi and M. Ghione, 1982. Academic Press, London and New
York.

the immunoperoxidase method (Accolla *et al.*, 1979). In addition, it was shown that one of these Mab (Mab-23) could be used very efficiently in immunoadsorbent columns to purify CEA from crude saline extract of colon carcinoma (Buchegger *et al.*, 1980).

Having established the specificity of these Mab for the CEA molecule, it was important to determine whether or not the new Mab could increase the tumour specificity of the CEA assay used to measure this marker in the serum of patients. The first report of a RIA for CEA suggested that only patients with gastrointestinal carcinoma had elevated circulating CEA levels (Thomson *et al.*, 1969). However, such highly specific results could never be reproduced and the question of tumour specificity of CEA remained a controversial issue (reviewed by Mach, 1979).

Another potential application of Mab against CEA is their use, after radioactive labelling, as tracer to detect CEA containing tumour. It was shown that immuno-absorbent purified polyclonal goat antibodies injected into nude mice bearing grafts of human colon carcinoma localized specifically in the tumours and could be detected by external scanning of the animal (Mach *et al.*, 1974a). More recently, tumour localization by radiolabelled goat anti CEA antibodies could be achieved in patients bearing different types of CEA producing tumour (Goldenberg *et al.*, 1978, 1980; Mach *et al.*, 1980a, b). One of the problems of this method of immunoscintigraphy is that when the patient has a high level of circulating CEA, it forms immune complexes with the injected labelled antibodies (Mach *et al.*, 1980b) which then have a tendency to localize non-specifically in the reticulo-endothelium, particularly in the liver. Therefore, we thought that Mab, which are non-precipitating antibodies because they react with a single determinant on the CEA molecule, would produce much smaller immune complexes and, consequently, less non-specific background in the reticulo-endothelium.

The purpose of this report is to briefly present some of the results obtained with Mab anti CEA both in immunoassay and in immunoscintigraphy. More detailed analysis of the results will be published elsewhere.

RESULTS

Monoclonal Anti CEA Antibodies in Solid Phase RIA

We first developed a solid phase RIA using immunoabsorbent purified goat CEA antibodies (Mach *et al.*, 1980a) physically coated to polystyrene balls (Precision Plastic Balls, Chicago, Illinois), in order to absorb the CEA present in the serum sample to be analysed. After thorough washing of the balls, the CEA immunoadsorbed to the solid phase was revealed by adding ^{125} I-labelled purified Mab-23 (2 ng = 40 nCi). The standard curve obtained with this solid phase RIA is shown in Fig. 1. The amount of standard CEA purified from metastases of a colon carcinoma (Fritsché and Mach, 1977) is shown in the abscissa, while the percentage of binding of labelled Mab bound to the plastic balls is shown in the ordinate. The sensitivity of the assay was in the range of 1-2 ng/ml of serum (Buchegger *et al.*, 1980). The disadvantage of this method was that 10-20% of interassay variations were observed when different batches of labelled Mab were used. Therefore, we developed an indirect enzyme immunoassay with the same Mab (M-EIA).

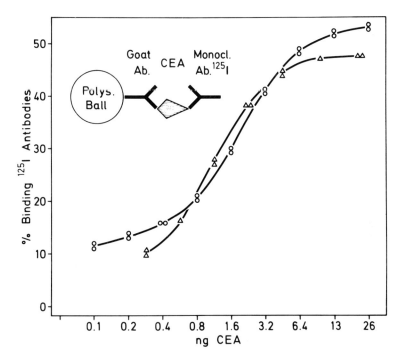

Fig. 1. Solid phase radioimmunoassay performed as described schematically on the left upper part of the figure: polystyrene balls coated with purified goat anti CEA antibodies were incubated with standard amounts of CEA (abscissa) diluted either in 0.3 ml of normal human serum (o—o) or in 0.02 M Tris–HCl buffer pH 7.4 (△—△). After washing, the balls were incubated with ^{125}I-labelled monoclonal anti CEA antibodies, washed again and the radioactivity bound to the balls was counted. The percentage of radioactivity bound to the balls is expressed in the ordinate. (Taken from Buchegger *et al.*, 1980.)

Monoclonal Anti CEA Antibodies in Solid Phase M–EIA

In this M–EIA the same plastic balls coated with purified goat anti CEA antibodies were used as a solid support. The balls were incubated with heat extracted patients' sera (70°C for 15 min in 0.2 M sodium acetate buffer, pH 5) followed by a second incubation with purified unlabelled Mab-23. The reaction was then revealed by a goat anti-mouse IgGl antiserum (Meloy, Springfield, Va.) coupled to alkaline phosphatase (Avrameas, 1969) and by the addition of the specific substrate (p-nitro-phenyl-phosphate). This assay was able to detect CEA in patient serum with a sensitivity of 1 ng/ml comparable to that of a classical inhibition RIA (Thomson *et al.*, 1969; Mach *et al.*, 1974b). Table 1 shows the correlation coefficients obtained in a comparison between M–EIA and classical RIA using polyclonal anti CEA antiserum on a series of 310 serum samples from patients known to have elevated circulating CEA. It can be seen that good correlation coefficients were obtained between the two assay systems in all groups of patients studied (Buchegger *et al.*, in prep.). However, the new M–EIA was not able to discriminate CEA molecules present in the serum of cancer patients from those present in serum of patients with non-malignant diseases.

Table I. Comparison between circulating CEA levels detected by enzyme immunoassay with Mab–23 (M–EIA) and classical radioimmunoassay (RIA)

Number of sera analysed	Type of diseases	M–EIA/RIA correlation coefficient
208	Colon and rectum carcinomas	0.88
28	Gastric and mammary carcinomas	0.83
15	Liver cirrhoses	0.86
59	Heavy smokers	0.92

The good correlation between M–EIA and RIA was confirmed at single patient level in follow-up studies of the serum CEA concentrations after surgical treatment. Figure 2 shows an example of sequential CEA measurements performed by the two assays in a patient who had two resections of tumour recurrences by surgical operations motivated exclusively by the results of the CEA assay. These findings indicate that monoclonal anti CEA antibodies can be employed as an excellent standard reagent in a sensitive enzyme immunoassay and can have clinical application in the follow-up of cancer patients.

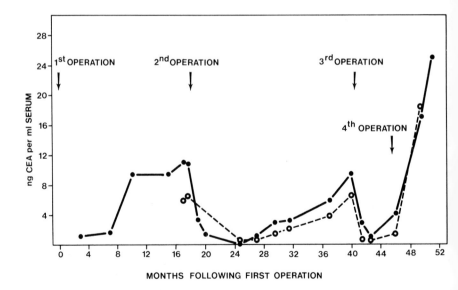

Fig. 2. Comparison of sequential CEA measurement performed either by conventional inhibition radioimmunoassay (•—•) or by solid phase enzyme immunoassay using monoclonal anti CEA antibodies (o---o). These sequential CEA assays were performed on the serum of a 56-year-old female patient who was operated for a carcinoma of the right colon and who developed three successive tumour recurrences which were detected exclusively by the elevation of circulating CEA. Three surgical operations were performed on the basis of the CEA results and in two of them the tumour recurrences could be macroscopically entirely removed. Note the good correlation of the results obtained by the two assays.

Use of ^{131}I-labelled Purified Mab for Tumour Localization by Immunoscintigraphy

After having shown that Mab anti CEA purified by DEAE 52 from ascites of hybridoma 23 (Buchegger *et al.*, 1980) and labelled with ^{131}I can also localize *in vivo* into human carcinomas grafted in nude mice (unpublished results), we injected a small series of patients bearing large bowel or pancreas carcinoma with ^{131}I-labelled purified Mab anti CEA in a similar protocol as the one described for injection of goat anti CEA antibodies (Mach *et al.*, 1980a, b). The results were encouraging in the sense that less non-specific accumulation of Mab in the reticulo-endothelium was observed as compared to polyclonal goat antibodies. Also a smaller percentage of injected Mab formed immune complexes with circulating CEA as determined by Sephadex G-200 filtration of serum sample obtained after injection (Mach *et al.*, 1980b).

Positive scans, in which increased radioactivity was observed in the region of known tumour deposit, were observed in eight out of 14 patients, doubtful scans in three patients and negative scans in the remaining three patients. A representative example of scanning results obtained in a 72-year-old man who had a carcinoma of the sigmoid is shown in Fig. 3. All the scans cover the abdomen and pelvis. This particular patient did not receive intact purified Mab anti CEA but $F(ab')_2$ fragments from Mab anti CEA. Panel A shows the total ^{131}I radioactivity 48 h after injection of 1 mCi of ^{131}I-labelled $F(ab')_2$, panel B the ^{99m}Tc radioactivity due to the injection of 500 μCi of ^{99m}Tc-labelled human albumin and 500 μCi of [99m]TcO$_4^-$. This injection is performed 15 min before scanning in order to detect blood pool and secreted radioactivity. The ^{99m}Tc radioactivity can be subtracted from ^{131}I radioactivity and this gives the results shown in panel C. The major information obtained from panel A is that there is relatively little non-specific accumulation of antibody associated ^{131}I radioactivity in the liver. In addition, there is a weak radioactive spot in the right lower part of the scan (arrow) corresponding to the sigmoid tumour. Unfortunately, there is a large amount of radioactivity in the urinary bladder (central lower part of the scan) due to the fact that the patient did not empty his bladder properly. Panel B shows the ^{99m}Tc radioactivity mostly in the liver and urinary bladder. After subtraction of ^{99m}Tc radioactivity from ^{131}I radioactivity, one sees in panel C, mostly the urinary bladder and on the right a definite asymmetric spot corresponding to the tumour (arrow). The tumour which was surgically removed 6 days after injection weighed 50 g. It was a well differentiated adenocarcinoma which infiltrated the sigmoid starting at a distance of 4 cm from the anus over a distance of 15 cm. The total ^{131}I radioactivity recovered in the tumour and measured in a gamma-counter was 897 nanoCuries (nCi) (this value was corrected for the physical half-life of ^{131}I during the six days period separating the injection from this measurement). This gave a concentration of 17.9 nCi/g of tumour. In comparison, the radioactivity was much lower in carefully dissected adjacent normal tissues, with values of 2.4 nCi/g for normal mucosa, 1.8 nCi/g of normal bowel wall after removal of the mucosa and 1.2 nCi/g of normal fatty tissues. One sees that the antibody associated radioactivity was 7-15 times more concentrated in tumour than in normal tissue. These factors of increased radioactivity in tumour are the highest that we obtained. Usually with polyclonal goat anti CEA antibodies (Mach *et al.*, 1980a, b) or with the same mouse Mab anti CEA these factors range between 2.5-10.

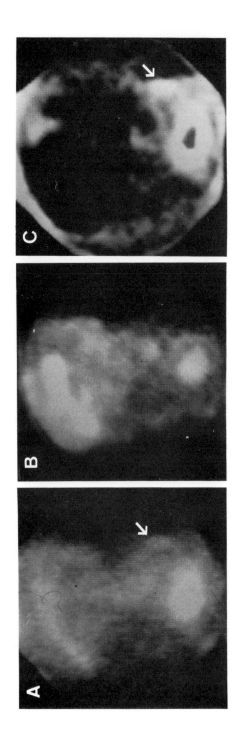

Fig. 3. Photoscans of the abdomen and pelvis from a 72-year-old patient who had an adenocarcinoma of the sigmoid and was injected 48 h before the scan with 0.5 mg of F(ab')$_2$ fragments from purified monoclonal anti CEA antibodies labelled with 1 mCi of ^{131}I. Panel A shows the total ^{131}I radioactivity with a weak radioactive spot corresponding to the tumour (arrow). Panel B shows the ^{99m}Tc radioactivity due to the injection, 15 min before the scanning, of 500 μCi of ^{99m}Tc linked to normal human serum albumin and 500 μCi of free ^{99m}TcO$_4$. Panel C shows the remaining ^{131}I radioactivity after computerized subtraction of the ^{99m}Tc radioactivity. Here, the radioactive spot corresponding to the tumour is more distinct (arrow) on the right of a marked radioactive area corresponding to the urinary bladder.

In conclusion, our results show that Mab-23 can be used as efficiently as the best goat anti CEA antibodies both in solid phase enzyme immunoassay for the measurement of CEA in patient serum and as radioactive tracer for the scanning localization of carcinoma in patients. Studies in progress in our laboratory and in others (Miggiano *et al.*, 1980; Rogers *et al.*, 1980) will determine whether or not other Mab directed against different epitopes of CEA can detect subpopulations of CEA molecules and further improve the tumor specificity of these methods.

REFERENCES

Accolla, R. S., Carrel, S., Phan, M., Heumann, D. and Mach, J. P. (1979). *In* "Protides of the Biological Fluids" (H. Peeters, Ed.), Vol. 27, 31–35. Pergamon Press, Oxford.

Accolla, R. S., Carrel, S. and Mach, J. P. (1980). *Proceedings of the National Academy of Sciences of USA* **77**, 563.

Avrameas, S. (1969). *Immunochemistry* **5**, 43.

Beihn, R. M., Damron, J. R. and Hafner, T. (1974). *Journal of Nuclear Medicine* **15**, 371.

Buchegger, F., Accolla, R. S., Carrel, S., Carmagnola, A., Girardet, Ch. and Mach J. P. (1980). *In* "Protides of the Biological Fluids" (H. Peeters, Ed.), Vol. 28, 511–515. Pergamon Press, Oxford.

Fritsché, R. and Mach, J. P., (1977). *Immunochemistry* **14**, 119.

Gold, P. and Freedman, S. O. (1965). *Journal of Experimental Medicine* **122**, 467.

Goldenberg, D. M., DeLand, F., Evishin, K., Bennett, S., Primus, F. J., van Nagell, J. R., Estes, N., De Simone, P. and Rayburn, P. (1978). *New England Journal of Medicine* **298**, 1384.

Goldenberg, D. M., Kim, E. E., DeLand, F. H., Bennett, S. and Primus, F. J. *Cancer Research* **40**, 2984.

von Kleist, S., Chavanel, G. and Burtin, P. (1972). *Proceedings of the National Academy of Sciences of USA* **69**, 2492.

Köhler, G. and Milstein, C. (1975). *Nature (London)* **256**, 495.

Mach, J. P. (1979). *In* "Tumor Markers: Impact and Prospects" (E. Boelsma and Ph. Rümke, Eds), Vol. 2, 117–149. Elsevier/North-Holland Biomedical Press, Amsterdam.

Mach, J. P., Carrel, S., Merenda, C., Sordat, B. and Cerottini, J. C. (1974a). *Nature (London)* **248**, 704.

Mach, J. P., Jaeger, Ph., Bertholet, M. M., Ruegsegger, C. H., Loosli, R. M. and Pettavel, J. (1974b). *Lancet* **II**, 535.

Mach, J. P., Carrel, S., Forni, M., Ritschard, J., Donath, A. and Alberto, P. (1980a). *New England Journal of Medicine* **303**, 5.

Mach, J. P., Forni, M., Ritschard, J., Buchegger, F., Carrel, S., Widgren, S., A. and Alberto, P. (1980b). *Oncodevelopmental Biology and Medicine* **1**, 49.

Miggiano, V., Stähli, C., Haring, P., Schmidt, J., Le Dain, M., Glatthaar, B. and Staehelin, T. (1980). *In* "Protides of the Biological Fluids" (H. Peeters, Ed.), Vol. 28, 501–504. Pergamon Press, Oxford.

Rogers, G. T., Rawlins, G. A. and Bagshawe, K. D. (1980). *In* "Protides of the Biological Fluids" (H. Peeters, Ed.), Vol. 28, 517–521. Pergamon Press, Oxford.

Thomson, D. M. P., Krupey, J., Freedman, S. O. and Gold, P. (1969). *Proceedings of the National Academy of Sciences of USA* **64**, 161.

MARKERS OF PROSTATE CANCER

J. E. Pontes

Urologic Oncology, Roswell Park Memorial Institute, Buffalo, New York, USA

The development of immunological assays for the measurement of biological markers has increased our capacity to detect small changes in these components in several biological fluids. As early as 1936, Gutman *et al.* (1936) using enzymatic determination established the relationship between an elevated serum acid phosphatase (SAP) and prostatic carcinoma. Since then, SAP has become the most common marker used in the diagnosis of prostatic carcinoma. The advent of immunological techniques for the measurement of serum prostatic acid phosphatase (SPAP), the isolation of prostate antigen (PA), a prostate specific protein, and the use of other non-specific markers in monitoring clinical changes in prostatic carcinoma are now part of the management of patients with this disease.

PROSTATE SPECIFIC MARKERS (PAP), (PA)

Prostatic Acid Phosphatase

Prostatic Acid Phosphatase (PAP) is a phosphohydrolase present in large amounts in normal prostatic secretions. The precise function of this enzyme in the semen is not fully known, although it may act upon several substrates such as phosphorylcholine producing important metabolites for the reproductive function of the spermatozoa. In the event of malignant transformation, PAP produced by the neoplastic cells will leak into the interstitium and event-

Serono Symposium No. 46, Markers for Diagnosis and Monitoring of Human Cancer, edited by M. I. Colnaghi, G. L. Buraggi and M. Ghione, 1982. Academic Press, London and New York.

ually will reach the intravascular space leading to the elevation in the serum commonly found in metastatic disease. Traditional methods for the assay of SAP have relied on an enzymatic reaction for the measurement of this enzyme. Since acid phosphatases are an ubiquitous group of enzymes present in almost every tissue, these methods lack the specificity for the measurement of PAP. A recent review of the subject by Yam (1974) illustrates the fact that traditional approaches such as the use of L-tartrate inhibition are inadequate for the separation of PAP from acid phosphatases present in other tissues. Early attempts to identify immunologically specific antigens to prostate are credited to Flocks *et al.* (1960). Shulman *et al.* (1964) were able to detect SPAP by immunological means using gel diffusion techniques. Antibodies to crude extracts of prostate were subsequently produced (Macalalag and Prout, 1967). Since then the purification and characterisation of PAP have been described extensively (Drechnin *et al.*, 1971; Luchter–Wasyl and Ostrowski, 1974; Choe *et al.*, 1978a). Initial methods for the immunological detection of serum PAP were relatively insensitive and semi-quantitative at best (Shulman *et al.*, 1964; Moncure *et al.*, 1972; Milasauskas and Rose, 1972). Presently used clinical methods for the detection of PAP in biological fluids fall into two categories: competitive binding assays and enzymoimmunoassays. Several competitive binding assays are presently available: they are either solid phase RIAs as described by Foti *et al.* (1975) or double antibody RIAs as described by Choe *et al.* (1978b), Vihko *et al.* (1978) and Mahan and Doctor (1979). Since these original descriptions a number of commercial assays have become available. Among the enzymoimmunoassays, the most frequently used clinically is the counterimmunoelectrophoresis (CIEP) as described by Chu *et al.* (1978), MacDonald *et al.* (1978) and Romas *et al.* (1978). More recently, new techniques with significantly increased sensitivity have become available. A solid phase fluorescent immunoassay (SPIF) has been described by Lee *et al.* (1980a); an enzymoimmunoassay (EIA) by Choe *et al.* (1979), a solid phase immunoabsorbent assay (SPIA) by Lee *et al.* (1980b). Techniques to localise PAP in histological sections have also become available. They are either immunofluorescent techniques as described by Pontes *et al.* (1977) or immunoperoxidase techniques as proposed by Jobsis *et al.* (1978). With the availability of techniques that are specific for determination of SPAP, a number of clinical studies using such techniques have become available, with contradictory results. Such conflicting results are due to differences in the specificity and sensitivity of various assays, poorly defined staging procedures and inadequate clinical trials (Pontes, 1981). Consensus of opinion is finally emerging on the value of these new immunochemical methods as a screening technique for prostatic carcinoma, the percentage of patients with localised prostatic disease and elevated serum PAP levels, and the use of such methods as a parameter of response to therapy in patients with disseminated disease. Because of the low prevalence of the disease in the general population combined with the relatively high percentage of false positive elevations in RIAs, it is obvious that despite the high sensitivity of these assays, their positive predictive value would be very low (Watson and Tang, 1980). This fact would lead to an unusually high percentage of patients with positive results (elevation) without disease (Kiesling and Watson, 1980). As mentioned above, a wide variation of positive results exists among patients with localised disease. Initial trials with RIA detected SPAP elevations in 33% of patients with stage A and 79% of patients with stage B prostatic carcinoma (Foti *et al.,* 1977). Subsequent trials yielded much lower results, only slightly superior to those obtained by colorimetric techniques (Mahan and Doctor, 1979; Bruce *et al.,* 1979; Griffiths, 1980; Quinones *et al.,* 1981). In a recent study of a group of patients with clinically localised prostatic carcinoma all elevations in SPAP were found in patients with microscopically disseminated disease at surgery (Pontes *et al.,* 1981a). It is clear that only a small percentage of patients with prostatic carcinoma localised to the prostate may show elevated values of SPAP in the absence of disseminated disease. Unfortunately, such information rather than being helpful, may actually be confusing as the clinician will be unsure if he is dealing with localised or disseminated disease. The use of SPAP determination by immunochemical methods as a parameter of response in patients with disseminated disease is an attractive concept as it is difficult in prostatic carcinoma to evaluate response to therapy objectively. Since in patients with extensive bony metastasis SAP determination may be influenced by acid phosphatase of other sources, it would be helpful if the measurement of SPAP would give a true extent of the disease. In several reports, there is a high percentage of patients with elevated SPAP by immunochemical methods as compared with colorimetric assays (Foti *et al.,* 1977; Mahan and Doctor, 1979; Bruce *et al.,* 1979; Griffiths, 1980). However, such differences have yet to be proven valuable since they are usually in good correlation with determinations of SAP by colorimetric techniques (Pontes *et al.,* 1981a). Acid phosphatase determination in the bone marrow samples (BMAP) were popularised in the mid-1970s as another parameter of early detection of disseminated disease. Although early reports showed this technique to be of value (Chua *et al.,* 1970; Sy *et al.,* 1973; Gursel *et al.,* 1974; Pontes *et al.,* 1975; Veneema *et al.,* 1977), it became clear that the number of false positive results using colorimetric assays were exceedingly high (Khan *et al.,* 1976; Boehme *et al.,* 1978). Comparison of BMAP determination by colorimetric assay and immunochemical methods was able to distinguish the false positive elevations found in the spectrophotometric assays (Pontes *et al.,* 1978, 1979; Belville *et al.,* 1978, 1979; Romas *et al.,* 1980). At the present time, although this test is no longer being used as an assay for detection of early disseminated disease, it appears of value in predicting patients at risk to develop disseminated prostatic carcinoma (Belville *et al.,* 1980). The development of immunohistochemical techniques for the localisation of PAP in tissue histological sections has proven valuable in clinical practice to identify metastatic prostatic carcinoma (Pontes *et al.,* 1977). This technique has also been helpful in the identification of prostatic epithelial cells in culture (Pontes *et al.,* 1977). Recently, attempts to correlate the histological grade with PAP production in tissue sections of patients with prostatic carcinoma and the relationship of such an association with hormonal responsiveness in these cases are being investigated with encouraging results (Pontes *et al.,* 1981b).

Prostate Antigen (PA)

The isolation and characterisation of a tissue specific protein from prostate having a molecular weight of 36,000 daltons has been accomplished by Wang

et al. (1979). Further studies led to the development of an assay for clinical
use in serum samples and an immunoperoxidase technique for localisation of
this antigen in histological sections (Papsidero *et al.*, 1980; Kuriyama *et al.*,
1980). This new marker has been found present in prostate tissue (both benign
and malignant) and found absent in a large number of other organs tested as
well as in a variety of tumors (Papsidero *et al.*, 1980). Using an immunoperoxidase
technique, metastasis of prostatic carcinoma has been identified in 100% of
the cases (Papsidero *et al.*, 1981). This marker has also been used to identify
cell lines of prostatic origin (Papsidero *et al.*, 1981) and has served as another
marker for the proper isolation of prostate epithelial cells. Work in progress
at our institution (Roswell Park Memorial Institute) in evaluating PA in serial
serum samples in patients with localised prostatic carcinoma treated either by
radical prostatectomy or by external radiation therapy is encouraging in the
detection of an association between the rise of serum PA and the development
of metastatic disease (Pontes *et al.*, 1981c).

NON-SPECIFIC MARKERS IN PROSTATE CANCER

A series of non-specific serum markers such as alkaline phosphatase and its
isoenzymes, polyamines (spermine and spermidine) and creatine kinase BB has
shown to be elevated in metastatic prostatic carcinoma. Such markers are helpful
in conjunction with other parameters to evaluate the progress of the disease
or response to therapy.

Alkaline Phosphatase and its Isoenzymes

The elevation of serum alkaline phosphatase occurs in a variety of diseases
with bone or liver involvement. Since prostatic carcinoma often metastasises
to the bone, producing osteoblastic lesions, total alkaline phosphatase (TAP)
in the serum is often elevated. Previous studies (Wajsman *et al.*, 1978) demonstrated a good relationship between bone metastasis and an elevated TAP. However, using the bone isoenzyme form of alkaline phosphatase (TAP) they noted
that 44% of patients with normal TAP had an elevated BAP. There was also
an excellent correlation to the decrease of TAP and BAP in response to therapy.
A more recent study (Killian *et al.*, 1981) correlated levels of TAP and its
isoenzymes with tumor burden in 98 patients with metastatic prostatic carcinoma.
A quantitative association between these enzymes and tumor mass was evident.
These markers were particularly valuable in evaluating progression or response
to therapy in a group of patients with extensive metastatic disease and normal
serum prostatic acid phosphatase. Noted in both of these studies was the fact
that highly elevated levels of TAP and its isoenzymes indicated poor prognosis,
probably reflecting the relationship of tumor burden and elevated alkaline phosphatase. In a recent study, another isoenzyme of alkaline phosphatase, the Regan
isoenzyme, was evaluated in a group of 148 patients, part of the clinical trials
of the National Prostatic Cancer Project (Slack *et al.*, 1981). Although 18%
of the patients demonstrated elevated values of this enzyme, no firm relationship
could be established regarding such values in progression or regression of the
disease.

Polyamines

The elevation of polyamines in the serum and urine of patients with malignant disease has been previously demonstrated (Bachrach, 1976). The value of such determinations, however, appears to be limited owing to lack of specificity (Russell, 1977). Because of this low specificity and lack of sensitivity, the measurement of erythrocyte polyamines may represent a better way to assess the value of these markers as these cells serve as carriers for both spermine and spermidine in the serum. Recently at our institute, Killian *et al.* (1981) have developed a method for the measurement of erythrocyte polyamines (spermidine and spermine) using a high pressure liquid chromatography (HPLC). In a study of sequential samples of 20 patients with disseminated prostatic carcinoma, an excellent relationship of the levels of polyamines in response to therapy was observed. The elevation of these markers, as alkaline phosphatase, appears to be related to tumor burden.

Other Markers

A variety of other non-specific markers are presently under study in patients with prostatic carcinoma. Chu *et al.* (1977) reported elevated ribonuclease (RNase) levels in about 70% of patients with prostatic carcinoma. No correlation was observed between RNase activity and acid phosphatase activity. Silverman *et al.* (1981) recently evaluated creatine kinase BB in the serum of patients with prostatic carcinoma. They reported a consistent relationship of elevated levels of CK–BB with the degree of tumor differentiation. Additionally, they reported significant differences between CK–BB purified from prostatic fluid from CK–BB of brain origin. The pattern of lactic dehydrogenase (LDH) isoenzymes in the semen has been extensively studied by Grayhack *et al.* (1980). The patterns of LDH as well as the presence of other components of prostatic fluid appear to be different between patients with benign and malignant conditions.

SUMMARY

The combined used of specific and non-specific markers are of tremendous importance in the diagnosis and follow-up of patients with prostatic carcinoma. Prostatic acid phosphatase (PAP) as measured by immunochemical assays may prove to be a good marker for objective measurement of response to therapy. Immunohistochemical techniques will aid the identification of metastatic lesions of prostatic origin. The use of serum PA as another specific marker in prostatic carcinoma will improve our capabilities to diagnose early metastatic disease. The concomitant use of non-specific markers as part of the evaluation and follow-up of those patients are particularly important in a small group of patients with prostatic carcinoma with normal levels of serum prostatic acid phosphatase. Further evaluation of new markers may improve the diagnosis and follow-up of prostatic cancer.

REFERENCES

Bachrach, U. (1976). *Italian Journal of Biochemistry* **25**, 77.
Belville, W., Cox, H. D., Mahan, D. E., Olmert, J. P., Mittenmeyer, B. T. and
Bruce, A. W. (1978). *Cancer* **41**, 2286.
Belville, W., Cox, H. D., Mahan, D. E., Stutzman, R. E. and Bruce, A. W. (1979).
Journal of Urology **121**, 422.
Belville, W., Mahan, D. E., Sepulveda, R. A., Bruce, A.W. and Miller, C. F. (1980).
American Urological Association Abstract No. 231.
Boehme, W. M., Augspurger, P. R., Wallner, S. F. and Dobohue, R. E. (1978).
Cancer **41**, 1433.
Bruce, A. W., Mahan, D. E., Morales, A., Clark, A. F. and Belville, W. D. (1979).
Journal of Urology **51**, 213.
Choe, B. K., Pontes, J. E., McDonald, I. and Rose, N. R. (1978a). *Preparative
Biochemistry* **8**, 73.
Choe, B. K., Pontes, J. E., Morrison, M. K. and Rose, N. R. (1978b). *Archives
of Andrology* **1**, 227.
Choe, B. K., Rose, N. R., Korol, M. and Pontes, J. E. (1979). *Proceedings of
the Society for Experimental Biology and Medicine* **162**, 396.
Chu, M., Wang, M. C., Kuciel, P., Valenzuela, L. A. and Murphy, G. P. (1977).
Cancer Treatment Reports **61**, 193.
Chu, T. M., Wang, M. C., Scott, W. W., Gibbons, R. P., Johnson, D. E., Schmidt,
J. D., Leoning, S. A., Prout, G. R. and Murphy, G. P. (1978). *Investigative
Urology* **15**, 319.
Chu, T. M., Wang, M. C., Lee, C. L., Killian, C. S., Valenzuela, L. A., Wajsman, Z.,
Slack, N. and Murphy, G. P. (1979). *Cancer Detection and Prevention* **2**, 693.
Chua, D. T., Veenema, R. J., Muggia, F. and Graff, A. (1970). *Journal of Urology*
103, 462.
Derechin, M., Ostrowski, W., Galka, M. and Barnard, E. A. (1971). *Biochimica
et Biophysica Acta* **250**, 143.
Flocks, W. H., Urich, C., Patel, C. A. and Opitz, J. M. (1960). *Journal of Urology*
84, 134.
Foti, A. G., Herschman, H. and Cooper, J. F. (1975). *Cancer Research* **35**, 2446.
Foti, A. G., Cooper, J. F., Herschman, H. and Malvaez, R. (1977). *New England
Journal of Medicine* **297**, 1357.
Grayhack, J. T., Lee, L., Oliver, L., Schaeffer, J. and Wendel, E. F. (1980).
The Prostate **1**, 227.
Griffiths, J. C. (1980). *Clinical Chemistry* **26**, 433.
Gursel, E. D., Rezvan, M., Sy, F. A. and Vennema, R. J. (1974). *Journal of
Urology* **111**, 53.
Gutman, E. B., Sproul, E. E. and Gutman, A. B. (1936). *American Journal of
Cancer* **28**, 485.
Jobsis, A. C., DeVries, G. P., Anholt, R. R. H. and Saunders, G. T. B. (1978).
Cancer **41**, 1788.
Kiesling, V. J. and Watson, R. A. (1980). *Urology* **16**, 242.
Khan, R., Turner, B., Edson, M. and Dolan, M. (1976). *Journal of Urology* **117**, 79.
Killian, C. S., Vargas, F. P., Pontes, J. E., Beckley, S., Wajsman, Z., Slack, N. H.,
Murphy, G. P. and Chu, T. M. (1981). *The Prostate* **2**, 187.
Kuriyama, M., Wang, M. C., Papsidero, L. D., Killian, C. S., Shimano, T., Valenzuela,
L., Nishiura, T., Murphy, G. P. and Chu, M. T. (1980). *Cancer Research* **40**,
4658.
Lee, C. L., Chu, T. M., Wajsman, L. Z., Slack, N. H. and Murphy, G. P. (1980a).
Urology **15**, 338.
Lee, C. L., Killian, C. S., Murphy, G. P. and Chu, T. M. (1980b). *Clinica Chimica
Acta* **101**, 209.

Luchter–Wasyl, E. and Ostrowski, W. (1974). *Biochimica et Biophysica Acta* **365**, 349.

Macalalag, E. V., Jr and Prout, G. R., Jr (1967). *Investigative Urology* **4**, 321.

Mahan, D. E. and Doctor, B. P. (1979). *Clinical Biochemistry* **12**, 10.

McDonald, I., Rose, N. R., Pontes, J. E. and Choe, B. K. (1978). *Archives of Andrology* **1**, 234.

Milisuaskas, V. and Rose, N. R. (1972). *Clinical Chemistry* **18**, 1529.

Moncure, C. W., Johnston, C. L., Jr, Smith, M. V. and Koontz, W. W., Jr (1972). *Journal of Urology* **108**, 609.

Papsidero, L. D., Wojcieszyn, J. D., Horoszewicz, J. S., Leong, S. S., Murphy, G. P. and Chu, T. W. (1980). *Cancer Research* **40**, 3032.

Papsidero, L. D., Kuriyama, M., Wang, M. C., Horoszewicz, J., Leong, S. S., Valenzuela, L., Murphy, G. P. and Chu, T. M. (1981). *Journal of National Cancer Institute* **66**, 37.

Pontes, J. E. (1981). *Journal of Urology* **125**, 375.

Pontes, J. E., Alcorn, S. W., Thomas, A. J. and Pierce, J. M., Jr (1975). *Journal of Urology* **114**, 422.

Pontes, J. E., Choe, B. K. and Rose, N. R. (1977). *Journal of Urology* **117**, 459.

Pontes, J. E., Choe, B. K., Rose, N. R. and Pierce, J. M., Jr (1978). *Journal of Urology* **119**, 772.

Pontes, J. E., Choe, B. K., Rose, N. R. and Pierce, J. M., Jr (1979). *Journal of Urology* **122**, 178.

Pontes, J. E., Choe, B. K., Rose, N. R., Ercole, C. and Pierce, J. M., Jr (1981a). *Journal of Urology* **126**, 363.

Pontes, J. E., Rose, N. R., Ercole, C. and Pierce, J. M., Jr (1981b). *Journal of Urology* **126**, 187.

Pontes, Y. E., Chu, T. M., Slack, N., Karr, J. and Murphy, G. P. (1981c). *Journal of Urology*. (In press.)

Quinones, G. R., Rohner, T. J., Drago, J. R. and Demers, L. M. (1981). *Journal of Urology* **125**, 361.

Romas, N. A., Hus, K. C., Tomashefsky, P. and Tannenbaum, M. (1978). *Urology* **12**, 79.

Romas, N. A., Veenema, R. J., Hsu, K. C., Tomashefsky, P., Lattimer, J. K. and Tannenbaum, M. (1980). *Journal of Urology* **123**, 392.

Russell, D. H. (1977). *Clinical Chemistry* **23**, 22.

Shulman, S., Manrod, L., Gonder, M. and Soanes, W. A. (1964). *Journal of Immunology* **93**, 474.

Silverman, L. M., Chapman, J. F., Jones, M. E., Dermer, G. B., Pullano, T. and Tokes, Z. A. (1981). *The Prostate*. (In press.)

Slack, N. H., Chu, T. M., Wajsman, L. Z. and Murphy, G. P. (1981). *Cancer* **47**, 146.

Sy, F. A., Gursel, E. D. and Veenema, R. J. (1973). *Urology* **2**, 125.

Veenema, R. J., Gursel, E. D., Romas, N., Wechsler, M. and Lattimer, J. K. (1977). *Journal of Urology* **117**, 81.

Vihko, P., Sajanti, E., Janne, O., Peltonen, L. and Vihko, R. (1978). *Clinical Chemistry* **24**, 1915.

Wajsman, Z., Chu, T. M., Bross, D., Saroff, J., Murphy, G. P., Johnson, D. E., Scott, W. W., Gibbons, R. P., Prout, G. P. and Schmidt, J. E. (1978). *Journal of Urology* **119**, 244.

Wang, M. C., Valenzuela, L. A., Murphy, G. P. and Chu, T. M. (1979). *Investigative Urology* **17**, 159.

Watson, R. A. and Tang, D. B. (1980). *New England Journal of Medicine* **303**, 497.

Yam, L. T. (1974). *American Journal of Medicine* **6**, 604.

HUMAN OVARIAN CANCER MARKERS AND ANTIGENS

K. O. Lloyd

Memorial Sloan-Kettering Cancer Center, New York, USA

HUMAN OVARIAN CANCER MARKERS AND ANTIGENS

Because the initial diagnosis of ovarian cancer is often fatally delayed, considerable efforts have been expended in attempts to develop an immunodiagnostic method for the early detection of this disease. In addition to examining the use of general markers such as CEA, investigators have attempted to identify antigens that are specific for ovarian cancer. Some of the markers and antigens that have been developed for ovarian epithelial cancer are listed in Table I. Many of these antigens have been comprehensively reviewed by Bhattacharya and Barlow (1979) and will not be discussed in detail here. Most of the putative markers that have been developed come under the heading of inappropriately expressed components, particularly those normally associated with placental or embryonic tissue or with pregnancy. To date, no antigen or marker that is capable of detecting very early ovarian cancer has emerged. A number of markers have possible use for monitoring tumor burden and a few others have potential use for early diagnosis but have not yet been fully analyzed.

Our early efforts in this area involved the immunisation of rabbits with extracts of ovarian adenocarcinomas in an attempt to determine the range of ovarian cancer related antigens that could be detected (Imamura *et al.*, 1978). Five antigens that could be detected in ovarian tumor extracts but not in normal ovary were identified. Three of these proved to be previously recognised antigens (CEA, NGP and PZP) and were not further investigated. Two others (OvC-1 and -2) appeared to be new antigens and were selected for further study. The distribution of these antigens in tumor extracts is given in Table II and in sera in Table III.

Serono Symposium No. 46, Markers for Diagnosis and Monitoring of Human Cancer, edited by M. I. Colnaghi, G. L. Buraggi and M. Ghione, 1982. Academic Press, London and New York.

Table I. Markers for epithelial ovarian tumors.

Marker	Reference
Embryonic	
CEA	Khoo and MacKay (1973)
BOFA	Goldenberg *et al.* (1978)
Prealbumin	Tatarinov *et al.* (1978)
Fetal sulfoglycoprotein	Hakkinen (1974)
Embryonic antigen	Tatarinov and Kalishnikov (1977)
OvC-2	Imamura *et al.* (1978)
Pregnancy associated	
PAM (PZP)	Stimson (1975); Bohn (1973); Lin and Halbert (1975)
OvC-1 (OCAA-1)	Imamura *et al.* (1978); Bhattacharya and Barlow (1976)
Placental	
Regan isoenzyme	Nathanson and Fishman (1971)
D-phenotype PAP	Inglis *et al.* (1973)
Placental lactogen	Weintraub and Rosen (1971)
Enzymes	
Urokinase	Astedt and Holmberg (1976)
Glycosyl transferases	Bhattacharya *et al.* (1976)
Plasma ribonuclease	Sheid *et al.* (1977)
Aminopeptidases	Blum and Sirota (1977)
Other antigens	
Thermostable antigen	Burton *et al.* (1976)
OCAA	Bhattacharya and Barlow (1976)
OTAG	Bagshawe *et al.* (1980)
M1	Bara *et al.* (1977)
M4 (OCAA-3/4)	Bara *et al.* (1977)
Mucinous cyst antigen	Dawson *et al.* (1980)
OCA-b	Knauf and Urbach (1977, 1978)
Miscellaneous	
Secretory piece (SC)	Klein *et al.* (1978)
Fibrin and fibrinogen degradative products	Svanberg and Astedt (1975)
Fibronectin (MAD-2)	Todd *et al.* (1980)

Both antigens have been partially purified and they have also been identified in tumors by immunoprecipitation of ^{125}I-labeled extracts (Lloyd, 1980a, b). Our recent work has concentrated on OvC-1 and progress in this area will be described in detail.

OvC-1 appears to be a new pregnancy associated protein that is anomalously expressed in certain tumors. It was detected in three out of five pregnancy sera, in placenta and in amniotic fluid. Its detection in a number of sera from ovarian cancer patients, even using the relatively insensitive Ouchterlony double-diffusion technique, suggested that it may be useful as a diagnostic marker. Amniotic fluid has been used as a convenient source of material for isolating and purifying

Table II. Occurrence of OvC-1 and -2 in extracts of human tumors.

Tumor extract	No. of tumors positive for antigens		No. of tumors tested
	OvC-1	OvC-2	
Ovarian tumors			
Epithelial cancer			
Mucinous cystadenocarcinoma	5	0	6
Serous cystadenocarcinomas	3	0	7
Adenocarcinoma	38	8	77
Endometroid cancer	2	0	3
Leiomyosarcoma	0	0	1
Dysgerminoma	0	1	1
Benign cystadenocarcinoma	0	0	2
Culture cell lines			
(SK-OV-3 and SK-OV-4)	0	0	2
Other tumors			
Fallopian tube cancer	0	0	2
Cervical cancer	2	0	8
Breast cancer	3	0	8
Bladder cancer	0	0	5
Gastric cancer	1	0	3
Colon cancer	5	0	10
Pancreatic cancer	2	0	4
Choriocarcinoma	0	0	1
Malignant melanoma	0	0	4

Table III. Occurrence of OvC-1 and -2 in sera of normal individuals and of patients with cancer.

Serum source	No. of sera positive for antigens		No. of sera tested
	OvC-1	OvC-2	
Cancer patients			
Ovarian cancer	4	0	22
Cervical cancer	0	0	16
Breast cancer	0	0	10
Colon cancer	0	0	11
Pancreatic cancer	0	0	3
Malignant melanoma	0	0	15
Normal individuals			
Male	0	0	25
Female	1[a]	0	20
Cord serum[b]	2	0	5
Pregnancy serum[c]	3	0	5

[a]Positive serum is from individual receiving contraceptive pills. [b]From full-term pregnancy. [c]From 6 to 9 months pregnancy.

this antigen. The procedure developed is shown in Fig. 1. This sequence of fractionation steps separates OvC-1 from OvC-2 by taking advantage of the larger size
of OvC-2 and its ability to bind to blue Sepharose. OvC-1 was finally purified
by affinity chromatography with *Lens culinaris* hemagglutinin (Lloyd, 1980a).
As the yield is rather low in this final step, however, we have recently developed
a procedure for isolating more antigen from the unbound fraction by CM-Biogel
chromatography. OvC-1 purified by this scheme is a glycoprotein of approximately 50,000 daltons molecular weight. Radioimmunoprecipitation experiments
using ^{125}I-iodinated samples confirmed that the antigen present in ovarian tumor
extracts was the same as the component detected in amniotic fluid (Lloyd,
1980a). Interestingly the 50,00 dalton glycoprotein seemed to be associated

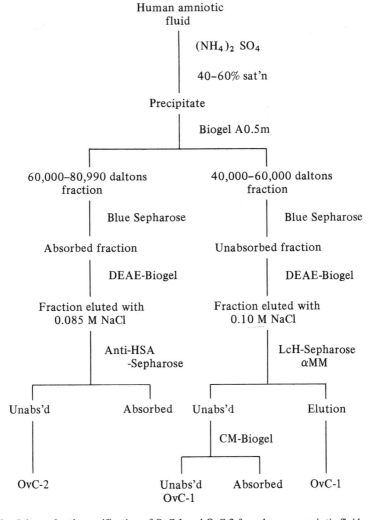

Fig. 1.   Scheme for the purification of OvC-1 and OvC-2 from human amniotic fluid.

with a 20,000 dalton component in tumor extracts, whereas only the higher molecular weight form was detected in amniotic fluid.

Current efforts are concerned with a detailed examination of the homogeneity of purified OvC-1 using 2-D polyacrylamide gel electrophoresis and with the development of mouse monoclonal antibodies OvC-1. As shown in Fig. 2, precipitation of ^{125}I-iodinated, partially purified OvC-1 by a specific rabbit antiserum results in the identification of one major and several minor components when the products are analyzed by 2-D electrophoresis. The major component, which corresponds to OvC-1 identified previously (Lloyd, 1980a), is a very acidic component with a pI of less than 4.0. In fact the pI is so low that OvC-1 is best analyzed by non-equilibrium pH gradient electrophoresis (NEPHGE). Our recognition of the highly acidic nature of OvC-1 will be extremely helpful in future studies on this antigen.

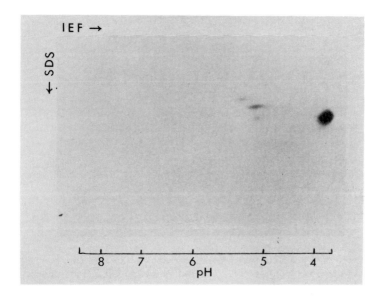

Fig. 2. Analysis of ^{125}I-labeled OvC-1 immunoprecipated by rabbit anti-OvC-1 serum by 2-D polyacrylamide gel electrophoresis.

Since the detection of OvC-1 would be greatly facilitated by the availability of monoclonal antibodies to this antigen, mice have been immunized with partially purified OvC-1. After fusion of spleen cells with NS-1 myeloma, antibody producing clones were surveyed using the radioimmunoprecipitation method. Preliminary results indicate that clones producing antibodies to 3 different components having molecular weights of 70,000, 52,000 and 48,000, respectively, were identified. The third antibody seems to be the one identifying the OvC-1 but further work is needed to confirm this and to determine whether this reagent is capable of detecting the antigen in tumor extracts and patients' sera.

ACKNOWLEDGEMENTS

This work is supported by National Institute grants (CA-08748 and CA-26184).

REFERENCES

Astedt, B. and Holmberg, L. (1976). *Nature* **261**, 595.
Bagshawe, K. D., Wass, M. and Searle, F. (1980). *In* "Ovarian Cancer, Proc. Int. Symp. On Ovarian Cancer" (C. E. Newman, C. H. J. Ford and J. A. Jordan, Eds), Adv. Bioscience, Vol. **26**, 57. Pergamon, Oxford.
Bara, J., Malarewicz, A., Loisillier, F. and Burtin, P. (1977). *British Journal of Cancer* **37**, 49.
Bhattacharya, M. and Barlow, J. J. (1976). *National Cancer Institute Monograph* **42**, 25.
Bhattacharya, M. and Barlow, J. J. (1979). *Int. Adv. Surg. Oncol.* **2**, 155.
Bhattacharya, M., Chatterjee, S. K. and Barlow, J. J. (1976). *Cancer Research* **36**, 2096.
Blum, M. and Sirota, P. (1977). *Israel Journal of Medical Science* **13**, 875.
Bohn, H. (1973). *Blut* **XXVI**, 205.
Burton, R. M., Hope, N. J. and Lubbers, L. M. (1976). *American Journal of Obstetrics and Gynecology* **125**, 472.
Dawson, J. R., Kutteh, W. H., Whitesides, D. B. and Gall, S. A. (1980). *Gynecologic Oncology* **10**, 6.
Goldenberg, D. M., Garner, T. F., Pant, K. D. and Van Nagel, J. R. (1978). *Cancer Research* **38**, 1246.
Hakkinen, I. P. T. (1974). *Transplantation Review* **20**, 61.
Imamura, I, Takahashi, T., Lloyd, K. O., Lewis, L. J. and Old, L. J. (1978). *International Journal of Cancer* **21**, 570.
Inglis, N. R., Kirley, S. and Stolbach, L. L. (1973). *Cancer Research* **33**, 1657.
Khoo, S. K. and MacKay, E. V. (1973). *Australian and New Zealand Journal of Obstetrics and Gynecology* **13**, 1.
Klein , J. L., Gall, S. A. and Dawson, J. R. (1978). *Journal of the National Cancer Institute* **61**, 57.
Knauf, S. and Urbach, G. I. (1978). *American Journal of Obstetrics and Gynecology* **131**, 780.
Knauf, S. and Urbach, G. I. (1978). *Journal of Obstetrics and Gynecology* **131**, 780.
Lin, T. M. and Halbert, S. P. (1975). *International Archives of Allergy* **48**, 101.
Lloyd, K. O. (1980a). *In* "Serological Analysis of Human Cancer Antigens" (S. A. Rosenberg, Ed.), pp. 515–524. Academic Press, New York.
Lloyd, K. O. (1980b). *In* "Serological Analysis of Human Cancer Antigens" (S. A. Rosenberg, Ed.), pp. 651–653. Academic Press, New York.
Nathanson, L. and Fishman, W. H. (1971). *Cancer* **27**, 1388.
Stimson, W. H. (1975). *Journal of Clinical Pathology* **28**, 868.
Sheid, B., Lu, T., Pedrinan, L. and Nelson, J. H. (1977). *Cancer* **39**, 2204.
Svanberg, L. and Astedt, B. (1975). *Cancer* **35**, 1382.
Tatarinov, V. S. and Kalashnikov, V. V. (1977). *Nature* **265**, 638.

Tatarinov, Y. S., Kalashnikov, V. V., Yu, M., Vasiliev, S. G., Voloshuk, S. G., Kraevsky, N. A. and Vorsanova, S. G. (1978). *Lancet* ii, 1122.
Todd, H. D., Coffee, M. S., Waalkes, T. P., Abeloff, M. D. and Parsons, R. G. (1980). *Journal of the National Cancer Institute* **65**, 901.
Weintraub, B. D. and Rosen, S. W. (1971). *Journal of Clinical Endocrinology and Metabolism* **32**, 94.

TUMOUR MARKERS AND TESTICULAR CANCER

P. Monaghan, D. Raghavan, R. A. J. McIlhinney, V. Moshakis, A. Sullivan,
E. Dinsdale and A. M. Neville

*Ludwig Institute for Cancer Research (London Branch), Royal Marsden
Hospital Sutton, Surrey, UK*

The appreciation that human tumours may express, elaborate and release a wide variety of products, i.e. the so-called tumour markers, has created new avenues of oncological study aimed at assessing their biological significance and clinical utility (Laurence and Neville, 1981).

Tumour markers may be grouped into several different categories; some are examples of oncofoetoplacental products with hormonal or enzymic properties. For others, functional properties remain to be ascribed. Many have been detected by immunological means and so are referred to as "antigens" (Neville *et al.*, 1978).

The recent advent of the monoclonal antibody technique (Kohler and Milstein, 1975) and the availability of other immunological reagents has resulted in the description of several antigens on the cell surfaces of both murine and human germ cell tumours (see McIlhinney, 1981). Little is, as yet, known of their biological significance or whether they are released into the circulation. Nonetheless, this approach to the study of these tumours may have important scientific, clinical and therapeutic implications for the future.

A list of some of the presently recognized products of human germ cell tumours, to which form of testicular cancer this paper will be limited, is shown in Table I. It may be seen that hormones, enzymes and antigens are all well represented. Most work to date has been carried out with human chorionic gonadotrophin (HCG) and α-fetoprotein (AFP), as they would appear at present to have most clinical relevance (Kohn, 1978; Lange and Fraley, 1977; Thompson and Haddow, 1979; Mann *et al.*, 1980; Laurence and Neville, 1981).

Serono Symposium No. 46, Markers for Diagnosis and Monitoring of Human Cancer, edited by M. I. Colnaghi, G. L. Buraggi and M. Ghione, 1982. Academic Press, London and New York.

Table I.   Some products of human germ cell tumours.

Placental type moeties	Human chorionic gonadtrophin (HCG)
	Human placental lactogen (HPL)
	Pregnancy specific β_1-glycoprotein (SP1)
	Fibronectin
Yolk sac products	α-Fetoprotein (AFP)
	Prealbumin, transferrin, α_1-antitrypsin
Oncofoetal antigens	Carcinoembryonic antigen (CEA)
Enzyme and isoenzymes	Placental alkaline phosphatase, lactate
	dehydrogenase

This paper will be devoted to a discussion of the role of tumour markers in improving our knowledge and appreciation of the pathology and histogenesis of human germ cell tumours and to examining their clinical role in facilitating tumour diagnosis, detection and monitoring.

PATHOLOGICAL ASPECTS

The production of HCG is classically associated with the trophoblastic elements which comprise choriocarcinomas (Bagshawe, 1969). However, elevated plasma levels of HCG have been noted in association with germ cell tumours. One recent survey reports that pre-operative HCG levels were raised in 15% of subjects with seminomas and 46% of those with non-seminomatous germ cell tumours (Mann *et al.*, 1980). This is generally regarded as being due to the presence of teratomatous or choriocarcinomatous elements in those tumours. Nonetheless, despite a meticulous search, it is frequently not possible to demonstrate such elements. The application of immunocytochemical methods for HCG has shown that not infrequently seminomas and non-seminomatous germ cell tumours contain HCG positive cells (Neville *et al.*, 1978). Generally, these cells are giant in type, often forming syncitia in relation to blood vessels or large, irregularly shaped groups (Neville *et al.*, 1978). Occasionally, isolated single cells of varying size may also contain HCG. The importance of these observations in both seminomas and non-seminomatous germ cell tumours is that HCG production can be associated with a cell type which does not necessarily have the characteristic structural form of trophoblast elements.

Studies of AFP, both in the plasma and at the cellular level also raise doubts about the accuracy of current classifications of germ cell tumours. AFP is a product of the normal yolk sac carcinomas (endodermal sinus tumours). Recent studies have drawn attention to the fact that embryonal cell carcinomas (MTU) in the absence of classical yolk sac elements may be associated with raised plasma AFP levels (Grigor *et al.*, 1977; Parkinson and Beilby, 1980; Mann *et al.*, 1980). Similarly, rare examples of "pure seminomas" may be found to have raised AFP values (Raghavan *et al.*, 1981a, b).

We have attempted to start to unravel this problem of classification and histogenesis and, thereby, to improve our understanding of these lesions by establishing human germ cell tumour xenografts in immune suppressed mice (Raghavan *et al.,* 1981a, b, c; Raghavan and Neville, 1981).

We have succeeded in establishing a series of six germ cell tumours in immune deprived mice (Table II) and have demonstrated that the histological and func-

Table II. Human germ cell tumour xenografts: patient, marker and histological details.

Xenograft designation	Patient details			Xenograft details		
	Histology	AFP	HCG	Histology	AFP	HCG
		production			production	
HX 39	E	±[a]	±[a]	E	±[a]	±[a]
HX 53	S/Y	+	−	S/Y	+	−
HX 57	Y	+	−	Y	+	−
HX 84	E	+→−[b]	−	E	−	−
HX 111	E	+	+	E	+	−
HX 112	Y	+	−	Y	+	−

Abbreviations E: embryonal cell carcinoma; S: seminoma; Y: yolk sac tumour; AFP: α-feto-protein; HCG: human chorionic gonadotrophin. "Both tumour products were present in raised amounts intermittently in the patient. Similarly raised levels occurred sporadically in the plasma of the xenograft bearing mice. [b]Raised serum AFP before treatment; subsequent relapse without detectable serum AFP levels.

tional properties of such xenografts are similar to those of the human tumours from which they were derived (Monaghan *et al.,* 1981). Moreover, these properties can be maintained through many serial passages. Unfortunately, no lesion classified as a pure seminoma was established as a xenograft in our immune deprived rodents.

The xenograft designated HX 53 (Table II) is of particular interest. Histo-logically, the primary testicular tumour was a classical seminoma. Tumour markers were not assayed at this time. The patient later developed raised AFP levels (6,600 μg/1) and was found to have abdominal lymph node metastases. These were removed and histological examination revealed that once again the lesion was a seminoma. In both the primary and, more especially, the metastatic tumours, small cystic spaces in which there are PAS positive eosinophilic globules were also noted. The lymph node lesion was the one from which a successful xenograft was derived. The xenograft maintained through numerous passages the same pattern of a seminoma (Fig. 1); cystic spaces were also found and in some of the passages became more prominent forming quite large cysts and occasionally Schiller–Duval bodies, thereby showing overt morphological features in keeping with the diagnosis of yolk sac-type differentiation. Using suitable immunocyto-chemical methods, AFP was demonstrated in the serum, in the cysts and their surrounding cells and, to a lesser extent, in some of the cells in the solid "seminoma" areas of the tumour (Raghavan *et al.,* 1981b). Fibronectin was also produced by this lesion (Ruoslahti *et al.,* 1981).

Ultrastructural examination revealed that the solid areas consisted of cells with features of classical seminoma cells, whereas in the cystic areas the tumour cells were more akin to yolk sac carcinoma cells (Figs 2 and 3). Between those two extremes there were intermediate cells showing gradations of structure

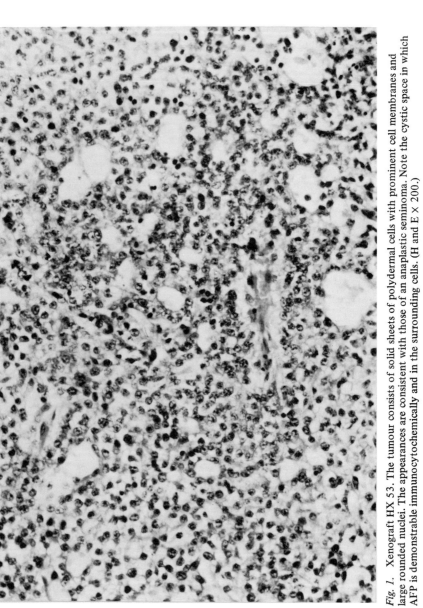

Fig. 1. Xenograft HX 53. The tumour consists of solid sheets of polydermal cells with prominent cell membranes and large rounded nuclei. The appearances are consistent with those of an anaplastic seminoma. Note the cystic space in which AFP is demonstrable immunocytochemically and in the surrounding cells. (H and E × 200.)

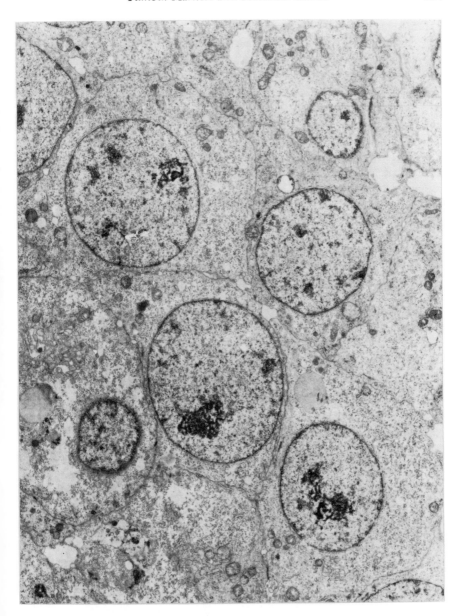

Fig. 2. Xenograft HX 53. Electron micrograph. Cells of the solid region resemble seminoma, with round nuclei, complex nucleoli and accumulations of glycogen. Desmosomes are rare. (× 4,500.)

between seminoma and yolk sac (Monaghan *et al.*, 1981). There is, therefore, an apparent ultrastructural and functional continuum between "seminoma" and yolk sac tumours. Moreover, the xenograft is not unique, as our further studies have confirmed that there is a group of tumours which at light micro-scopic level have the appearance of seminoma but which in fact are more properly classified as yolk sac tumours (Raghavan *et al.*, 1981a, b, c).

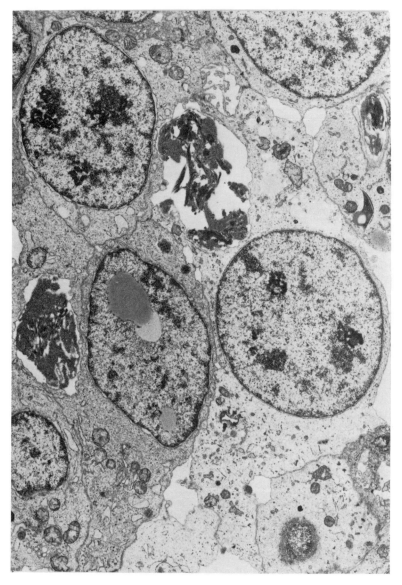

Fig. 3.   Xenograft HX 53. Electron micrograph. Cells of the cystic region form small lumina
lined by microvilli. Large areas of extracellular electron dense material are present. (× 6,500.)

The embryonal cell carcinoma xenografts (Table II) also suggest that a continuum may exist between embryonal cell carcinoma and yolk sac carcinoma.
Three xenografts are of particular interest, namely HX 84, 111 and 39. They
show a range of varying degrees of differentiation with HX 111 being the best
differentiated, 84 the poorest and 39 intermediate between those two (Figs
4, 5 and 6). Of interest is that HX 111 is associated with AFP production (Fig. 7),

while AFP is occasionally produced by HX 39 but not at all by HX 84. At the ultrastructural level all the tumours show marked heterogeneity (Figs 8 and 9). However, HX 111 expresses features in many areas akin to yolk sac, while HX 39 expresses such features only in some areas. In HX 84, these structures are not seen. There is, therefore, once more a continuum between embryonal cell carcinoma and yolk sac carcinomas.

These conclusions regarding homology between different germ cell tumour types helps to explain how seminoma and teratoma may co-exist; why non-seminomatous metastases may occur from tumours diagnosed as pure seminomas; why seminomatous and teratomatous elements may occur together in extragonadal sites; and the association of marker proteins such as HCG and AFP with lesions not showing the classical histological patterns associated with their production.

On this basis, therefore, it would appear not unreasonable to propose a modified scheme for the evolution of germ cell tumours (Raghavan and Neville, 1981). In this scheme (Fig. 10) morphologically recognizable seminomas of germ cell origin are considered to be the precursor for a series of stages of further differentiation forming a continuum and which can result in various forms of teratomatous and extra embryonic-type tumours. The present scheme has been shown in part, namely the continuum between seminoma and seminoma with yolk sac and for HCG differentiation and the equation of certain embryonal cell carcinomas with yolk sac carcinomas. While other aspects of the proposals remain to be fully substantiated, this putative classification is potentially more accurate and could have biological and clinical importance.

DIAGNOSTIC AND MONITORING ASPECTS

Many studies have been conducted regarding the clinical role of HCG and AFP (for a comprehensive review see Norgaard–Pederson and Raghavan, 1981). There is now little doubt that their sequential measurement in plasma and/or urine after initial diagnosis and treatment can result in the earlier detection of metastases with therapeutic advantage. Their sequential assay can also serve to give an indication of the efficacy of the various therapies. Nonetheless, it is important to realize that metastases may develop in the presence of normal levels of either marker, and marker levels may decline with therapy, yet the metastases persist or continue to grow. This may be because the therapy has a greater effect on the HCG and/or AFP producing clones than on other cell types present (Willemse et al., 1981a, b). In some, chemotherapy has been reported to induce maturation to form in differentiated teratoma.

While the assay of plasma HCG and AFP is of little value in the detection of primary germ cell tumours, it may be of assistance with the more accurate staging of disease at or before operation (Barzell and Whitmore, 1979). This is particularly true when elevated levels are present at the time of initial presentation. It has now been shown by several workers (Lange and Fraley, 1977; Kohn, 1978; Mann et al., 1980) that to estimate the plasma half-life of these marker proteins has clinical merit. When there is a delay in their decline to normal with various therapies, it indicates either the persistence of disease because of complete surgery or the relative inadequacy of other therapies.

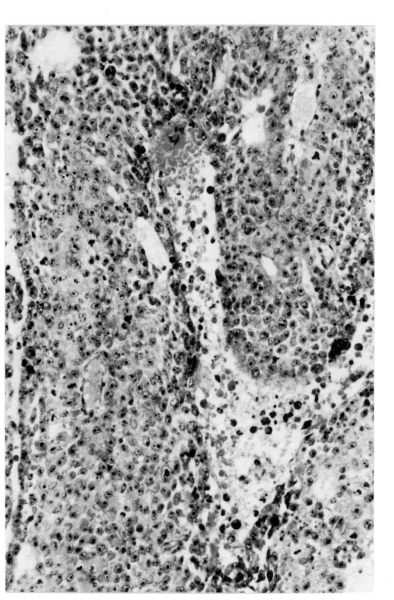

Fig 4. Xenograft HX 84. The tumour cells which form solid sheets and cords, are pleomorphic and contain enlarged vescicular nuclei with a prominent nucleolus. Necrosis is marked. The appearances are consistent with those of an embryonal cell carcinoma. (H and E × 250.)

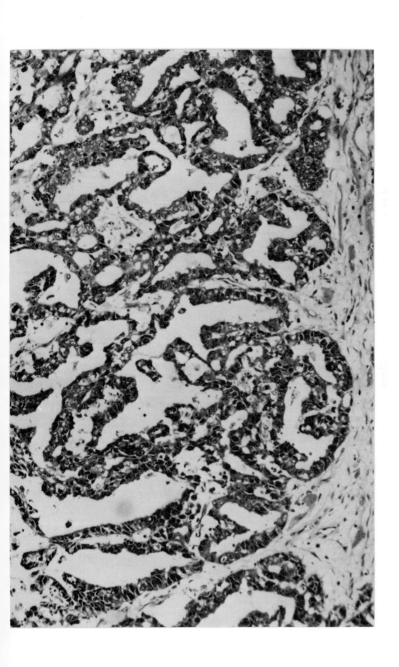

Fig. 5. Xenograft HX 111. The tumour consists of a series of cystic spaces into which adenopapillary projections abut. (H and E × 200.)

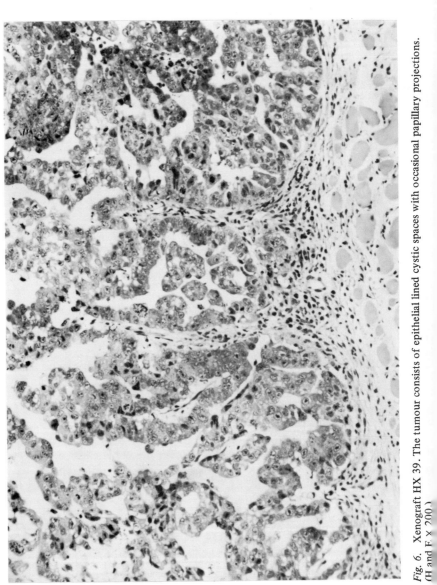

Fig. 6. Xenograft HX 39. The tumour consists of epithelial lined cystic spaces with occasional papillary projections. (H and E x 200.)

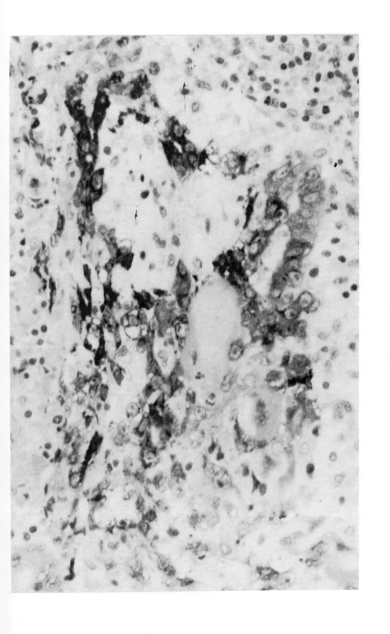

Fig. 7. Xenograft HX 111. An immunocytochemical stain for AFP using antibody linked alkaline phospharase as the indicator. Note that AFP is present in the cytoplasm of some cells and absent from others. (H and E × 250.)

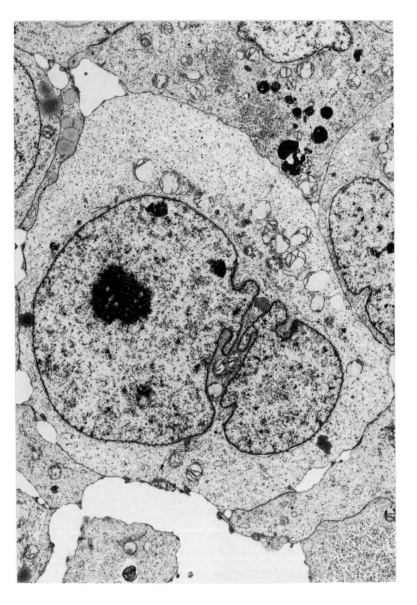

Fig. 8. Xenograft HX 84. Electron micrograph. The cells show few differentiated features, lacking desmosomes and microvilli on their cell membranes. (× 3,600.)

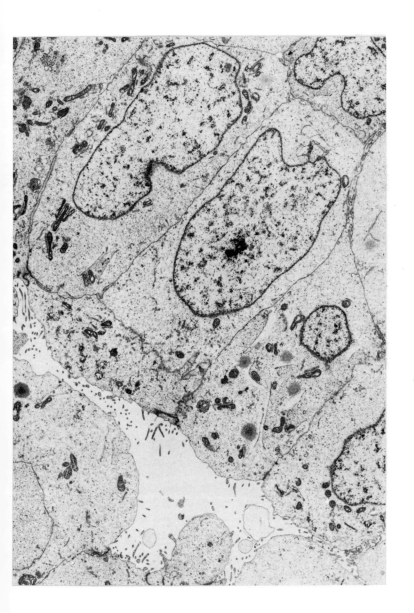

Fig. 9. Xenograft HX 111. Electron micrograph. The cells show an organized growth pattern with microvilli lined lumina. Junctional complexes are present at the luminal borders of the cells. (× 4,635.)

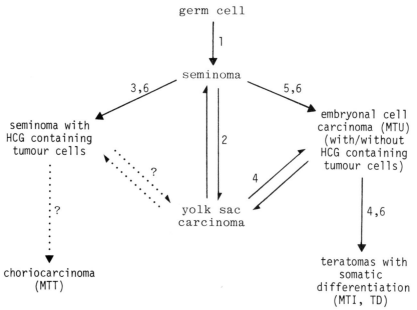

Fig. 10. Tentative scheme for the evolution of germ cell tumours.

Nevertheless, HCG and AFP represent only certain types of tumour cell and there is a need to derive markers for the other cell types in such tumours. While enzymes such as lactate dehydrogenase, alkaline phosphatase and the placental proteins have been proposed, none, has proved to be as good as either AFP or HCG in a clinical setting (Norgaard–Pederson and Raghavan, 1981). The recent demonstration that certain germ cell tumours may produce a different form of fibronectin (Ruoslahti *et al.*, 1981) may provide us with a further useful marker.

CELL SURFACE MARKERS AND GERM CELL TUMOURS

The introduction of the monoclonal antibody technique (Köhler and Milstein, 1975) is proving to be an important source of reagents for the examination of the cell surface with respect to differentiation and development. In addition, this approach may provide a series of new markers and reagents which may have clinical applicability enabling the better classification and detection of germ cell tumours.

There is evidence to suggest that murine embryonal cell carcinomas may possess unique cell membrane components. Preliminary evidence from studies of human teratoma would suggest that they possibly share certain cell surface antigens in common with the murine system and that the human systems may express unique cell membrane determinants (McIlhinney, 1981). This may make it possible to derive monoclonal antibodies to these unique cell surface components and, thereby, provide markers with a degree of specificity for germ cell tumours not hitherto seen.

Accordingly, we have been using a cell line derived from one of the xeno-grafts, HX 39 (Table II), to prepare a series of monoclonal antibodies. Some of these have been examined at the histopathological level using formalin fixed paraffin embedded tissues and have been found to react with the parent cell line used to raise the antibody and with various testicular germ cell tumours. Indeed, some of these monoclonal antibodies preferentially react with certain tumour structures such as those showing acinar patterns, papillary or endodermal sinus-type differentiation. Further study is needed, but it is possible that with this approach we will derive markers of value at a pathological level and with a degree of tissue type specificity which will further our understanding of the various cell types which comprise these lesions.

More experience has been gained with one particular monoclonal antibody, LICR-LON-HT13, and it has been used in a series of radioimmunodetection experiments *in vivo* employing xenografts of both human germ cell and non-germ cell tumours (Table III) (Moshakis *et al.*, 1981). Other workers have achieved

Table III. Localization[a] of teratoma and non-teratoma xenografts with the monoclonal antibody LICR-LON-HT13.

Xenograft tumour		Localization index[b]	
		48 h	96 h
HX 39	ECC[c] with yolk sac elements	7.0	10.9
HX 112	Yolk sac carcinoma	6.5	7.7
HX 111	ECC	3.8	5.6
HX 53	Seminoma with yolk sac elements	4.0	3.6
HX 57	Yolk sac carcinoma	2.8	2.9
HX 99	Breast adenocarcinoma	1.1	1.1
HX 65	Bronchial adenocarcinoma	1.2	1.1
LICR-LON/HN.BR	Squamous cell carcinoma	1.6	1.4
XK1	Renal adenocarcinoma	8.7	27.1

[a]Mean of 4–8 tumours at each time point. Tumour weight ranged between 15 and 22 mg.

[b]Localization index: $\dfrac{\text{tumour or tissue }^{125}I/^{131}I}{\text{Blood }^{125}I/^{131}I}$

[c]Embryonal cell carcinoma (malignant teratoma undifferentiated).

success with the *in vivo* localization of tumours in patients and experimental animals making use of antibodies to the carcinoembryonic antigen and colon specific antigen for epithelial tumours (Goldenberg *et al.*, 1978, 1980a, b, c; Dykes *et al.*, 1980; Gaffar *et al.*, 1981; Mach *et al.*, 1979) and of antibodies to HCG or AFP to detect germ cell tumours (Goldenberg *et al.*, 1980b, c). However, as pointed out before, there is a need to derive reagents which will in fact outline and react with cell types other than those that produce HCG or AFP. In this context a monoclonal antibody to a murine teratoma has been used by Ballou *et al.* (1979) and success in the radioimmunodetection of the tumour was achieved.

We have examined the localizing potential of LICR-LON-HT13 (Table III). This particular antibody exhibits a high degree of specificity for germ cell tumours and, with the exception of renal cell carcinoma, does not localize in other tumour cell types studied so far. Localization occurs in viable parts of the tumour xeno-graft, especially at its periphery. By autoradiography, the antibodies have been shown to be associated with the cell membrane of the tumour cells. The precise distribution of specific radioactivity is predominantly dependent on the blood supply of the tumour (Moshakis *et al.*, 1981). On the basis of these experiments on animals, this particular antibody and other related monoclonal antibodies are being tested in a clinical situation.

CONCLUSIONS

Germ cell tumours represent an area of human oncology where, to date, markers such as HCG and AFP have been shown to have clinical and pathological usefulness. However, such products are frequently derived from minority cell populations in such lesions. There remains a need, therefore, to develop markers for the other cell types in germ cell tumours. If markers which express specificity for the various different cell lineages and types can de derived, they will be of biological interest with respect to differentiation and development, and may well have clinical and pathological value in the detection, diagnosis, classification and treatment of germ cell tumours.

REFERENCES

Bagshawe, K. D. (1969). *In* "The Clinical Biology of the Trophoblast and its Tumours". Edward Arnold Ltd., London.

Ballou, B., Levine, G., Hakala, R. J. and Solter, D. (1979). *Science* **206**, 844–847.

Barzell, W. E. and Whitmore, W. F., Jr (1979). *Seminars in Oncology* **6**, 48–52.

Dykes, P. W., Hine, K. R., Bradwell, A. R., Blackburn, J. C. *et al.* (1980). *British Medical Journal* **280**, 220–222.

Gaffar, S. A., Pant, K. D., Shochat, D., Bennett, S. J. and Goldenberg, D. J. (1981). *International Journal of Cancer* **27**, 101–105.

Goldenberg, D. M., DeLand, F., Euishin, K. and Bennett, S. (1978). *New England Journal of Medicine* **298**, 1384.

Goldenberg, D. M., Ki, E. E., DeLand, F. H., Bennett, S. and Primus, F. J. (1980a). *Cancer Research* **40**, 2984–2992.

Goldenberg, D. M., Kim, E. C., DeLand, F., Spremulli, E., Nelson, M. O., Gockerman, J. P., Primus, F. J., Corgan, R. L. and Alpert, E. (1980b). *Cancer* **45**, 2500–2505.

Goldenberg, D. M., Kim, E. E., DeLand, F., Van Nagell, J. R., Jr and Javadpour, Nasser (1980c). *Science* **208**, 1284–1286.

Grigor, K. M., Detre, S. I., Kohn, J. and Neville, A. M. (1977). *British Journal of Cancer* **35**, 52.

Köhler, G. and Milstein, C. (1975). *Nature* **256**, 495–497.

Kohn, J. (1978). *Scandinavian Journal of Immunology* **8** (Suppl. 8), 103–107.

Lange, P. H. and Fraley, E. (1977). *Urologic Clinics of North America* **4**, 393–405.

Laurence, D. J. R. and Neville, A. M. (1981). *Clin. Biochem. Reviews* **2**, 135–161.

McIlhinney, R. A. J. (1981). *International Journal of Andrology* (Supp. 4). (In press.)

Mach, J. P., Forni, M., Ritschard, J. and Carrel, S. (1979). *In* "Peptides of Biological Fluids." (H. Peeters, Ed.), pp. 205–209. Pergamon, Oxford.

Mann, K., Lamerz, R., Hellman, Th., Kumper, H. J., Staehler, G. and Karl, H. J. (1980). *Oncodevelopmental Biology and Medicine* 1, 301.

Monaghan, P., Raghavan, D. and Neville, A. M. (1981). *Cancer* (In press.)

Moshakis, V., McIlhinney, R. A. J., Raghavan, D. and Neville, A. M. (1981). *Journal of Clinical Pathology*. (In press.)

Neville, A. M., Grigor, K M and Heyderman, F. (1978). *In* "Recent Advances in Histopathology" (P. P. Anthony and N. Woolf, Eds), p. 1. Churchill Livingstone, Edinburgh.

Norgaard–Pederson, B. and Raghavan, D. (1981). *Oncodevelopmental Biology and Medicine* 1, 327.

Parkinson, C. and Beilby, J. O. W. (1980). *Investigative and Cell Pathology* 3, 135.

Raghavan, D. and Neville, A. M. (1981). *Sci. Found. Urology*. (In press.)

Raghavan, D., Heyderman, E., Gibbs, J., Neville, A. M. and Peckham, M. (1981a). *In* "Thymus Aplastic Nude Mice and Rats in Clinical Oncology." (G. Bastert, H. Schmidt-Mathiesson and H. P. Fortimeyer, Eds). Fischer-Verlag, Berlin. (In press.)

Raghavan, D., Heyderman, E., Monaghan, P., Gibbs, J., Ruoslahti, E., Peckham, M. J. and Neville, A. M. (1981b). *Journal of Clinical Pathology*. (In press.)

Raghavan, D., Sullivan, A. L., Peckham, M. J. and Neville, A. M. (1981c). *Cancer* (In press.)

Ruoslahti, E., Jalanki, H., Comings, D. E., Neville, A. M. and Raghavan, D. (1981). *International Journal of Cancer*. (In press.)

Thompson, D. K. and Haddow, J. E. (1979). *Cancer* 43, 1820–1829.

Willemse, P. H. B., Sleijfer, D. Th., Schraffordt Koops, H., de Bruijn, H. W. A., Oosterhuis, J. W., Brouwers, Th. M., Ockhuizen, Th. and Marrink, J. (1981a). *Oncodevelopmental Biology and Medicine*. (In press.)

Willemse, P. H. B., Sleijfer, D. Th., Schraffordt Koops, H., de Bruijn, H. W. A., Oosterhuis, J. W., Brouwers, Th. M., Ockjuisen Th. and Marrink, J. (1981b). *Onco. Biol. Med.* (In press.)

MARKERS OF UROGENITAL TRACT TUMOURS:
A DISCUSSION

K. D. Bagshawe

Charing Cross Hospital Medical School, London, UK

I have assumed that my role as a discussant on the preceding papers is to make comment rather than to present new data so I shall take each of the topics in turn.

The introduction of more sensitive and specific assays for prostatic acid phosphatase was attended by claims, at least, in the lay press in the USA, that it could be used for screening as the "male PAP test" and for the detection of non-metastatic disease. Subsequent experience is well reflected in the paper which Dr Pontes has given. The original results reported by Foti *et al.* (1977) with 79% of patients in stage II having abnormal levels have not been confirmed and we must suppose that their early optimism was attended by inadequate staging of the clinical material.

There is, however, no doubt that the development of immunological methods for PRAP, as we prefer to designate it to distinguish it from placental alkaline phosphatase (PLAP), provides greater specificity compared with the earlier spectrophotometric methods. Validation of the specificity of sensitive immunoassays is more secure when indicated by tests which employ a sensitive assay for binding experiments and which, therefore, provide for tests of parallelism, rather than by simple gel diffusion. Thus, the dilution curves of a preparation of PRAP and sera from various prostatic carcinoma patients show parallelism, whereas acid phosphatase from other sources has no response in the system.

Given a reasonably specific assay, does it follow that an elevated PRAP value indicates the presence of prostatic carcinoma? It seems clear from Dr Pontes's

Serono Symposium No. 46, Markers for Diagnosis and Monitoring of Human Cancer, edited by M. I. Colnaghi, G. L. Buraggi and M. Ghione, 1982. Academic Press, London and New York.

studies and others, including our own, that elevated values are found in a few cases with apparently benign prostatic hypertrophy and in a few patients with other cancers.

As with other markers one problem is that of the cut-off value. A high cut-off value minimizes false positives in other diseases but reduces the incidence of positives in the specific disease group. Lowering the cut-off value has the opposite effect. In general, however, false positives are the greater problem.

The correlation of immunoassay and spectrophotometric analysis of PRAP is, however, sufficiently close to ask just where the advantages of immunoassay lie. This is illustrated with a group of patients where the same samples were estimated by radioimmunoassay in our laboratory and independently in our Chemical Pathology Department by a spectrophotometric method. From this it seems clear that the main advantage of RIA lies in the range 0–20 μg/l where the immunoassay frequently indicates small elevations of PRAP which were consistent with the patient's disease status but which were not detected by the spectrophotometric method (Dass et al., 1980).

One curious aspect of the RIA of PRAP, at least in the UK, is the reluctance of urologists to make use of it. It may be that those treating prostatic cancer generally have not yet tuned into the value of tumour markers, and the publicity given to the "male PAP test" in the USA at least served the purpose of drawing the attention of urologists to it without undue delay.

The bone marrow phosphatase measurements described by Dr Pontes are very interesting. There is, I think, a need to determine whether this approach or immunoperoxidase demonstration of PRAP positive cells is the more consistent guide. Perhaps both methods need to be used but if the assay method is of comparable sensitivity and reliability a comparison of cost/effectiveness will be necessary.

The work with a prostate specific antigen is also interesting. There are perhaps more precedents for organ specific antigens than for tumour specific antigens — but not many and there is always a need for caution about specificity claims. We await with interest further studies with this substance. As with other tumours, we need markers with better sensitivity and preferably ones capable of reflecting a limited tumour burden.

Some markers only reflect changes at the peak of the tumour mountain and non-biochemical methods may provide the clinician with an adequate view of such changes. Indeed, this may be the problem with all our methods for monitoring prostatic cancer. The rapidity with which PRAP values fall to the normal range when oestrogens are used and the rapid change from normal to abnormal values when disease progresses may reflect changes in tumour burden, but the possibility of changes in secretory and synthesizing activity by the tumour cells are factors we need to bear in mind.

Turning to ovarian epithelial tumours and Dr Lloyd's paper, one is impressed by the number of putative markers already described. For diagnostic purposes, of course, we need markers that match in their breadth the spectrum of ovarian epithelial tumours and we need to detect disease before it is far advanced. For the most part we seem to be identifying substances that can be detected in a proportion of ovarian cancers and even then only in their advanced stages. But, as Dr Lloyd has pointed out, we may have to make use of multiple markers and some may be more suitable for diagnostic purposes while others may be more suitable for monitoring. It is, one suspects, a consideration that will demand more attention as monoclonal antibodies impinge increasingly on this area. Already we can group ovarian antigens under several headings.

The antigen we formerly described as OTAG (Bagshawe *et al.*, 1980) has now been re-named CXl since we know it to be widely distributed in non-ovarian tissues. It has been detected in the serum of 49% of 700 samples from patients with ovarian cancer and in some patients with other cancers. Dr Melica Wass who identified CXl and developed a radioimmunoassay for it has spent much effort in trying to relate this glycoprotein to other tumour enzymes or antigens but so far without success. Since CXl is widely expressed in normal adult tissues as well as the foetus, it cannot be described as "oncofoetal".

Although the antigen CXl was extracted from ovarian cystadenocarcinoma (Bagshawe *et al.*, 1980), it is present in normal adult serum up to about 70 µg/l. It is also present in increased amounts in the sera of some patients with carcinoma of the breast, lung, prostate, teratoma and some leukaemias. Clearly it is very non-specific and one may ask whether such a marker is of any use at all. Furthermore, some patients die from advanced ovarian adenocarcinoma without CXl increasing significantly in the serum.

Nevertheless, in the absence of better markers it is not without interest; so far we have found it to be a fairly reliable marker of ovarian cancer in ascitic fluid. We have had a few false negatives but so far the only "false positive" was a mesothelioma. It will be interesting to know the status of Dr Lloyd's OvC-1 and OVC-2 in this respect when suitable assays have been developed.

In addition, when the concentration of CXl in the serum of patients with ovarian cancer is increased it does show a good correlation with the course of the disease. We can see the effect of debulking very clearly and in some instances values increase ahead of clinical relapse, but this is not always the case.

I suspect that with this marker we are at present detecting about 10^9 – 10^{12} ovarian tumour cells. To have something comparable to HCG for choriocarcinoma we need another four to seven orders of magnitude improvement in sensitivity.

Turning to the teratoma field I would preface my remarks by saying that if one had the job of designing a tumour for which marker measurements would seem to present insurmountable difficulties one would design a malignant teratoma. No two tumours appear to be identical, the morphological spectrum is vast and the bio-chemical spectrum is almost certainly just as wide. Yet we have a situation where in reality two markers prove to be of great value provided their limitations are recognized.

In 1930 Zondek described HCG production by a testicular teratoma and since then it has become clear that a high proportion of these tumours produced HCG and that even about 20% of seminomas do also. More than 15 years ago I attempted to interest the Testicular Tumour Panel in the UK in determining the frequency and usefulness of HCG measurements in teratoma patients but it was thought to be unnecessary because the incidence of trophoblast in testicular cancer was very low. Subsequently, when we reported that 85% of testicular tumour patient blood samples contained AFP or HCG or both, this also aroused little interest from our histopathology colleagues. Fortunately, however, histo-chemical techniques came along and now histopathologists are interested because they can demonstrate these markers to their own satisfaction.

Clearly, new markers may be expected and, therefore, it would be premature to introduce new classifications of malignant teratoma. Pathologists, of course, love classifications. We already have three systems of classification for the germ cell tumours and we can only express the hope that we have no repetition of the lymphoma situation.

Professor Neville has suggested that HCG and AFP assays are of little value in the diagnosis of primary germ cell tumours. Although I have pointed out for many years that their main role lies in monitoring the course of the disease, they do have an important diagnostic role. It still happens that young men present with a swelling in the testis or gynaecomastia and get reassurance of antibiotics for long periods. It still happens that unexplained back pain may result from para-aortic nodes and the primary in the testis is too small to palpate, but marker measurements provide a diagnosis — a point we first made in 1968. It can still happen that patients with unsuspected testicular or ovarian teratomas go to thoractomy, craniotomy or laparatomy before serum is sent for marker measurements. Mediastinal teratoma may be diagnosed on radiographic appearances coupled with marker measurements, and thoracotomy may be best reserved for the removal of residual disease after chemotherapy, but too often, thoracotomy is the initial, and sometimes unnecessary, procedure.

It is also worth noting that brain metastases are most likely to occur with HCG producing tumours and that these can be detected by plasma/spinal fluid HCG measurements although not as reliably as in gestational choriocarcinoma. AFP measurements in spinal fluid have not proved useful.

Reference should also be made to the prognostic significance of HCG and AFP. A recent analysis of our data at Charing Cross has related survival to various prognostic factors (Germa-Leuck *et al.*, 1980). The data show that taking cut-offs of 100,000 IU/l for HCG and 1,000 ng/l for AFP, the malignant teratoma population fall into groups with relatively good and bad prognosis more clearly than by any other factor or set of factors that we have been able to define. The advantage of a marker based prognostic scoring system is that, within the limits of quality control for assays, it provides a clearly defined numerical basis for comparison between different series of cases.

Of course we do need markers for the non-HCG and non-AFP producing components. Fortunately, in some instances, these components are benign or at least less malignant than those producing HCG or AFP. After successful eradication of the HCG and AFP producing components surgical removal of non-marker producing elements is often possible. Where residual disease after chemotherapy contains HCG or AFP producing elements the technique of radioimmunolocalization, described by Goldenberg and his colleagues, may provide a useful tool for localizing surgically resectable disease and may help to distinguish viable from necrotic tumour masses (Begent *et al.*, 1980).

REFERENCES

Bagshawe, K., D., Wass, M. and Searle, F. *Archives of Gynaecology* **229**, 303–310.

Begent, R. H. J., Searle, F., Stanway, G. *et al.* (1980). *Journal of the Royal Society of Medicine* **73**, 624–630.

Dass, S., Bowen, N. L. and Bagshawe, K. D. (1980). *Clinical Chemistry* **26** (11), 1583–1587.

Foti, A. G., Cooper, A. F., Herschman, H. and Malvaez, R. R. (1977). *New England Journal of Medicine* **297**, 1357–1361.

Germa-Lluch, J. R., Begent, R. H. J. and Bagshawe, K. D. (1980). *British Journal of Cancer* **42**, 850–855.

MARKERS IN DIAGNOSIS AND MONITORING OF GENITAL TRACT TUMOURS: A DISCUSSION

G. Pizzocaro[1], E. Bombardieri[2] and S. Pilotti[3]

Section of Urological Oncology[1], Department of Nuclear Medicine[2], and Department of Pathology[3], Istituto Nazionale per lo Studio e la Cura dei Tumori, Milan, Italy

GENITAL TRACT TUMOUR MARKERS

Genital tract markers producing tumours are represented by cancer of the prostate and of both the female and male gonads. Biological markers in prostatic and testicular cancer have been available for about 40 years (Gutman and Gutman, 1938; Lacquer, 1946), but it was only during the last decade that tumour marker studies grew to clinical relevance and common use when radioimmunoassay became widely available (Vaitukaitis *et al.*, 1972; Waldmann and McIntire, 1974, Foti *et al.*, 1977). Today, techniques to detect specific surface antigens are developing and new specific markers are being found.

Markers of Prostate Cancer

Dr Pontes gave an excellent paper on the actual status of markers in prostate cancer. Besides showing us his wide experience and the recent progress which has been made at Roswell Park Memorial Institute, he masterly taught how marker studies should be articulated.

Very little needs to be added to Pontes' lesson. He voluntarily restricted his paper to the most important classic and new markers of prostatic cancer. However, many other techniques which attempt to identify biologically patients

Serono Symposium No. 46, Markers for Diagnosis and Monitoring of Human Cancer, edited by M. I. Colnaghi, G. L. Buraggi and M. Ghione, 1982. Academic Press, London and New York.

with carcinoma of the prostate have been developed in recent years. Some of them are promising and deserve a short report.

Serum Studies

Denis and Prout (1963) reported observations on *lactic dehydrogenase* (LDH) isoenzyme levels in the serum of 21 patients with advanced carcinoma of the prostate. The 16 patients with untreated or relapsed disease had elevated levels of LDH-4 and LDH-5 in the serum. The five patients with disease in remission showed only traces of LDH-4 and LDH-5.

Carcinoembryonic antigen (CEA) has been evaluated in patients with carcinoma of the prostate (Reynoso *et al.*, 1972). Although CEA is present in increased amounts in some patients with carcinoma of the prostate, including a few who have normal serum acid phosphatase levels, the test is too non-specific to be diagnosticably valuable.

Prostatic Fluid

The prostatic fluid is easily obtained at the time of routine rectal examination and prostatic secretions would be expected to reflect the metabolic activity of the prostatic epithelial cell. In the case of prostate cancer, the evaluation of prostatic fluid composition provides a unique opportunity to analyse a concentrated sample of cytoplasmic metabolic products.

A reversal of the isoenzyme pattern of lactic dehydrogenase from the normal predominance of LDH-1 to the predominance of LDH-5 has been demonstrated in malignant prostatic tissue (Oliver *et al.*, 1970). A consistently increased ratio of LDH-5/LDH-1 in the prostatic fluid of about 80% of patients with carcinoma, regardless of stage, has been observed by Grayhack *et al.* (1980). About 12% of men in whom a histological diagnosis of BPH has been established and 44% of men with an inflammatory change in the prostate have an elevated LDH-5/ LDH-1 ratio. Di Silverio (1980) confirmed these data: he found a LDH-5/LDH-1 ratio >2 in 59/70 patients with prostatic cancer (84.3%) vs 20/140 suffering from BPH (14.3%). Prostatis, however, led to frequent false positive findings.

Both concentration of *proteins C3 complement* and *transferrin* are present in much higher concentrations in the prostatic fluid of patients with carcinoma of the prostate than in those with BPH or prostatic inflammatory disease (Grayhack *et al.*, 1979). At present, it seems that combinations of these observations of lactic dehydrogenase isoenzyme pattern and C3 and transferrin concentration in the prostatic fluid hold promise for identifying patients with prostatic carcinoma early in their course; their usefulness in following patients with prostatic cancer has yet to be established.

Markers of Ovarian Cancer

In striking contrast with testicular tumours, germ cell tumours of the ovary are rare and epithelial cancers predominate. Of course, markers of germ cell tumours are the same in the ovary as in the testis. In particular, AFP is very sensitive for yolk sac tumours (Mann, 1981) and malignant ovarian teratoma

(Scott, 1981) and its half-life after initial treatment correlates well with both the extent of the disease and the response to therapy. However, false alarm may occur in the following of β HCG levels, owing to inadequate specificity of antisera and cross-reactivity with LH.

Markers of Epithelial Cancer

As reported by Lloyd in his extremely interesting paper, work by many investigators in this field has resulted in the development of a series of markers. None of the reagents yet studied is capable of detecting early ovarian cancer, but a number have potential in monitoring the disease. Early detection of ovarian cancer remains a challenge in practical oncology; further improvement is expected in the field of ovarian tumour antigens and Lloyd has shown the progress he is making.

To confirm the low reliability of markers in epithelial cancer of the ovary, we report the results of a recent study which was carried on in our institute (Turrin *et al.*, 1981). CEA levels were studied in free and in washed peritoneal fluid of 15 and 96 patients, respectively, with or without epithelial cancer of the ovary. CEA was above 15 ng/ml in 90% of patients with ovarian cancer and in 20% of patients with benign disease in the group of patients with free peritoneal fluid. Cytology was positive in all cancer patients. With the exception of two patients with mucinous cancer involving the peritoneum, there was no significant difference in CEA levels in fluids obtained by peritoneal washing in patients with or without ovarian cancer, even in the case of documented peritoneal involvement. Cytology performed on peritoneal washing gave positive results in 50% of cases with ovarian cancer involving the peritoneum.

There are recent reports on AFP production by ovarian cystadenocarcinoma in about 25% of cases (Buamah *et al.*, 1981). These findings could be interpreted as questioning the epithelial origin of cystadenocarcinoma of the ovary.

Markers of Testicular Cancer

Dr Neville has presented a very interesting and original paper on markers of testicular cancer. Of primary interest are his studies on xenografts of human derived germ cell tumours in immune deprived mice and the demonstration that a continuum exists between either seminoma or embryonal carcinoma and yolk sac tumour. The modified scheme he proposed for the evolution of germ cell tumours is very exciting. The heterogenicity of germ cell tumours, the difficulty of clearly defining several histological patterns, the questions surrounding the classification of tumours containing solitary giant cells producing HCG and the morphological basis for AFP production, the experimental evidence that embryonal carcinoma may be initiated by ectopic transplantation of early embryos and that transplantation of embryonal carcinoma cells from *in vitro* tissue cultures back into embryos can result in efficient re-incorporation of the malignant cells into a normal embryo (Evans, 1981) all suggest that a circle concept of germ cell tumours with possible equations between histotypes is more in evidence than the rigid Teilum's (1976) dicotomy (Fig. 1). Germ cell can give rise to both embrioyd bodies and clusters of undifferentiated cells (Parkinson, 1981).

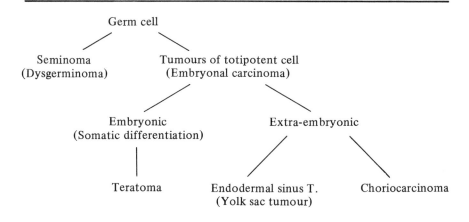

Fig. 1.   Traditional concept of germ cell tumours.

Further differentiation toward embryonic and extra-embryonic tissue has been demonstrated from both structures, and equations exist between different histo-types. The difficulty, however, is to fit seminoma into this circle concept. A necessary compromise is to continue with classifications in routine practice and to correlate them with descriptive systems including different morphological patterns and their biochemical features.

Diagnostic and Monitoring Aspects of AFP and HCG

α-Fetoprotein (AFP) and human chorionic gonadotrophin (HCG) have proved to be the most reliable markers of testicular tumours. AFP is measured by a double antibody radioimmunoassay, using an antibody raised against AFP extracted from pooled foetal plasma (Waldmann and McIntire, 1974). Pathological levels exceed 15–40 ng/ml. We considered as abnormal, levels above 15 ng/ml. HCG is measured in a double antibody radioimmunoassay, using an antibody raised against the β subunit of HCG—that part of the HCG molecule which is immuno-logically different from luteinizing hormone (LH). This assay reliably measures 1 ng/ml (5 mIU/ml) of HCG (Vaitukaitis et al., 1972) and levels exceeding this are considered pathological. The AFP half-life is 5 days and it is yolk sac derived (foetal liver and intestine, regenerative liver, epatoma, yolk sac tumour, yolk sac elements in germ cell tumours). HCG has a 1-day half-life and it is produced by the trophoblastic cells of placenta, choriocarcinoma and isolated syncitial giant cells in germ cell tumours. It cross-reacts with FSH, LH and TSH. Both AFP and HCG can be identified in 5 μm thick serial sections of formaldehyde fixed tumours using an indirect immunoperoxidase technique (Kurman et al., 1977). Blocks of tissue, decades old, may be sectioned and examined. With the use of counterstains the histology may be readily and simultaneously assessed; the results are reproducible and permanent.

Serum HCG and AFP in Non-seminoma

Over a period of 2 years (1978–1979) 83 patients were studied in our institute for both HCG and AFP. As 27 patients had no tumour present when first examined (usually stage I disease after orchidectomy), they were excluded. HCG was positive in 26 of the remaining 56 patients (46.4%), AFP in 32 (57.1%) and 40 patients (71.4%) were positive to either or both HCG and AFP. Our figures are lower than those reported by Scardino *et al.* (1977) and by Javadpour (1980), even though a lower threshold for AFP was used. However, 10–30% of non-seminomatous germ cell tumours of the testis are not marker producing. It makes assays of serum HCG and AFP of little value in the detection of primary testicular tumours.

Table I shows the correlation between serum HCG and AFP and TNM categories (UICC, 1974). Two remarks can be made: only positivity to HCG increased at increasing stages of disease and 42.3% of patients with pathologically proven retroperitoneal disease showed negative pre-lymphadenectomy serum markers. Nevertheless, pre-operative HCG and AFP are useful in reducing the staging error by lymphangiography (LAG) as reported by Barzell and Whitmore (1979) and Javadpour (1980). In addition, in our case series the staging error was reduced to only 10% in pathological stages I and II disease by combining LAG and pre-operative serum markers (Table II).

Table I. Serum HCG and AFP in non-seminoma and TNM categories.

TNM categories	No. cases	(%) positive		
		HCG	AFP	HCG or AFP
N– MO	2	(50.0)	(50.0)	(50.0)
N+ MO	26	(23.1)	(57.7)	(57.7)
N3 ; N4 ; M1	28	(67.8)	(57.1)	(85.7)
TOTAL	56	(46.4)	(57.1)	(71.4)

Table II. Comparison of LAG, serum HCG and AFP and pathological staging.

Pathological staging	No. cases	Staging error (%)		
		LAG	HCG or AFP	Both
Stage I	24	(29.1)	(4.1)	(4.1)
Stage II	26	(26.9)	(42.3)	(15.4)
TOTAL	50	(28.0)	(24.0)	(10.0)

It is commonly believed that patients with positive serum markers have a bad prognosis. This could have been true before the present sophisticated multi-disciplinary treatment modalities were developed. Begent (1981) was able to demonstrate that only patients with very high serum marker levels (AFP above 1×10^3 ng/ml or HCG above 1×10^5 mIU/ml) have a significantly worse prognosis ($P = 0.001$) despite treatment, as well as patients with bulky disease (any mass larger than 5 cm and more than 8 lung metastase). In our case series we were unable to find any correlation between pre-treatment serum markers levels and the fate of patients at any stage of the disease except for patients with bulky advanced disease and high levels of either HCG or AFP.

Both HCG and AFP are very useful in monitoring therapy. Interpretation of falling levels of serum markers requires consideration of their biological half-lives. Patients showing initial half-lives for AFP of < 5 days and for HCG of < 1 day showed complete remission (Milford–Ward, 1981). A second group showed half-lives of 5–10 days for AFP and of 1–3 days for HCG; these patients showed evidence of relapse after apparent remission. Patients with half-lives for AFP greater than 10 days and for HCG greater than 3 days, or rising levels after initial therapy, all had extensive and residual disease recalcitrant to therapy. On the other hand, in patients with bulky disease on chemotherapy we have observed a number of patients with a remnant of disease in spite of the return of the markers to normal (Table III). It appears that chemotherapy can eradicate the clones of marker producing tumour cells selectively, and normal markers in partial responders (PR) may be followed by either complete response (CR) or progression. Progression was accompanied or preceded by a return to elevated serum levels.

Table III. Behaviour of serum HCG and AFP, and outcome after therapy in patients with advanced non-seminoma.

Serum markers	No. cases	Outcome	
Returned to normal	19	CR	6
		PR ► CR	3
		PR (%)	6
		PR ► progr.	4
Persisted elevated	5	Progression	3
		PR ► progr.	2

CR: complete remission. PR: partial remission.

The problem in following patients for complete response is a false positive rise in serum HCG or AFP. We observed this phenomenon once for each marker. In one case a rise of AFP was due to hepatic toxicity from post-operative chemotherapy. Another patient had an unexplained and transient rise of HCG up to 20 mIU/ml which returned to normal in 40 days; he had negative markers before surgery. Of course, the sole rise of serum HCG or AFP in the follow-up of patients in otherwise complete remission needs critical consideration and marker revaluation before starting chemotherapy.

Markers can also help in localizing tumour desposits. Javadpour *et al.* (1978) have been able to detect a recurrence in iliac lymph nodes by selective venous catheterization and assaying for the α subunit of HCG. This subunit has a half-life of 20 min and it allows one to detect a step-up when venous blood draining the tumour is sampled. Markers with longer half-lives, such as AFP and intact HCG, are not suitable for tumour localization by this technique. Radioisotope localization of germ cell tumours is now possible. Bradwell (1981) was able to localize tumour deposits by external scanning after injection of radiolabelled antibody of AFP in all of nine patients with elevated serum AFP. All abnormal areas were confirmed by CT scans and lymphangiography, although four secondary deposits were missed and two areas of anti-AFP uptake over the stomach were not confirmed. By analogy, Begent (1981) succeeded in localizing tumour deposits in seven of eleven patients with elevated HCG using ^{131}I-labelled antibody direct against human chorionic gonadotrophin. These preliminary results show that it is possible to identify tumour deposits using antibody to either AFP or HCG and positive results probably indicate the presence of viable AFP or HCG producing tumour, which promises to be of value in discriminating between necrotic deposits and living tumour before surgery.

HCG and AFP in Seminoma

Javadpour (1980) found elevated levels of serum HCG in only 11 of 130 patients with seminoma (7.7%) and one of these patients had an element of choriocarcinoma in subsequent histological sections of the primary tumour. He also found elevated AFP in two patients with seminoma: one had liver metastases, and elevated AFP may be explained on the basis of regenerative changes of liver parenchyma secondary to metastase; the other one had elements of embryonal carcinoma in subsequent histological sections. It seems, therefore, that seminoma cannot produce AFP and very few secrete HCG. A different therapeutic approach (surgery and chemotherapy, instead of classical radiotherapy) is also suggested for HCG positive seminomas.

Over 4 years (1976–1979) we studied 98 patients with testicular seminoma for *serum HCG*. Thirty-eight patients were disease-free when first examined and they were excluded. Seventeen of the remaining 51 patients had elevated levels of serum HCG (33.3%). In Table IV patients are distributed according to clinical categories. There seems to be no correlation between stage and serum HCG levels in our case series. In another five stage I patients elevated

Table IV. Elevated serum HCG in testicular seminoma.

TNM categories	No. cases	Elevated HCG	
		No.	%
N0 M0	20	7	(35.0)
N1–2, M0	14	3	(21.4)
N3, N4, M1	17	7	(41.2)
TOTAL	51	17	(33.3)

HCG was found only in the blood of the spermatic vein. Histology was reviewed in 18 of 22 patients and new histological sections were taken. In only one patient was an area of embryonal carcinoma found and in 11 of the remaining 17 (64.7%) syncytial giant cells were optically recognized (Fig. 2). Morphological aspects different from typical seminoma were found in 15 of 17 patients in whom the diagnosis of seminoma was confirmed. Absence or only minimal amounts of lymphocytic stromal reaction, focal aggregations of numerous capillaries with or without interstitial haemorrhage, areas of focal necrosis, increased mitotic activity and cellular pleomorphism with anaplasia were all characteristic features.

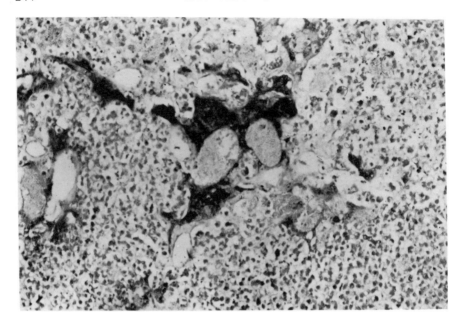

Fig. 2. Seminoma with syncytiotrophoblastic giant cells in 38-year-old male; the dark areas represent the immunoperoxidase staining for HCG. (× 100.)

We were aware of these findings but things became clear at the Germ Cell Tumours Conference which was held in Leeds on March 24-26, 1981. Milford-Ward (1981) reported elevated pre-orchidectomy HCG in the sera of 50% of patients with histological diagnosis of pure seminoma. Slides were not reviewed and new sections were not done, but this figure is very high indeed. Besides, Heyderman (1981) reported a 17% positive indirect immunoperoxidase staining for HCG in seminoma showing syncytial giant cell elements which could not be classified as choriocarcinoma on conventional morphological grounds. Javadpour (1981) himself reported elevated levels of serum HCG in 32% of stage II and in 50% of stage III seminoma. Only five of 132 stage I patients had elevated HCG, but orchidectomy had been usually performed before serum markers so these data are not reliable.

In conclusion, there is a growing body of evidence to show that an appreciable percentage of patients with seminoma do have elevated serum HCG and syncytial giant cell elements can be identified in a great proportion of these cases both optically and with the indirect technique. Other morphological features are present in a great majority of these seminomas and further studies are needed to identify these tumours better. From a clinical point of view, our patients have been treated as pure seminomas, regardless of HCG serum levels, and no significant difference in prognosis could be found at any stage between patients with and without elevated HCG. However, a more careful evaluation is necessary in a larger case series.

We succeeded in finding elevated serum AFP in four patients with seminoma. All had advanced disease. One patient had liver metastases and another one received 2,000 rad to a large abdominal field encompassing half of the liver, so liver regeneration could explain elevated AFP in both patients. In the other two cases histology was reviewed and new sections made. One had an area of embryonal carcinoma, the other one had a pure atypical seminoma, with positive staining to AFP immunoperoxidase and with the same morphological features as described by Neville (Fig. 3)

It seems, therefore, that there is a need to modify our classical concept on seminoma. There is obviously a need to determine the relationship between seminoma and HCG or AFP secreting cells. However, further studies are necessary to give some frank explanation.

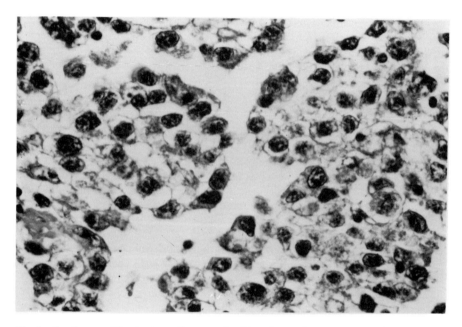

Fig. 3. Seminoma with minute cystic spaces lined by a layer of cuboidal cells in 31-year-old male. This patient had a detectable amount of serum AFP. (H and E, × 400.)

Other Markers in Testicular Tumours

In testicular tumours, AFP and HCG are specific markers of two different clones of malignant cells which are widely represented in non-seminomatous germ cell tumours. However, nearly 20% of non-seminoma and 70% of seminoma do not have these elements and, therefore, there is a consistent proportion of testicular tumours which is not marker producing. New or different markers are needed to identify these tumours.

Lactic Dehydrogenase

Cancer cells have increased glycolysis, leading to an increased synthesis of lactate. LDH may be utilized as a non-specific tumour marker in several cancers including that of testicular germ cells. Usually LDH levels correlate with the tumour bulk and Friedman *et al.* (1980) were able to demonstrate a correlation between higher LDH levels and a lower response rate to chemotherapy in patients with advanced non-seminoma. We found elevated LDH levels in several cases with bulky disease, but only in one such patient were neither AFP nor HCG elevated.

Pregnancy Specific Glycoprotein

SP1 is a product of syncytiotrophoblastic cells as well as HCG, and it is detectable by radioimmunoassay. Serum levels above 1 ng/ml in the male can be considered abnormal. Lange *et al.* (1980) studied 91 patients with testicular cancer reporting 100% specificity and 52% sensitivity. In one patient with seminoma and in two with non-seminomatous tumours SP1 was the only elevated marker. In another two patients the SP1 levels appeared to reflect the clinical course better than did the levels of either AFP or HCG.

Multiple Markers in Seminoma

Javadpour (1981) studied the role of γ-glutamyl transpeptidase (GGT), placental alkaline phosphatase (PLAP) and HCG in 89 seminoma patients with negative AFP. Thirty patients had active tumour and HCG was positive in six of them (20%), PLAP in 12 (40%) and GGT in ten (33%). When these three serum markers were considered together, over 80% of the patients with clinically active tumour had detectable serum levels of one or more of these biochemical serum markers. However, it should be emphasized that the false positive, false negative rates of these markers, especially false positive rates for GGT in liver disease, and their biological half-lives should be taken into consideration. Besides, a majority of bulky stage II and stage III seminoma seen at the National Cancer Institute have had elevated serum levels of LDH which have been useful in monitoring this tumour.

New Marker Possibilities

There are different ways of searching for new markers in germ cell tumours. For example, pragmatic serial measurement of the serum levels of compounds associated with pregnancy, or with a malignant condition, in general, has led to the current evaluation of pregnancy specific glycoprotein SP1, lactate dehydrogenase and immunocomplexes as serum markers. Alternatively, germ cell models can be studied *in vitro* or in animal species. Many such studies identify membrane constituents which may be useful as markers. Current examples are the F9 antigen, glycerolipids and plasminogen activator. Neville introduced us to the field of monoclonal antibodies to cell surface components which promise to provide markers with a degree of specificity for germ cell tumours not hitherto seen. All these approaches require a considerable investment of time and effort before the merit of the marker is finally proved or disproved by sensitive assays in a clinical situation. The justification of this expensive work is the need to determine the presence of malignant cells which do not secrete AFP or HCG.

REFERENCES

Barzell, W. E. and Whitmore, W. F. Jr. (1973). *Seminars in Oncology* **6**, 48.
Begent, R. H. J. (1981). *In* "Proceedings of the Germ Cell Tumour Conference"
(C. K. Anderson and W. G. Jones, Eds). Taylor & Francis, Leeds. (In press.)
Bradwell, A. R. (1981). *In* "Proceedings of the Germ Cell Tumour Conference"
(C. K. Anderson and W. G. Jones, Eds). Taylor & Francis, Leeds. (In press.)
Buamah, P. K., Bates, G. and Milford-Wards, A. (1981). *In* "Proceedings of the
Germ Cell Tumour Conference" (C. K. Anderson and W. G. Jones, Eds).
Taylor & Francis, Leeds. (In press.)
Denis, L. J. and Prout, G. R., Jr (1963). *Investigations in Urology* **1**, 101.
Di Silverio, F. (1980). *In* "Valori e Limiti dei Markers Biologici nei Tumori
Urologici", Atti 53° Congresso Nazionale Soc. It. Urol. (In press.)
Evans, M. (1981). *In* "Proceeding of the Germ Cell Tumours Conference" (C. K.
Anderson and W. G. Jones, Eds). Taylor & Francis, Leeds. (In press.)
Foti, A. G., Cooper, J. F., Hirschman, H. and Malvaez, P. R. (1977). *New England
Journal of Medicine* **297**, 1357.
Friedman, A., Vugrin, D. and Golbey, R. B. (1980). *American Society of Clinical
Oncology Abstracts* 323.
Grayhack, J. T., Wendel, E. F., Oliver, L. and Lee, C. (1979). *Journal of Urology*
121, 295.
Grayhack, J. T., Lee, C., Kolbusz, W. and Oliver, L. (1980). *Cancer* **45**, 1896.
Gutman, A. B. and Gutman, E. D. (1938). *Journal of Clinical Investigation*
17, 473.
Heyderman, E. (1981). *In* "Proceedings of the Germ Cell Tumour Conference"
(C. K. Anderson and W. G. Jones, Eds). Taylor & Francis, Leeds. (In press.)
Javadpour, N. (1980). *Cancer* **45**, 1755.
Javadpour, N. (1981). *In* "Proceedings of the Germ Cell Tumour Conference"
(C. K. Anderson and W. G. Jones, Eds). Taylor & Francis, Leeds. (In press.)
Javadpour, N., McIntire, K. R., Waldman, T. P., Scardino, P. T., Bergman, S.
and Anderson, T. (1978). *Journal of Urology* **119**, 759.
Kurman, R. J., Scardino, P. T., McIntire, K. R., Waldmann, T. A. and Javadpour,
N. (1977). *Cancer* **40**, 2136.
Lacquer, G. L. (1946). *Stanford Medical Bulletin* **4**, 67.
Lange, P. H., Bremner, R. D., Horne, C. H. W., Vessella, R. L. and Fraley, E. E.
(1980). *Urology* **15**, 251.
Mann, J. R. (1981). *In* "Proceedings of the Germ Cell Tumour Conference"
(C. K. Anderson and W. G. Jones, Eds). Taylor & Francis, Leeds. (In press.)
Milford-Ward, A. (1981). *In* "Proceedings of the Germ Cell Tumour Conference"
(C. K. Anderson and W. G. Jones, Eds). Taylor & Francis, Leeds. (In press.)
Oliver, J. H., Elhilali, M. N., Belitsky, P. and Mackinnon, K. J. (1970). *Cancer*
25, 863.
Parkinson, C. (1981). *In* "Proceedings of the Germ Cell Tumour Conference"
(C. K. Anderson and W. G. Jones, Eds). Taylor & Francis, Leeds. (In press.)
Reynoso, G., Chu, M. T., Guiman, P. and Murphy, G. P. (1972). *Cancer* **30**, 1.
Scardino, P. T., Cox, H. D., Waldmann, T. A., McIntire, K. R., Mittermeyer,
B. and Javadpour, N. (1977). *Journal of Urology* **118**, 994.
Scott, I. V. (1981). *In* "Proceedings of the Germ Cell Tumour Conference"
(C. K. Anderson and W. C. Jones, Eds). Taylor & Francis, Leeds. (In press.)
Teilum, G. (1976). *In* "Special Tumours of Ovary and Testis" J. B. Lippincott
Co., Copenhagen.
Turrin, A., De Palo, G., Spinelli, P., Bombardieri, E., Pilotti, S., Ringhini, R.
and Buraggi, G. L. (1981). *International Journal of Cancer*. (In press.)

UICC (1974). "TNM Classification of Malignant Tumours", 2nd Ed., pp. 88–91. Geneva.

Vaitukaitis, J. L., Brannstein, G. D. and Ross, G. T. (1972). *American Journal of Obstetrics and Gynecology* **113**, 751.

Waldmann, T. A. and McIntire, K. R. (1974). *Cancer* **34**, 1510.

MARKERS OF ENDOCRINE TUMOURS OF THE
GASTROINTESTINAL TRACT

P. Vezzadini[1], M. Cecchettin[2], A. Albertini[2], G. Bonora[1], G. L. Ferri[1] and
G. Labò[1]

*I° Clinica Medica dell'Università di Bologna, Bologna[1], and
Istituto di Chimica della Facoltà Medica di Brescia, Brescia[2], Italy*

With advances in radioimmunoassay and immunohistochemical techniques, the
list of endocrine tumours of the gastrointestinal tract (gut, pancreas and biliary
system) is growing rapidly. It has recently been appreciated that many gastro-
enteropancreatic (GEP) endocrine tumours contain a mixture of cells as defined
immunochemically and secrete several different hormonal peptides. As a rule, the
peptides originate from different endocrine cell types, but in a few cases it has
been shown that the same neoplastic cell produces two peptides simultaneously
(Fiocca *et al.*, 1980; Galmiche *et al.*, 1980). In several reported series, the
frequency of multiple hormone producing tumours, as determined by immuno-
histology, was greater than 50%, but the clinical symptoms of mixed tumours
were nearly always explained by hypersecretion of only one of the products
(Larsson *et al.*, 1975; Arnold *et al.*, 1976). The other hormones secreted by the
tumour generally remain clinically and metabolically silent, but may serve as
tumour markers as well as the hormone responsible for the syndrome.

The clinical features of GEP endocrine tumours producing gastrin (Zollinger-
Ellison syndrome), insulin (hypoglycaemic syndrome), vasoactive intestinal
polypeptide (Verner-Morrison syndrome), glucagon (glucagonoma syndrome),
somatostatin (somatostatinoma syndrome) and serotonin (carcinoid syndrome)
have been relatively well defined. Overt hyperfunctional syndromes resulting

Serono Symposium No. 46, Markers for Diagnosis and Monitoring of Human Cancer, edited
by M. I. Colnaghi, G. L. Buraggi and M. Ghione, 1982. Academic Press, London and New
York.

from secretion of other peptides have yet to be defined. As regards the clinically silent GEP endocrine tumours, the failure to recognize a hyperfunctional syndrome may in part be due to the fact that the function of normal cells from which the tumour takes origin is at present unknown.

There are no epidemiological data on the incidence of GEP endocrine tumours. The fact that the majority of the cases have been reported during the last 10 years probably does not indicate an increasing frequency but rather depends on the availability of radioimmunological methods for the detection of hormone markers and on the increased information about the tumour syndromes. An estimate based upon the 10 years experience of Rehfeld (1979) in the Danish population (5 million inhabitants) suggests that GEP endocrine tumour syndromes are rare, appearing with an incidence of about one patient per year per syndrome per million.

The peptide or peptides produced by the neoplastic tissue and the other non-peptide secretory products have been proven to be good markers for diagnosis and monitoring of GEP endocrine tumours. The radioimmunoassay technique has played a crucial role in the identification of these hormone tumour markers. Diagnostically valuable radioimmunoassays for GEP hormones include those for gastrin, insulin, vasoactive intestinal polypeptide (VIP), pancreatic polypeptide (PP), glucagon, somatostatin and, presumably, also substance P (Rehfeld, 1979).

The peptides produced by the tumour are generally immunologically similar, if not identical, to the corresponding physiological hormone. In order to obtain reliable results with the radioimmunoassay technique, it is necessary to evaluate the specificity of each assay towards the different molecular forms of a given hormone. In fact, like other secretory peptides and proteins, normal and tumour GEP hormones are heterogenous, i.e. they exist in a number of molecular forms that differ greatly in immunological and biological activity.

The importance of specificity testing is illustrated by the following example. Essentially all gastrin radioimmunoassays are established with antisera against G-17 (component III), using G-17 as tracer and as standard. Some assays measure G-17 and G-34 (component II) with equimolar potency, but most assays measure G-17 with full potency and G-34 with low or no potency. If the antiserum is specific only for G-17, the assay fails to recognize the cases of Zollinger-Ellison syndrome in which the larger gastrin component constitutes almost all the gastrin released by the tumour (Fig. 1).

Secretion of different molecular forms of a hormone may be of diagnostic significance if the component pattern changes in a pathognomonic way. Such change has been observed between proinsulin and insulin in insulinomas (Hayashi *et al.*, 1977). Thus, a large percentage of proinsulin in serum supports diagnosis of the insulinoma.

Fractionation of the serum of tumour patients with raised peptide levels frequently reveals the presence of pro-hormones of high molecular weight which are not detectable in significant amounts in serum from normal subjects. These peptides may have less biological activity than the normal hormones. The determination of total serum hormone-like immunoreactivity may not, therefore, reflect the biological activity. This could explain the lack of clinical symptoms in some patients with incidentally found endocrine tumours associated with elevated levels of immunoreactive hormone markers.

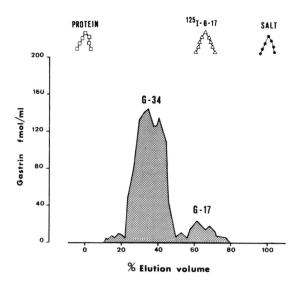

Fig. 1. Elution profile of immunoreactive gastrin in serum from a patient with Zollinger-Ellison syndrome. In this case almost all the gastrin immunoreactivity emerged with an elution volume typical of that for G-34. Column: Sephadex G-50, 1 × 100 cm, flow rate: 10 ml/h; buffer: 0.02 M sodium barbital, pH 8.4. The fraction number of the eluates is described in terms of percentage elution volume from protein (0%) to salt peaks (100%). The gastrin immunoreactivity was measured according to the method of Vezzadini *et al.* (1975).

Several peptides, in addition to the hormones responsible for the well defined syndromes, have been proposed as markers of GEP endocrine tumours.

Polak *et al.* (1976) found that PP is produced in an unusually high frequency by all types of endocrine pancreatic tumours and suggested that raised circulating concentration of PP is a specific marker for the endocrine tumours of the pancreas. PP cells have been demonstrated in the neoplastic tissue (Polak *et al.*, 1976), but many tumours are associated with a more or less pronounced hyperplasia of extratumoral pancreatic PP cells and elevated serum PP levels may persist following tumour extirpation (Schwartz, 1979). PP can, therefore, be considered a useful marker for the diagnosis but not for the monitoring of pancreatic endocrine tumours. Elevated serum PP levels are more frequent in patients with Zollinger-Ellison syndrome as a component of multiple endocrine adenomatosis than in sporadic cases (Bloom *et al.*, 1978). Friesen *et al.* (1980) have proposed PP as a specific marker for the pancreatic component in patients with multiple endocrine adenopathies, type I, and as a screening test for the disease in family members. Recently the specificity of PP as a marker of the endocrine tumours of the pancreas has been questioned. In fact, PP related peptides may also work as markers of non-argentaffin rectal carcinoids, as demonstrated by recent immuno-histochemical studies (Fiocca *et al.*, 1980). We have observed high serum PP levels in a patient with Verner-Morrison syndrome due to an extrapancreatic endocrine tumour producing VIP (Labò *et al.*, 1980).

Increased circulating immunoreactive calcitonin, which was initially reported in medullary carcinoma of the thyroid, has been observed in patients with non-thyroid tumours, including GEP endocrine tumours (Abe *et al.*, 1977). Elevated levels of serum calcitonin have been found in 21% of our patients with Zollinger-Ellison syndrome.

The production of ACTH has been demonstrated in a variety of tumours, including some gastrointestinal carcinoids and islet cell carcinomas of the pancreas (Goodwin, 1975; Marcus *et al.*, 1980). In many cases the neoplastic serum ACTH-like immunoreactivity does not seem to cause any characteristic clinical symptoms. We have measured the serum levels of ACTH in 28 patients with endocrine pancreatic tumours. An elevated concentration (144 pmol/l, upper limit of normal range 29 pmol/l was found in a case of malignant gastrinoma with Zollinger-Ellison syndrome, not associated with Cushing syndrome. ACTH does not seem to be a clinically useful marker of GEP endocrine tumours.

The production of human chorionic gonadotrophin (HCG) by malignant non-trophoblastic tumours has been demonstrated by several groups. It is well known that HCG, one of the glycoprotein hormones, is composed of two non-covalently bound α and β subunits, the latter being responsible for biological and immunological specificities. Free HCG-α and HCG-β subunit production as well as the whole molecule of HCG has been demonstrated in 7–19% of patients with endocrine GEP tumours (Rosen and Weintraub, 1974, Kahn *et al.*, 1977; Polak *et al.*, 1977). Abnormal concentrations of HCG-β were found in two out of 30 endocrine GEP tumours examined in our laboratory (7% of cases). Kahn *et al.* (1977) noted that elevated levels of HCG or one of its subunits were present in one-half of the patients with malignant islet cell tumours, suggesting that these markers may be specific indicators for malignancy. Stabile *et al.* (1978) confirmed this suggestion by showing that approximately one-third of the patients with malignant gastrinomas have elevated serum α subunit levels compared to patients with benign gastrinomas. These observations are certainly interesting since it is often impossible to distinguish benign from malignant forms of the disease by the hormonal findings or even by the cytological characteristics of the tumours.

A multiplicity of serum enzymes have been associated with cancer, but circulating enzyme markers have not been associated with GEP endocrine tumours. Of particular interest is a cytochemical enzyme marker first isolated from mammalian nervous tissue (Pickel *et al.*, 1974) and found to be a neuron specific form of the glycolytic enzyme enolase (Bock and Dissing, 1975). This protein has, therefore, been denominated neuron specific enolase (NSE). Recently, the presence of NSE-like immunoreactivity has been demonstrated by immunocyto-chemical analysis in the peripheral diffuse neuroendocrine system (Schmechel *et al.*, 1978) and related tumours (Tapia *et al.*, 1981). NSE-like immunoreactivity was present in all of ten gastrinomas, in all of nine insulinomas, in 13 out of 15 VIP producing tumours, and in six out of eight gut carcinoids (Tapia *et al.*, 1981). Although further investigation will be needed, NSE seems to be a useful cyto-chemical marker for neuroendocrine tumours. No data are available on the presence of this protein in the blood of patients with such tumours.

MARKERS OF GEP ENDOCRINE TUMOURS ASSOCIATED WITH CLINICALLY WELL DEFINED SYNDROMES

Zollinger-Ellison Syndrome

Gastrin has proven to be the most reliable marker of the GEP endocrine tumours associated with Zollinger-Ellison syndrome, both in the diagnosis and in the monitoring of the therapy. Using an antiserum with similar reactivity against the different molecular forms (Vezzadini *et al.*, 1975), we have found levels of fasting immunoreactive gastrin within the normal range only in 5% of cases (Fig. 2). Using a radioimmunoassay with similar characteristics, the serum concentration of total gastrin-like immunoreactivity can be considered a sufficiently valid marker of the disease. Gastrin secretory response to various stimuli (secretin, calcium, protein meal, glucagon, bombesin) can confirm the diagnosis in borderline cases (Vezzadini *et al.*, 1980).

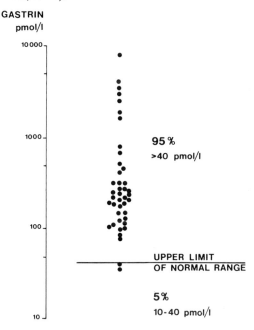

Fig. 2. Serum gastrin levels in 42 patients with Zollinger-Ellison syndrome (normal range: 10–40 pmol/l).

The diagnosis of Zollinger-Ellison syndrome is late, as is confirmed by the observation of our 42 cases in which the interval between the initial symptoms and surgery was less than 1 year in only one-quarter of cases and greater than 5 years in one-third of cases (Labò *et al.*, 1980). For the early diagnosis of gastrinoma, gastrin radioimmunoassay should be indicated as a screening test in all patients with peptic ulcer. Of 670 unoperated patients with duodenal and/or gastric ulcer, screened in our laboratory, three (0.45%) were shown to have a gastrinoma.

P. Vezzadini et al.

Gastrin has proved of special value in the follow-up of patients after surgery. In fact, metastases or the primary lesion may often be overlooked during surgery. Only if high concentrations of serum gastrin decrease to normal levels after extirpation of the tumour can metastases be excluded. Three out of our 41 operated patients had normal gastrin levels after surgery and they did not have recurrent tumours for more than 5 years after the radical operation. If the elevated gastrin levels persisted after treatment, recurrent tumours were found months or years later and before the patients were symptomatic or before recurrence was detectable by any other clinical tests. Consequently, gastrin proved to be a sensitive indicator of the presence of otherwise undetectable metastases. Gastrin is also useful in the monitoring of the chemotherapy (Fig. 3).

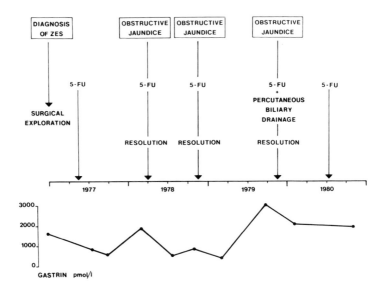

Fig. 3. Serum gastrin concentrations following chemotherapy in a patient with hepatic metastases from a primary duodenal gastrinoma (case 32: Labò *et al.*, 1980). Treatment with 5-fluoruracil invariably resulted in marked reductions in gastrin levels and these reductions were associated with the resolution of the obstructive jaundice on three different occasions.

Several peptides (PP, calcitonin, parathyroid hormone, insulin) have been proposed as markers for GEP tumours with Zollinger-Ellison syndrome (Kahn *et al.*, 1977; Bloom *et al.*, 1978), but they appear to be much less sensitive markers than gastrin. High serum concentrations of PP, parathyroid hormone and insulin were found respectively in 18, 19 and 24% of patients with gastrin producing tumours (Labò *et al.*, 1980). Zollinger-Ellison syndrome can readily be diagnosed by radioimmunoassay of gastrin, which is the marker of choice, and there is no evidence that measurement of other peptides in equivocal cases is helpful in establishing or excluding the diagnosis.

Hypoglycaemic Syndrome

Insulin producing tumours (insulinomas) and neonatal nesidioblastosis of the pancreas are characterized by their ability to produce insulin and related peptides and to cause hypoglycaemia. Whereas patients with Zollinger-Ellison syndrome who frequently have fasting immunoreactive gastrin levels ten fold higher than in normals, patients with hypoglycaemic syndrome rarely have elevated fasting serum insulin levels. Insulin secretory responses are well established as aids in the diagnosis (Fajans *et al.*, 1975). Proinsulin levels are abnormally high in most patients with proven insulinoma (Hayashi *et al.*, 1977; Turner Heding, 1977) and are strongly indicative of organic hyperinsulinism where cirrhosis of the liver, uraemia and thyrotoxicosis have been ruled out. Insulinomas can produce other peptides, such as glucagon, gastrin or PP (Hayashi *et al.*, 1977; Adrian *et al.*, 1978), but these peptides are less sensitive indicators of the disease.

Verner-Morrison Syndrome

VIP is the marker of a substantial number of cases with Verner-Morrison syndrome, characterized by watery diarrhoea, hypokalaemia, hypochlorhydria or achlorhydria (Bloom, 1978). The problem of whether VIP is, in fact, the major mediator of the syndrome is far from clarified (Gardner and McCarthy, 1978). In fact, it appears that several secretory products of GEP endocrine tumours (prostaglandins, serotonin, calcitonin, gastrin, substance P and, perhaps, PP, secretin, glucagon associated with gastrin) are capable of determining severe diarrhoea (Holst, 1979). Furthermore, this clinical feature may be a prominent part of other syndromes associated with GEP endocrine tumours. Elevated serum concentrations of PP have been observed in 60–80% of the patients with VIP producing pancreatic tumours (Schwartz, 1979). We have observed high serum levels of gastrin in two patients with VIP producing tumours, but there was no association of an ulcerogenic syndrome with the diarrhoeagenic syndrome. If possible, VIP, PP and gastrin should all be measured in serum of the patients with diarrhoea (Schwartz, 1979). VIP has proven to be a good marker for monitoring tumour therapy (Bloom and Polak, 1979; Holst, 1979).

Glucagonoma Syndrome

The levels of circulating immunoreactive glucagon in patients with glucagon producing tumours exceed the levels reached under physiological circumstances (Holst, 1979). Cases of glucagonoma syndrome are more likely to be discovered by the dermatologist, who should suspect the existence of this syndrome in all patients with bullous dermatosis of not well defined aetiology.

Somatostatinoma Syndrome

Somatostatin producing GEP tumours were first observed in 1977 and circulating immunoreactive somatostatin has proven to be a valuable marker for the tumours so far described. Most tumours were mixed and the simultaneous production of a number of other peptides has been demonstrated (Kaneko *et al.*,

1979; Galmiche *et al.*, 1980). Somatostatin radioimmunoassay seems to be a promising screening test for GEP endocrine tumours producing somatostatin in patients with diabetes, steatorrhoea and perhaps gall stones.

Carcinoid Syndrome

Carcinoid tumours arise from enterochromaffin (or argentaffin) cells, which constitute the major site of synthesis and storage of the biogenic amine serotonin. Thus, an elevated serum concentration of serotonin and an increased urinary excretion of 5-hydroxyindolacetic acid are the most frequent biochemical characteristics of carcinoid syndrome. Besides serotonin, other secretory products such as bradikinin, histamine and catecholamines have been implicated in the pathogenesis of the carcinoid syndrome (Goedert *et al.*, 1980), but their role as tumour markers is not well defined. Prostaglandin E seems to be a sensitive marker of tumours with carcinoid syndrome, but elevated levels of this substance have also been found in other endocrine diarrhoeagenic syndromes (Jaffe and Condon, 1976). Great expectations are now attracted to the diagnostic value of immunoassayable substance P, since the observation of substance P production from carcinoid tumours (Rehfeld, 1979). GEP endocrine tumours displaying a typical carcinoid pattern may also produce peptides (e.g. gastrin and PP) not normally produced by argentaffin cells (Heitz, 1977). Secretion of HCG has been demonstrated in 16% of patients with malignant carcinoid syndromes (Rosen and Weintraub, 1974). A subgroup of carcinoid tumours, particularly those of the pancreas and stomach, produce ACTH in addition to vasoactive amines. associated with the classic carcinoid syndrome (Goodwin, 1975; Marchs *et al.*, 1980).

CONCLUSIONS AND FUTURE PROSPECTIVES

The use of hormone tumour markers in patients suspected of having a GEP endocrine tumour can be of considerable help in selecting those for whom extensive diagnostic procedures are indicated. At present it seems worthwhile to screen patients with peptic ulcer, chronic diarrhoea of unknown cause, hypoglycaemia, bullous dermatosis of not well defined aetiology, or flushing, whether or not associated with diarrhoea. The use of hormone markers for detection of GEP endocrine tumours in asymptomatic subjects is not justified, owing to the apparent rarity of the tumours.

When the diagnosis has already been carried out but the tumour has not been localized by current techniques, attempts can be made to localize the tumour by percutaneous transhepatic portal catheterization with selective venous sampling for radioimmunoassay of tumour markers (Reichardt and Ingemansson, 1980). The procedure is very interesting, but it is quite difficult to perform, and the localization is not precise if the venous drainage is aberrant or if there are multiple tumours. Significant progress will probably be achieved in the pre-operative tumour localization by portal venous sampling with the development of "fast" radioimmunoassays, which have already proved valuable for insulinomas (Turner *et al.*, 1978).

Owing to the frequency of tumours producing more than one hormone, once a tumour is suspected, the diagnosis and follow-up of the patients after surgical or other treatment should be monitored by determining as many peptides as possible, since they may serve as tumour markers even in the absence of overt clinical symptoms. Modifications of tumour markers with time or after chemotherapy, associated with transition from one type of syndrome to another (Broder and Carter, 1973; Hammar and Sale, 1975), can be observed in some mixed tumours. Furthermore, in some cases, primary tumours may give rise to metastases that contain only a part of the original types of cells and the hormone markers for the metastases after extirpation of the primary tumour may differ from the original main tumour product.

The advent of hormone tumour markers has already had a significant impact on the current management and will play an even more important part in the future management of GEP endocrine tumours. One can safely predict that over the next 10 years the need for radioimmunoassays of GEP hormones will rise sharply in order to assure proper diagnosis and monitoring of GEP endocrine tumours.

REFERENCES

Abe, K., Adachi, I., Miyakawa, S., Tanaka, M., Yamaguchi, K., Tanaka, N., Kameya, T. and Shimosato, Y. (1977). *Cancer Research* 37, 4190.

Adrian, T. E., Bloom, S. R., Besterman, H. S. and Bryant, M. G. (1978). *In* "Gut Hormones" (S. R. Bloom, Ed.), pp. 254–266. Churchill Livingstone, Edinburgh.

Arnold, R., Creutzfeldt, C. and Creutzfeldt, W. (1976). *In* "Proceedings of the Fifth Congress of Endocrinologists" (V. H. T. James, Ed.), Vol. 2, 448–452. Excerpta Medica, Hamburg, Amsterdam.

Bloom, S. R. (1978). *Digestive Diseases* 23, 373.

Bloom, S. R. and Polak, J. M. (1979). *In* "Gut Peptides. Secretion, Function and Clinical Aspects" (A. Miyoshi, Ed.), pp. 327–336. Elsevier North-Holland Biomedica Press, Amsterdam, New York, Oxford.

Bloom, S. R., Adrian, T. E., Bryant, M. G. and Polak, J. M. (1978). *Lancet* 1, 1155.

Bock, E. and Dissing, J. (1975). *Scandinavian Journal of Immunology* 4, 31.

Broder, L. E. and Carter, S. K. (1973). *Annals of Internal Medicine* 79, 101.

Fajans, S. S., Floyd, J. C. and Vij, S. K. (1975). *In* "Endocrinology and Diabetes" (L. J. Kryston and R. A. Shaw, Eds), p. 453. Grune and Stratton Inc., New York.

Fiocca, R., Capella, C., Buffa, R., Fontana, R. Solcia, E., Hage, E., Change, R. E. and Moody, A. J. (1980). *American Journal of Pathology* 100, 81.

Friesen, S. R., Kimmel, J. R. and Tomita, T. (1980). *American Journal of Surgery* 139, 61.

Galmiche, J. P., Chayvialle, J. A., Dubois, P. M., David, L., Descos, F., Paulin, C., Ducastelle, T., Colin, R. and Geffroy, Y. (1980). *Gastroentreology* 78, 1577.

Gardner, J. D. and McCarthy, D. M. (1978). *In* "Gut Hormones" (S. R. Bloom, Ed.), pp. 570–573. Churchill Livingstone, Edinburgh.

Goedert, M., Otten, U., Suda, K., Heith, P. U., Stalder, G. A., Obrecht, J. P., Holzach, P. and Allgower, M. (1980). *Cancer* 45, 104.

Goodwin, J. D. (1975). *Cancer* **36**, 560.
Hammar, S. and Sale, G. (1975). *Human Pathology* **6**, 349.
Hayashi, M., Floyd, J. C. Jr, Pek, S. and Fajans, S. S. (1977). *Journal of Clinical Endocrinology and Metabolism* **44**, 681.
Heitz, P. (1977). *Verhandlungen Der Deutschen Gesellschaft Fur Pathologie* **61**, 24.
Holst, J. J. (1979). *Clinics in Endocrinology and Metabolism* **8** (2), 413.
Jaffe, B. M. and Condon, S. (1976). *American Surgeon* **184**, 516.
Kahn, C. R., Rosen, S. W., Weintraub, B. D., Fajans, S. S. and Gorden, P. (1977). *New England Journal of Medicine* **297**, 565.
Kaneko, H., Yanaihara, N., Ito, S., Kusumoto, Y., Fujita, T., Ishikawa, S., Sumida, T. and Sekiya, M. (1979). *Cancer* **44**, 2273.
Labò, G., Vezzadini, P. and Gasbarrini, G. (1980). *In* "Sindromi cliniche con alterata secrezione di ormoni gastrointestinali". Relazione al 81° Congresso della Società Italiana di Medicina Interna, Vol. 1, pp. 43–202. Pozzi, Rome.
Larsson, L. I., Grimelius, L., Hakanson, R., Rehfeld, J. F., Stadil, F., Holst, J., Angervall, L. and Sundler, F. (1975). *American Journal of Pathology* **79**, 271.
Marcus, F. S., Friedman, M. A., Callen, P. W., Churg, A. and Harbous, J. (1980). *Cancer* **46**, 1263.
Pickel, V. M., Reis, D. J., Marangos, P. J. and Zomzelv-Neurath, C. (1974). *Brain Research* **105**, 184.
Polak, J. M., Bloom, S. R., Adrian, T. E., Heitz, P., Bryant, M. G. and Pearse, A. G. E. (1976). *Lancet* **1**, 328.
Polak, J. M., Bishop, A., Bloom, S. R. and Pearse, A. G. E. (1977). *Gut* **18**, A416.
Rehfeld, J. F. (1979). *Scandinavian Journal of Gastroenterology* **14** (53), 33.
Reichardt, W. and Ingemansson, S. (1980). *Acta Radiologica Diagnosis* **21**, 177.
Rosen, S. W. and Weintraub, B. D. (1974). *New England Journal of Medicine* **290**, 1441.
Schmechel, D., Marangos, P. J., Zis, A. P., Brightman, M. and Goodwin, F. K. (1978). *Science* **199**, 313.
Schwartz, T. W. (1979). *Scandinavian Journal of Gastroenterology* **14**, (53), 93.
Stabile, B. E., Braunstein, G. D., Hershman, J. M. and Passaro, E. (1978). *Surgical Forum* **24**, 488.
Tapia, F. J., Polak, J. M., Barbosa, A. J. A., Bloom, S. R., Marangos, P. J. and Pearse, A. G. E. (1981). *In* "Proceedings of the Pathological Society of Great Britain and Ireland" 142° Meeting, pp. 59–60. London.
Turner, R. C. and Heding, L. G. (1977). *Diabetologia* **13**, 571.
Turner, R. C., Lee, E. C. G., Morris, P. J., Harris, E. A. and Dick, R. (1978). *Lancet* **1**, 515.
Vezzadini, P., Tomassetti, P., Cipollini, F., Bonora, G. and Cavicchi, A. (1975). *In* "Metodi radioimmunologici in Endocrinologia", Serono Symposia, Milano, pp. 291–307.
Vezzadini, P., Tomassetti, P., Bagnoli, L., Sternini, C. and Bonora, G. (1980). *In* "Sindromi cliniche con alterata secrezione di ormoni gastrointestinali". Relazione al 81° Congresso della Societa Italiana di Medicina Interna, Vol. 1, pp. 50–73. Pozzi, Rome.

MARKERS OF THYROID TUMOURS

L. Baschieri[1], C. Giani[1], S. Mariotti[1], F. Pacini[1], B. Busnardo[2],
M. E. Girelli[2] and A. Pinchera[3]

*Cattedra di Patologia Medica II°, University of Pisa, Pisa[1], Istituto di Semeiotica
Medica[2] and Cattedra di Medicina Costituzionale ed Endocrinologia[3],
University of Padua, Padua, Italy*

INTRODUCTION

The possibility of identifying circulating substances indicative of neoplasia
can provide a useful tool for early diagnosis and follow-up of cancer. These
substances are generally called tumour "markers" and should satisfy some precise
requirements. First of all, markers should be produced by or strictly associated
with tumour cells; furthermore, these materials should be specific of neoplastic
tissue or, alternatively, major quantitative differences in the production of these
substances should be present between tumoral and normal cells. Moreover, marker
assays should be sensitive enough to allow an early diagnosis in the presence
of a small number of cells and the techniques employed should be relatively
simple and not very expensive. Potentially useful materials employed as tumour
markers are secretion products (including ectopic hormones), isoenzymes, oncofoetal antigens and tumour associated antigens. In this paper we shall review
the possible usefulness of some serological markers in the diagnostic evaluation
of thyroid tumours. In these tumours no specific tumour associated antigen has
been described so far; thus, determination of secretion products (like thyroglobulin
(Tg) and calcitonin (CT)) and oncofoetal antigens have been employed in clinical
investigation. Before discussing this topic in detail, it is useful to recall that
thyroid tumours have different histological and biological characteristics. Differ-

Serono Symposium No. 46, Markers for Diagnosis and Monitoring of Human Cancer, edited
by M. I. Colnaghi, G. L. Buraggi and M. Ghione, 1982. Academic Press, London and New
York.

entiated thyroid carcinomas (papillary and follicular) derive from follicular cells and maintain some properties of normal gland, such as TSH responsiveness, the ability to concentrate iodine and to synthesize Tg. In several instances this substance can be used as a very specific marker (Van Herle and Uller, 1975; Shlossberg *et al.*, 1979; Pacini *et al.*, 1980a). Similarly, CT is now widely employed in the diagnosis of medullary thyroid carcinoma which derives from parafollicular (C) cells producing this hormone (Williams, 1970; Goltzam *et al.*, 1974); carcino-embryonic antigen (CEA) determination is also very useful in this tumour (Ishikawa and Hamada, 1976; Cimitan *et al.*, 1979). Undifferentiated thyroid carcinoma lacks any specific characteristic of normal thyroid and no valuable marker is known, although CEA assay has been proposed by some authors (Madeddu *et al.*, 1980).

MARKERS OF THYROID TUMOURS

The presence of circulating abnormal iodine compounds in patients with differentiated thyroid cancer was reported several years ago. Robbins *et al.* (1955) found a constant elevation of PBI with respect to BEI in patients with metastatized thyroid tumours and considered this finding indicative of secretion by the tumour of iodoproteins different from normal iodothyronines. Baschieri *et al.* (1964) found high levels of circulating iodoproteins with the electrophoretic mobility of albumin in a patient with follicular thyroid carcinoma and spread lung metastases. Similar findings were reported by Robbins *et al.* (1959) in rats with a transplantable thyroid tumour. Thyroid neoplastic tissue produces Tg which seems to be abnormal under several aspects. Tumoral Tg has been shown to be less iodized than normal Tg (Monaco and Andreoli, 1977). Tg content of carbohydrates and sialic acid is reduced in a transplantable tumour of rats (Monaco and Robbins, 1973) and in some cases of human cancer (Monaco and Andreoli, 1977). These abnormalities do not seem to affect the immunoreactivity of Tg, and, until now, attempts to identify neoplastic Tg by specific antisera have not been successful. However, in one patient with metastatic follicular thyroid carcinoma Fenzi *et al.* (1976) found circulating iodoproteins having preferential reactivity with antisera raised to bovine Tg. This interesting finding needs further confirmation. In summary, although the above data suggest that some abnormalities may be present in the secretion products of thyroid tumours, so far no specific alteration of diagnostic value has been clearly demonstrated. In absence of a specific marker of thyroid cancer, the finding of elevated serum levels of some normal components of thyroid gland, such as Tg and CT, may lead to the specific identification of tumours.

THYROGLOBULIN

Identification and estimation of Tg in human sera by specific radioimmuno-assay (RIA) was first reported by Roitt and Torrigiani (1967). Increased levels of serum Tg have been reported in several benign and malignant thyroid disorders, including differentiated thyroid carcinoma, Graves' disease, toxic adenoma, non-toxic goitre and subacute thyroiditis (Torrigiani *et al.*, 1969; Van Herle *et al.*, 1973; Ochi *et al.*, 1975; Pezzino *et al.*, 1978; Izumi and Larsen, 1978; Pacini *et al.*, 1980a). Van Herle and Uller (1975) drew attention to the very low Tg levels observed in patients with differentiated thyroid carcinoma successfully treated by total thyroidectomy. In contrast, the same authors documented very high circulating Tg in patients with metastatic disease. This finding was late confirmed and extended by several investigations (LoGerfo *et al.*, 1977; Shlossberg *et al.*, 1979; Pacini *et al.*, 1980a). In our laboratory, we assayed serum Tg in a large series of patients with and without various thyroid diseases (Pacini *et al.*, 1980a, b) with particular regard to thyroid carcinoma in different clinical conditions. The Tg RIA employed in our study has been reported in detail elsewhere (Pacini *et al.*, 1980a). Briefly, the minimum detectable was 1.25 ng/ml and the normal range was < 1.25–27 ng/ml (mean $\pm$ SD = 9.5 $\pm$ 0.9). Sera with detectable anti-Tg autoantibody by passive haemagglutination ($\geqslant 1:10$) were excluded. In agreement with previous studies serum Tg levels were found clearly elevated in patients with untreated papillary or follicular thyroid carcinoma, while normal levels were observed in medullary or undifferentiated thyroid tumours. However, elevated Tg was also found in several benign thyroid disorders such as Graves' disease, toxic adenoma, toxic multinodular goitre, non-toxic goitre and subacute thyroiditis. Thus, serum Tg determinations were then performed in a large series of patients with differentiated thyroid carcinoma treated by total thyroidectomy. Figure 1 shows the results of serum Tg concentrations in 88 patients with papillary of follicular thyroid carcinoma after surgery. The mean serum Tg level was low (8.5 $\pm$ 2.2 ng/ml) in the 24 subjects, with no evidence of either a thyroid residue or metastic disease and moderately increased (56.7 $\pm$ 16.2 ng/ml) in the 27 patients with residual thyroid tissue. Elevated levels were found in most of the 28 cases with documented metastatic disease. Interestingly, the mean serum Tg concentration found in eight patients with bone metastases (4,004 $\pm$ 982 ng/ml) or in five with lung metastases (2520 $\pm$ 620 ng/ml) were much higher than in those with lymph node metastases (199 $\pm$ 50 ng/ml). Values above 500 ng/ml were found in all but one of the patients with either bone or lung metastases. Furthermore, when metastatic lesions were subdivided into functioning and non-functioning metastases, as assessed by ^{131}I whole body scan (WBS), the mean Tg concentration found in the two groups did not differ significantly. This finding prompted us to perform a comparison of results of the WBS with the levels of circulating Tg in a large series of patients with treated differentiated thyroid carcinoma. The results obtained are shown in Fig. 2. Serum Tg levels were above the normal range in all the 45 patients with positive WBS. Thirteen of the 56 subjects with negative WBS had clinical and/or radiological evidence of metastases: in this group serum Tg was elevated in 11 (84%) cases and the mean Tg Level (572 $\pm$ 442 ng/ml), although lower, did not significantly differ from the mean Tg concentration (1416 $\pm$ 350 ng/ml) observed in patients with positive WBS. These data, in agreement with other reports (Van Herle and Uller, 1975; LoGerfo *et al.*, 1977), clearly indicate that serum Tg measurement is of a great diagnostic value in the assessment of metastases from differentiated thyroid carcinoma after thyroidectomy. With respect to WBS, Tg determination has the clear advantage of also detecting metastases unable to concentrate radio-iodine. This finding has been recently reported also by Schlumberger *et al.*

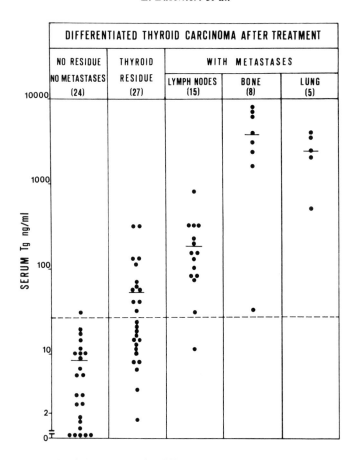

Fig. 1. Serum Tg levels in patients with differentiated thyroid carcinoma previously treated by total thyroidectomy, with or without subsequent radioiodine therapy. The number of subjects is indicated in parentheses. The solid horizontal lines indicate the mean concentration of serum Tg for each group. The broken horizontal line represents the upper limit of the normal range.

(1980). Since the radioiodine scan requires withdrawal of thyroid replacement therapy, we have investigated the possibility to use serum Tg determination as a marker of recurrences or metastatic disease in patients with differentiated thyroid carcinoma submitted to suppressive therapy with L-thyroxine. In Fig. 3 (part A) are illustrated the results obtained in 12 subjects: in five or six patients with bone or lung metastases Tg levels increased after withdrawal of therapy, but were also elevated during thyroid medication. In five patients with either thyroid residue or neck lymph node metastases serum Tg was within the normal range during the treatment, while it was clearly increased after discontinuation of therapy. No change was noted in one patient without any evidence of thyroid residue or metastases. A clear reduction of serum Tg levels during thyroid therapy was also observed in non-toxic diffuse goitre (Fig. 3, part B). These data indicate that serum Tg can also be used as marker of metastases during thyroid suppressive

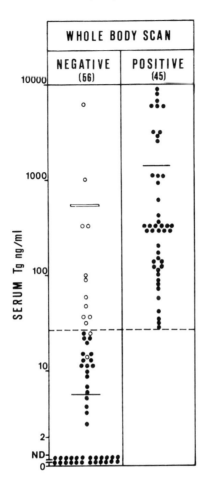

Fig. 2. Serum Tg concentrations and results of ^{131}I scanning in patients with differentiated thyroid carcinoma after surgical thyroidectomy and ^{131}I ablation of residue thyroid
tissue. The first column (•) indicates patients with no metastatic thyroid tissue, (○) indicates
patients with detectable non-functioning metastases. For each group the mean Tg levels
is indicated: ——, for solid circles ⊏⊐, for open circles. The broken horizontal line represents the upper limit of the normal range. (ND = not detectable.)

therapy, but only in patients with already spread disease. Similar effects of
thyroid treatment on serum Tg levels in differentiated thyroid carcinoma were
recently confirmed by Schlumberger *et al.* (1980). These authors also showed
that the effect of suppressive therapy on circulating Tg were similar in patients
with metastases able or not to concentrate radioiodine.

To further investigate the extent to which serum Tg determination can be
used for the identification of thyroid malignancies before thyroidectomy, Tg
was measured in 52 patients with single cold thyroid nodule and in 44 patients
with single cold thyroid nodule associated with diffuse non-toxic goitre. For
comparison, circulating Tg was evaluated in 23 patients with non-toxic goitre

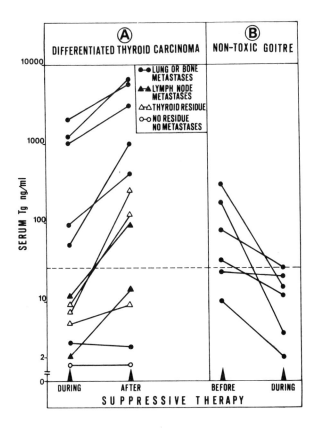

Fig. 3. Effect of suppressive therapy with thyroid hormone on serum Tg levels in patients with differentiated thyroid carcinoma (A) previously submitted to total thyroidectomy and in patients with non-toxic goitre (B). The broken horizontal line represents the upper limit of the normal range.

and in 27 patients with toxic adenoma. In subjects with single thyroid nodules, the mean Tg value was 59.0 ± 100.4 ng/ml and almost 50% of the patients had Tg levels significantly higher than normal subjects; 26 (58%) of 44 patients with nodular goitre showed elevated levels of circulating Tg (67.6 ± 100.9 ng/ml). Similary, elevated levels of Tg were found in toxic adenoma (98.7 ± 136 ng/ml) and in non-toxic goitre (61.0 ± 15.0 ng/ml). Twenty-one patients with single thyroid nodule were eventually operated on; in nine adenomas mean Tg level was 24.2 ± 27 ng/l and only one patient had serum Tg above the upper limit of the normal range (Fig. 4). Four cases of adenocarcinomas without metastases had elevated Tg levels (61.7 ± 17 ng/ml), which did not differ significantly from those observed in benign lesions. It is, however, conceivable that this finding is due to the limited number of cases examined. Eight patients with metastatic thyroid carcinoma had very high Tg concentrations (206 ± 180 ng/ml). It is to be pointed out that these values significantly differed from Tg levels observed in benign nodules and in carcinomas without metastases ($P < 0.0005$). These data indicated that high levels of Tg are found only in carcinomatous nodules and that very elevated values are suggestive of metastases. This observation is

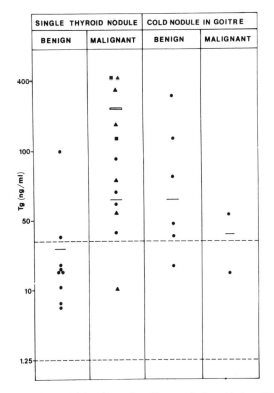

SINGLE THYROID NODULE		COLD NODULE IN GOITRE	
BENIGN	MALIGNANT	BENIGN	MALIGNANT

Fig. 4. Tg levels in patient with benign and malignant single cold thyroid nodule associated or not with goitre. The second column (•) represents patients without metastatic disease, (▲) indicates subjects with lymph node metastases and (■) patients with bone metastases. For each group the mean Tg concentration is indicated —— for • (in the second column the mean Tg level is indicated ⊏⊐ for ▲ and ■). The broken horizontal lines represent the upper and the lower limit of the normal range.

of particular interest because metastases are generally evident, but sometimes they may be casually discovered by routine X-ray examination. Similar data on circulating Tg levels in patients with thyroid nodules have been recently reported by Shlossberg *et al.* (1979).

CALCITONIN

Medullary thyroid carcinoma is a differentiated thyroid tumour deriving from parafollicular (C) cells of the thyroid producing CT (Milhaud *et al.*, 1968; Cunliffe *et al.*, 1968; Meyer and Abdelbari, 1968; Tashjian and Melvin, 1968). Serum CT determination by RIA is now considered the best index for the early diagnosis of this tumour and for follow-up after surgical treatment. In one study of Deftos (1974) abnormally elevated plasma CT levels were found in the large majority (26 of 33) of patients with medullary thyroid carcinoma before thyroidectomy. In the same report measurements of CT in the plasma obtained from veins draining the tumour showed a ratio to the peripheral levels ranging from 4.3 to 570, clearly indicating the tumour origin of plasma CT. Goltzam *et al.*

(1974) firstly evaluated the value of CT determination after surgery in thyroid medullary carcinoma. In four of nine patients the assay led to the identification of metastatic disease before its documentation on clinical or pathological grounds. CT assay in samples obtained by venous catheterization was found by these authors of value in the surgical management of metastases, being effective in estimating total tumour burden. Furthermore, CT determination confirmed the complete removal of the tumour in five cases.

We have recently performed serum CT determination by RIA in a large series of patients with medullary thyroid carcinoma. With the method employed in our laboratory basal CT levels of > 0.40 ng/ml were considered abnormally elevated. As reported in Fig. 5, all but one of 16 patients evaluated before thyroid surgery had increased levels of CT. This hormone was also elevated in 17 of 28 (61%) patients examined at least 2 months after thyroidectomy. In spite of some discrepancies a clear relationship was found between CT levels and the presence

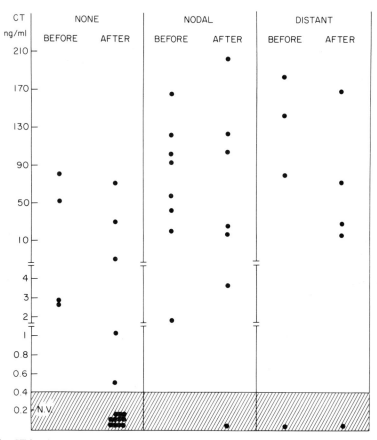

Fig. 5. CT levels in patients with and without metastases before and after surgery. NV = normal values.

of metastases. In fact, ten of twelve (83%) subjects with nodal or distant metastases showed high values of serum CT, while only five of 16 (31%) without
any clinical evidence of metastatic disease had elevated CT levels. In these latter
cases, residual tumour tissue and/or metastases undetectable on clinical grounds
were the most probable source of circulating CT.

In some cases the production of CT by the tumour may not be detectable
without a provocative test. For this purpose, calcium chloride infusion or pentagastrin injection are the most frequently used tests for clinical investigation,
but other procedures like glucagon infusion (Deftos, 1974) and ethanol ingestion
(Wells *et al.*, 1975a) have been also reported. Calcium chloride infusion is generally
performed for 2–4 h: increased serum CT is observed after a variable time interval
during administration of calcium. Using this provocative test, Deftos (1974)
found abnormally elevated CT levels in three patients with untreated medullary
carcinoma in whom basal CT concentrations were within the normal range.
Pentagastrin is a potent stimulator of CT secretion, as first reported in the pig
by Cooper *et al.* (1971). Injection of pentagastrin i.v. was found by Hennessey
et al. (1974) to be more effective than calcium infusion in stimulating CT secretion in patients with medullary thyroid carcinoma. Furthermore, with pentagastrin the peak response is obtained after a short time (1–5 min) interval than
that observed after calcium infusion. Pentagastrin provocative test has been
reported (Wells *et al.*, 1975b) to be of special value in the detection of small
tumours which are not clinically appreciated. Glucagon infusion was found
to have no consistent effect on plasma calcium concentration and it is therefore
considered an unreliable provocative test (Deftos, 1974). Ethanol is an effective substance in the stimulation of CT secretion, but it has been only rarely
employed as a diagnostic test in medullary thyroid carcinoma (Cohen *et al.*,
1973; Dymling *et al.*, 1976).

The determination of serum CT in the peripheral blood in basal conditions
and after secretory stimulation is also a very useful tool in the diagnostic screening
of the relatives of patients with the heritable variant of thyroid medullary carcinoma (Sipple, 1961). This tumour is generally associated with multiple endocrine neoplasias, such as pheochromocytoma, parathyroid adenomas, and mucosal
neuromas. A study on a large series of relatives of patients with medullary thyroid
carcinoma was carried out by Miller *et al.* (1972). Nine of 83 subjects were found
to have elevated basal circulating CT and three had abnormally high levels after
calcium infusion. In spite of the lack of any clinical evidence of thyroid abnormalities surgical exploration confirmed the presence of medullary thyroid carcinoma
in 11 of 12 patients with abnormally elevated serum CT. Similar results were
reported by Wells *et al.* (1975b) who found the pentagastrin stimulation test
very useful in the early diagnosis of thyroid neoplasia in children.

In summary, the data reported above, show that CT should be considered
a very specific and sensitive marker for thyroid medullary carcinoma. However,
some caution should be exercised in the interpretation of elevated serum CT
levels. In fact, high concentrations of CT have been described in subacute thyroid-
ities (Cervi–Skinner and Castleman, 1973) and in several non-thyroidal neoplasias
such as oat cell carcinoma of the lung, carcinoids, carcinoma of the breast and
in patients with the Zollinger–Ellison syndrome (Sizemore *et al.*, 1973; Coombes

et al., 1974). The evidence that CT is secreted by these tumours as an ectopic hormone is conflicting. At least in one case of lung carcinoma associated with hypercalcitonaemia, the origin of CT indentified by catheterization was from the thyroid and not from the tumour (Silva *et al.*, 1975).

CARCINOEMBRYONIC ANTIGEN

High concentrations of serum CEA have been frequently reported in patients with medullary thyroid carcinoma (Calmettes *et al.*, 1978; Cimitan *et al.*, 1979). CEA levels are generally well correlated with CT concentrations, although some patients with evolutive medullary carcinoma may show normal CEA levels in the presence of elevated circulating CT. (Cimitan *et al.*, 1979). In thyroid tumours different from medullary thyroid carcinoma, CEA determinations appear to be without practical value (DeGroot *et al.*, 1977).

In order to further evaluate the clinical usefulness of serum CEA determination as marker of thyroid carcinoma, we performed CEA radioimmunoassay in a large series of patients with untreated thyroid tumour. The results obtained are reported in Table I, and confirmed that high CEA levels ($<$ 6 ng/ml) were frequently

Table I. CEA levels in thyroid tumours before treatment.

Malignancy	Number of subjects	Number of patients with CEA $\geqslant$ 6 ng ml
Follicular or papillary	105	8 (7.6%)
Medullary	16	10 (62.5%)
Undifferentiated	12	—

but not constantly found in medullary carcinoma, while positive results were observed only in sporadic cases in other histological types. Previous studies carried out in patients with medullary thyroid carcinoma submitted to thyroidectomy (Cimitan *et al.*, 1979) showed that in the positive cases CEA levels appeared to be fairly well correlated with the effectiveness of the therapy, suggesting that CEA assay may be useful in the follow-up of this tumour. However, even if CEA determination may partially replace CT as marker of medullary thyroid carcinoma, it is clearly less specific and sensitive than CT. Furthermore, no clear advantage is present in measuring both CT and CEA with respect to CT alone.

Very recently, Madeddu *et al.* (1980) evaluated the diagnostic value of CEA measurements in a large series of patients with thyroid nodules. The results obtained showed that determination of CEA can be useful in the pre-operative diagnosis of thyroid malignancies, with particular regard to medullary and undifferentiated (giant cells) carcinomas. The latter finding has not been reported in previous studies and needs further confirmation.

CONCLUSIONS

In conclusion, the data reported above indicate that Tg and CT are respectively very useful markers of thyroid differentiated or medullary carcinoma. Measurement of serum CEA may also be of value in medullary tumours but, due to the lower sensitivity and specificity of this assay, CT determination should be preferred. Tg measurement is of paramount importance in the identification of recurrences of metastases during the follow-up of thyroid tumours after surgery. In particular, Tg assay shows clear advantages when compared with the WBS by ^{131}I, since elevated serum Tg may be also observed in patients with metastases unable to concentrate iodine which are not detected by the scan. Moreover, at least in subjects with spread disease, Tg measurements can be also performed without suspending the suppressive therapy with thyroid hormones. On the other hand, Tg assay is generally of little value in untreated patients, since Tg is elevated in several malignant or benign thyroid disorders. However, in subjects with single thyroid nodules, high levels of circulating Tg may represent the only clue to the identification of already metastatized cancer.

With few exceptions, elevated CT is indicative of thyroid medullary carcinoma before and after surgery. Thus, CT measurements are very useful both in the diagnostic evaluation of thyroid nodules and in the follow-up of patients submitted to total thyroidectomy. Furthermore, the studies carried out in the familiar variant of medullary tumours show that the presence of elevated serum CT in patients without clinically appreciated thyroid nodules but affected by other disorders such as Marphan syndrome, neurofibromatosis, pheocromocytoma or with familial history of medullary tumours, may be sufficient to indicate the surgical exploration of thyroid gland.

REFERENCES

Baschieri, L., Salabé, G. B. and Tonelli, S. (1964). *Folia Endocrinologica* 6, 676.

Calmettes, C., Mouktar, M. S. and Milhaud, G. (1978). *Cancer Immunology and Immunotherapy* 4, 251.

Cervi–Skinner, S. J. and Castleman, B. (1973). *New England Journal of Medicine* 289, 472.

Cimitan, M., Busnardo, B., Girelli, M. E., Casara, D. and Zanatta, G. P. (1979). *Journal of Endocrinological Investigation* 2, 241.

Cohen, S. L., MacIntyre, I., Graham–Smith, D. and Walker, J. G. (1973). *Lancet* 2, 1172.

Coombes, R. D., Hillyard, C., Greenberg, P. B. and MacIntyre, I. (1974). *Lancet* 1, 1080.

Cooper, C. W., Schwesinger, W. K., Mahgoub, A. M. and Ontjes, D. A. (1971). *Science* 172, 1238.

Cunliffe, W. J., Black, A. M., Hall, R., Johnston, I. D. A., Hugdson, P., Shuster, S., Gudmundsson, T. V., Joplin, G. F., Williams, E. D., Woodhose, N. J. Y., Galante, L. and MacIntyre, I. (1968). *Lancet* 2, 63.

Deftos, L. F. (1974). *Journal of the American Medical Association* 227, 403.

DeGroot, L. J., Hoye, K., Refetoff, S., Van Herle, A., Asteris, G. and Rochman, H. (1977). *Journal of Clinical Endocrinology and Metabolism* **21**, 699.
Dymling, J. F., Ljungberg, O., Hillyard, C. J., Greenberg, P. B., Evans, I. M. A. and MacIntyre, I. (1976). *Acta Endocrinologica* **82**, 500.
Fenzi, G. F., Refetoff, S., Asteris, G. and Vassart, G. (1976). *Acta Endocrinologica* (Suppl. 204), 63.
Goltzam, D., Potts, J. T., Jr, Ridgway, E. C. and Maloof, E. (1974). *New England Journal of Medicine* **290**, 1035.
Hennessey, J. F., Wells, S. A., Jr, Ontjes, D. A. and Cooper, C. W. (1974). *Journal of Clinical Endocrinology and Metabolism* **39**, 487.
Ishikawa, H. and Hamada, S. (1976). *British Journal of Cancer* **34**, 111.
Izumi, N. and Larsen, P. R. (1978). *Metabolism* **27**, 449.
LoGerfo, P., Stillman, T., Colacchio, D. and Feind, C. (1977). *Lancet* **1**, 881.
Madeddu, G., Langer, M., Dettori, G. and Costanza, C. (1980). *Cancer* **45**, 2607.
Meyer, J. S. and Abdelbari, W. (1968). *New England Journal of Medicine* **278**, 523.
Milhaud, G., Tubiana, M., Pommentier, C. and Coutris, C. (1968). *CR Academic Science* **266**, 608.
Miller, H. H., Melvin, K. E. W., Gibson, J. M. and Taschjian, A. H., Jr (1972). *American Journal of Surgery* **438**, 1972.
Monaco, F. and Andreoli, M. (1977). *American Radiology* **20**, 735.
Monaco, F. and Robbins, J. (1973). *Journal Biological Chemistry* **248**, 2535.
Ochi, Y., Hachiya, T., Yoshimura, M., Miyazaki, T., Majima, T., Kaimatsu, I. and Takahashi, H. (1975). *Endocrinological Japonica* **22**, 351.
Pacini, F., Pinchera, A., Giani, C., Grasso, L., Doveri, F. and Baschieri, L. (1980a). *Journal of Endocrinological Investigation* **3**, 283.
Pacini, F., Pinchera, A., Giani, C., Grasso, L. and Baschieri, L. (1980b). *Clinical Endocrinology* **13**, 107.
Pezzino, V., Vigneri, R., Squatrito, S., Filetti, S., Camus, M. and Polosa, P. (1978). *Journal of Clinical Endocrinology and Metabolism* **46**, 653.
Robbins, J., Rall, J. E. and Rawson, R. W. (1955). *Journal of Clinical Endocrinology and Metabolism* **15**, 1315.
Robbins, J., Wolf, J. and Rall, J. E. (1959). *Endocrinology* **64**, 1959.
Roitt, I. M. and Torrigiani, G. (1967). *Endocrinology* **81**, 421.
Schlumberger, M., Charbord, P., Fragu, P., Lumbroso, J., Parmentier, C. and Tubiana, M. (1980). *Journal of Clinical Endocrinology and Metabolism* **51**, 513.
Shlossberg, A. H., Jacobson, J. C. and Ibbertson, H. K. (1979). *Clinical Endocrinology* **10**, 17.
Silva, O. L., Becker, K. L., Primack, A., Doppman, J. L. and Smider, R. H. (1975). *Journal of the American Medical Association* **234**, 183.
Sipple, J. H. (1961). *American Journal of Medicine* **31**, 163.
Sizemore, G. W., Go, V. L. W., Koplan, E. L., Sanrebacher, L. J., Holtermuller, K. H. and Armand, C. D. (1973). *New England Journal of Medicine* **268**, 641.
Tashjian, A. H., Jr. and Melvin, K. E. W. (1968). *New England Journal of Medicine* **279**, 279.
Torrigiani, G., Doniach, D. and Roitt, I. M. (1969). *Journal of Clinical Endocrinology and Metabolism* **29**, 305.
Van Herle, A. J., Uller, R. P., Matthews, N. L. and Brown, J. (1973). *Journal of Clinical Investigation* **52**, 1320.
Van Herle, A. J. and Uller, R. P. (1975). *Journal of Clinical Investigation* **56**, 272.
Wells, S. A., Cooper, C. W. and Ontjies, D. A. (1975a). *Metabolism* **24**, 1215.
Wells, S. A., Jr, Ontjies, D. A., Cooper, C. W., Hennessey, J. F., Ellis, G. J., McPherson, H. T. and Sabiston, D. C., Jr. (1975b). *Annals of Surgery* **182**, 370.
Williams, E. D. (1970). *In* "Calcitonin 1969 Proceedings of the 2nd International Symposium", London, pp. 485–486.

CURRENT STATUS AND PROSPECTS FOR CLINICAL
USE OF TUMOR MARKERS

R. B. Herberman

*Laboratory of Immunodiagnosis, National Cancer Institute,
National Institutes of Health, Bethesda, Maryland, USA*

Attending a meeting like this, I am torn between feelings of strong pessimism and sustained optimism. The problem is, which attitude is more realistic and in line with the scientific evidence? To assess this, I have tried to remain as objective as possible. This is perhaps considerably easier for me than for most of speakers in this conference, since I do not work directly on tumor markers and am more an interested bystander.

Firstly, particularly because it may reflect the feelings of many of you, I would like to state some of the reasons for my feeling of pessimism or discouragement.

(1) There seems to be a general inverse correlation between the amount of knowledge and the extent of investigation about a particular marker and the level of enthusiasm or optimism that is experienced. In many, probably most, cases, as we gain more insight into the actual value of a marker, we become increasingly aware of its limitations. There appear to be several phases through which the work on tumor markers go. (a) Initial examination of its ability to discriminate between cancer and non-cancer; this is most often, for the circulating markers, a limited examination of readily available serum specimens, involving obvious cancer, usually advanced, and healthy controls, usually considerably younger than the cancer patients. There are a large number of reports in this category. (b) Unfortunately, there are far fewer studies that go on to a second phase, to determine more clearly the discriminatory value of a marker and to assess

Serono Symposium No. 46, Markers for Diagnosis and Monitoring of Human Cancer, edited by M. I. Colnaghi, G. L. Buraggi and M. Ghione, 1982. Academic Press, London and New York.

thoroughly the levels of markers in the whole spectrum of health and disease. For
this, it is necessary to use age matched normal controls, patients with relevant
benign diseases, other cancers, and various other appropriate controls. Most of the
markers discussed at this meeting have reached this point and although the results
are not as promising in most cases as in the initial studies, a considerable portion
of these assays have survived this stage. (c) The next stage relates to the determination of the actual value of a marker for a particular clinical application. This is
usually dependent on time consuming, expensive, and logistically difficult, well
designed clinical studies and, therefore, is approached only in a handful of cases.
Even among the highly selective series of markers discussed at this meeting, only a
portion have undergone this type of rigorous evaluation.

(2) Because of some major problems in the adequate evaluation of markers,
coupled with the growing availability of tests for various tumor markers, there is a
rather widespread and uncontrolled utilisation of tumor markers. CEA is the best
known and most widely used example of tumor markers, and millions of assays
are now being done each year, at an estimated cost of many millions of dollars,
probably well in excess of 30–50 million dollars. A large portion of this testing is
probably being performed for ill defined reasons or with results that are not
reliable, because of technical problems in the testing laboratory or because their
application for management is not adequately understood by the clinicians who
ordered the tests.

(3) Progress in this field appears quite slow. As a personal milestone, I have
reflected back on a meeting at NIH in late 1978 that was designed to assess
critically the status of tumor markers and the available documentation regarding
their value for particular clinical applications. Relatively little, additional solid
information has come forth at this meeting that was not known, or at least
anticipated, two-and-a-half years previously.

With these points being mentioned, why do I still have a feeling of sustained
optimism?

(1) Although the number of advances and new insights into tumor markers
has been rather small, some have occurred and appear very promising. One
example is the development and practical demonstration of radioimmunodetection
at a clinical level, which had been predicted, from many earlier studies, to be
almost hopeless or unfeasible. The successful demonstration of some value of this
procedure has come despite the main use of an antibody to a marker, CEA, which
is clearly not tumor specific or as selective as desired or as are some other, already
available markers. Another important success in this field relates to the use of the
assays for α-fetoprotein for screening for primary liver cancer among high risk
populations. In a large-scale study in mainland China, the feasibility of mounting
such a large-scale screening project has been demonstrated, and the results have
shown an ability of the marker to detect at least a small number of cases of
primary liver cancer at early, treatable, and perhaps curable stages. Yet another
important example of an important practical application of tumor markers is the
increased documentation of the value of AFP and HCG for the management of
patients with choriocarcinoma and for testicular cancer. Yet another impressive
success has been the demonstration of the value of the radioimmunoassay for
calcitonin, particularly after provocative stimulation, in the screening of families

with medullary carcinoma of the thyroid. In a somewhat different area, the rapid application of the expanding body of information on markers for subpopulations of normal lymphoid cells to the classification of leukemias and lymphomas has already resulted in considerable revision of the classification of these diseases. In several instances, this is being shown to be important for adequate management. For example, acute lymphocytic leukemia of the T cell type (T-ALL) has been shown to have a considerably poorer prognosis than common acute lymphocytic leukemia and it seems likely that a different form of therapy will be needed for T-ALL.

There have also been some recent impressive advances in technology. For this field, monoclonal antibodies have been rapidly recognised as offering the potential for a whole new generation of tumor markers and perhaps even for new approaches to the use of tumor markers. However, I must introduce a note of caution at this point. It remains unclear as to just how much more powerful or selective the monoclonal antibodies will be. It is proving quite difficult to find monoclonal antibodies that detect specific antigens on tumor cells. Thus, the problems that are being encountered are similar to those which have been experienced for many years with the conventionally produced antisera. Although the monoclonal antibodies will clearly provide better defined reagents, for more consistent and standardised results, it is not clear that they will allow definitive discrimination between cancer and all normal tissues. There is a continuing need for experienced sereologists to evaluate thoroughly the specificity of each new monoclonal antibody that appears promising. A good example of such extensive evaluation has come at the meeting from the work of Dr Maria Colnaghi and her colleagues, who, on the one hand, have demonstrated a monoclonal antibody which appeared to be highly selective for breast cancer, but on the other hand, by very extensive evaluation of normal tissues, have demonstrated the presence of the detected marker on some normal tissues. It is possible that one of the main limitations with the current generation of monoclonal antibodies is that they are being produced in rodents, which may lack the ability to detect the small variations in specificities between tumor cells and normal tissues. More selective and hopefully tumor specific reagents may come from the new attempts to make human monoclonal antibodies, by fusion of human B cells with human B cell lymphomas. In any event, the monoclonal antibodies and other reagents for detection of tumour markers can now be used for more refined and careful examination of cells and tissues, because of the increasing availability of cell sorters, for objective and large scale utilisation of markers and because of the development of sensitive and relatively simple, enzyme linked immunoassays. Certainly, the widespread experience with immunohistochemical techniques also represents considerable progress with a promising approach.

(2) More generally, the potential ability of immunological procedures to detect very few molecules on a cell or materials released from a cell continues to provide a very strong set of tools for approaching the problem of identification of markers associated with a tumor.

(3) Furthermore, the widespread experience, although largely disappointing, over the past few years with the current generation of markers, has provided an excellent learning experience for investigators in the field, who are now

considerably more sophisticated and aware of the potential pitfalls and difficulties in going from the initial findings of a promising marker to the critical evaluation of its utility. It certainly should not take as long now to make this transition as it did for CEA, HCG, and AFP.

After this long introduction, let us now consider where we stand and where we should be going in this field.

(1)   Clearly most of the definite progress in this field has been with the use of markers for management of patients with malignant disease. This can be subdivided into several particular aspects.

(a)   The improved classification of disease, particularly into subgroups which vary in their prognosis and responsiveness to certain treatments. This includes the already widespread use of lymphoid cell markers for the classification of leukemias and lymphomas; the use of AFP and HCG for improved staging with testicular tumors; and the demonstrated potential for CEA and a few other markers to divide a particular stage of disease into prognostic categories. The information from the last example is still awaiting adoption by clinicians to help in the stratification of patients for clinical therapy trials.

(b)   There are an increasing number of markers for more accurate assessment of the efficacy of primary therapy. For example, the persistence of marker elevation after operation or chemotherapy, the increased ability to search for occult metastases, the search for residual tumor cells by cytological or immuno-histochemical examination of lymph nodes, bone marrow, even blood, particularly by the use of such selective markers as monoclonal antibodies, with the possible use of a fluorescence activated cell sorter. For most of these applications, it is important to note the usual need for tissues and/or pre-therapy serum specimens, to evaluate adequately the presence of a particular marker. Such specimens can be screened for the presence of a variety of markers and one that is found can then be used for further follow-up of the patient. For this application, it is also important to consider the possible value of assays for immune responses; even relatively non-specific immune response assays may reflect the tumor burden in the patient. For example, in recent studies performed in my laboratory it has been possible to demonstrate that depressed mixed lymphocyte culture reactivity in the early post-operative period in stage I lung cancer patients is associated with a particularly poor prognosis. Similarly, by performing mixed lymphocyte-tumor interactions with post-operative breast cancer patients, it has been possible to show that patients with strong reactivity to their autologous tumors have significantly better prognosis than do patients with the same pathological stage of disease who have low or undetectable reactivity. Radioimmunodetection also appears to be quite promising for detection of occult metastases. However, this procedure has yet to be shown able to detect very small foci of tumor. The present ability seems to be limited to the localisation of tumors at least 1–2 cm in diameter; yet, even this could be very helpful for the management of various types of tumors. In a more experimental way, there is the potential to use markers to identify possible new types of effective chemotherapy or other treatments. One could sequentially screen a series of drugs in a particular patient, looking for early changes in the levels of circulating marker. Very soon after treatment, one might expect an increase in tumor marker levels, related to necrosis of tumor cells if the tumor is responsive. A bit later, one would expect to find falling levels of the circulating marker associated with some response of the tumor to the agent. Such changes in marker levels should allow much more rapid identification of potentially useful drugs than can now be accomplished by following the usual clinical parameters. It is surprising that this approach has not been utilised more by chemotherapists. It has been well demonstrated, as discussed by Professor Bagshawe, to be a very potent approach for choriocarcinoma and testicular cancer. This approach should be particularly valuable in the search for new and more effective drugs for solid tumors, where currently only a limited number of useful agents are available. Perhaps investigators in the tumor marker field have been somewhat negligent in bringing the potential of this approach to the attention of clinical oncologists.

(c)   Assays for tumor markers can also be quite useful in following patients in regard to their response to continued treatment and regarding early detection of recurrent disease. Successes with this approach include the application of radioimmunoassays for HCG and AFP for choriocarcinoma and testicular cancer, radioimmunoassays for CEA in colorectal cancer, and some of the assays for ectopically produced hormones, which we heard about during the course of this meeting.

In regard to all of the above applications, it is important to note that the real determinant of successful utilisation of the markers will be their leading to improved survival of the patients. I was rather concerned by the comment of Professor Bagshawe that it is difficult to get the cooperation of clinicians to directly couple such studies of tumors with the randomised clinical trials that are being performed for therapy. As proposed by Dr Serrou, this approach seems to be the most reasonable and economical way to obtain solid documentation of the value of markers in management in cancer patients. The main problem may be adequate explanation by investigators in the tumor marker field to the clinicians, as to how the markers may actually be of value.

It is likely that the markers that will be useful for the above management applications will be mainly those associated with metastatic tumor cells, since this is the main problem in this area, the early detection of occult metastases at the time of initial treatment or upon follow-up. We continue to face real problems of both sensitivity and specificity with the markers. In regard to the circulating markers, a critical question is how many tumor cells are needed to make enough molecules to enter the circulation and be detected, even by the highly sensitive radioimmunoassays or enzyme immunoassays. Professor Bagshawe has estimated that the radioimmunoassays for HCG can detect about 10^4 tumor cells and at this level a marker can be very helpful. However, if detection of the marker is only seen when 10^7 or 10^8 tumor cells are present, this may not provide sufficient lead time to be really valuable. There is clearly a need to develop more sensitive approaches to the detection of small numbers of tumor cells. The assays for circulating markers may not, in general, turn out to be sufficiently sensitive for this problem. In any situations where tumor cells themselves can be looked at, or where one can obtain secretions or blood from the region of tumor growth, one might anticipate considerably more sensitive detection of a marker.

I would now like to turn to the more difficult, but the potentially more important, application of markers to the initial detection and diagnosis of cancer.

In general, I suspect that markers which prove to be best for management of cancer patients will also be particularly useful for diagnosis. However, I would like to point out that there may well be markers for local tumors which will not be well expressed or applicable to metastases. This is of particular importance because it is obviously desirable to detect tumors accurately at a local stage. For both detection and diagnosis, an important measure of success should be: does the marker provide additional information beyond that of the available established techniques or does it help to identify those individuals who should be evaluated by difficult or potentially dangerous diagnostic procedures? The real criterion for success is, how do the markers make a difference in the ultimate survival of the patients or do they provide an increased chance for curative therapy? In this context, it is of interest to consider the possible use of markers for breast cancer relative to the established use and demonstrated value of mammography. Mammography clearly has some limitations, both in its inability to detect all small breast cancers and in its considerable rate of false positive results. It should be noted that among women with positive mammograms, only one out of four to one out of ten who are biopsied can be shown to have breast cancer as opposed to benign breast disease. However, such a screening test can still be very helpful to identify subpopulations of individuals who are much more likely to have malignant disease. We can then accept the increased risk of surgery or other procedures to make a more definitive diagnosis. The radioimmunodetection procedure might be useful to complement or possibly even replace mammography, since it might be expected to distinguish accurately cancer lesions from various benign lesions in the breast.

A central question is, what type of technique is likely to have sufficient sensitivity and specificity? As commented on before, it may be unlikely that circulating markers in general will allow very early detection of small numbers of locally growing tumor cells. Again, if it is possible to obtain cells, either by biopsy or by cytology, one would expect to have a much better chance of finding small numbers of tumor cells in the specimens. However, an alternative approach, as illustrated by Dr Thomson's presentation on the leukocyte adherence inhibition assay, is the potentially high sensitivity of assays for immune responses to tumor associated antigens. It seems likely that immune responses to tumor antigens could occur very early in the course of disease, substantially earlier than one would expect to have a release of sufficient quantities of tumor products into the circulation. However, most of these assays for immune responses are still in early stages of development. It will be necessary to develop assays which are considerably more sensitive and reproducible and suitable for large-scale application than is the current generation of assays.

Clearly workers in this field still have much to do, but I am optimistic that continued real progress can be made and that markers will become established as parts of the armamentarium for diagnosis and management of cancer. Hopefully, subsequent meetings on this topic will demonstrate the verification of my continued optimism for progress in this important field of research.

SUBJECT INDEX

A

Acid ferritin assay, 119
ACTH, 85–88, 252, 256
  ectopic, 87
ADH, 86, 89
  inappropriate secretion, 86
AFP
  in lung cancer, 99
  in urogenital tract tumours, 213–
    215, 219, 226, 233, 234, 238–
    245, 272, 274
Alkaline phosphatase, 200
Alpha-1 Antitrypsin, 101
Amylase, 103
Arachidonic Acid
  effect on LAI, 165

B

BCA, 28–32, 51
β-2 microglobulin
  in breast cancer, 67
  in colorectal cancer, 176, 177
  in lung cancer, 101
  structure, 67
BMAP, in prostate cancer, 199, 232
BOFA, 60, 206
Breast cancer markers, 21, 35, 51, 75,
  81
  in detection, 81
  in prevention, 81
  in prognosis, 81

C

Calcitonin
  ectopic, 90, 268
  in breast cancer, 67, 82
  increase after pentagastrin, 267
  in endocrine tumours, 252, 254
  in lung cancer, 90
  in thyroid tumours, 259, 265, 272
Carbohydrates, 105
Carcinoid tumours, 256
Casein, 35
Ceruloplasmin, 101
CEA, 130, 131, 272, 274
  CEA-like, 25, 55
  in breast cancer, 21, 35, 37, 51, 76, 82
  in colorectal tumours, 26, 28, 141–
    144, 146–151
  in combined assay, 117, 139
  in lung cancer, 98, 115–117
  in ovarian cancer, 206, 239
  in thyroid tumours, 268
  in urogenital tract tumours, 238
  monoclonal antibody anti-, 189
  radioimmunodetection, 147–151,
    193
CG, in lung cancer, 90
Circulating immune complexes, 9,
  132, 190
  in breast cancer, 14, 76
  in cancer progression, 16, 17
  in leukaemia, 10
  in lung cancer, 17, 102, 132
  in prognosis, 13–15, 19
  in relapse, 13